CARING FOR OLDER

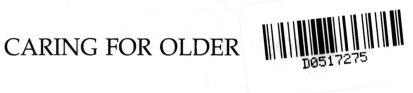

CARING FOR OLDER PEOPLE

PEOPLE

Developing Specialist Practice

Edited by

Jim Marr
MA (Gerontology), BA (Education Studies)
Diploma in Clinical Nurse Education, RGN, RMN, RCNT, RNT
Director of Nursing, Westminster Healthcare, London, UK

and

Dr Betty Kershaw
RGN, MSc (Nursing), RNT
Director of the Centre for Professional Policy Development
of the School of Nursing, Midwifery and Health Visiting,
University of Manchester, UK
President of the Royal College of Nursing, UK (1994–98)

A member of the Hodder Headline Group
LONDON • SYDNEY • AUCKLAND

First published in Great Britain 1998 by
Arnold, a member of the Hodder Headline Group
338 Euston Road, London NW1 3BH
http://www.arnoldpublishers.com

British Library Cataloguing in Publication Data
A catalogue record for this book is available from the British Library

Library of Congress Cataloging-in-Publication Data
A catalog record for this book is available from the Library of Congress

Publisher: Clare Parker
Production Editor: Liz Gooster
Production Controller: Rose James
Cover design: Terry Griffiths

ISBN 0 340 61374 2

Typeset in 10/12 Palatino by Photoprint Typesetters, Torquay, Devon
Printed and bound in Great Britain by J W Arrowsmith, Bristol

Contents

List of contributors

Ken Barker
Lecturer in Nursing, University of Manchester, School of Nursing,
Midwifery and Health Visiting

Marilyn Cartwright
Formerly Nurse Teacher, currently Community Health Nurse,
Queensland Health, Australia

Alan Crump
Charge Nurse, Leeds Community and Mental Health Trust

Pauline Ford RGN, CMS, DHMS, MA (Gerontology)
RCN Advisor on Nursing and Older People

Ann Hayes
Lecturer, School of Physiotherapy, Manchester Royal Infirmary, Central
Manchester NHS Trust

Hazel Heath MSc Advanced Clinical Practice (Care of Older People),
BA (Hons), DipN (London), Cert.Ed, FETC, ITEC, RGN, RCNT, RNT
Chair, Royal College of Nursing Forum for Nurses Working with Older
Peple and Independent Nurse Advisor

Kevin Hope
Lecturer in Nursing, University of Manchester, School of Nursing,
Midwifery and Health Visiting

Ian Jacques RMN, DipN (London), MA (Gerontology)
Practice Support Manager, Anchor Trust, Manchester

Betty Kershaw RGN, MSc (Nursing), RNT, PhD
Director, the Centre for Professional Policy Development, School of
Nursing, Midwifery and Health Visiting, University of Manchester;
President, the Royal College of Nursing (1994–98)

Jim Marr MA (Gerontology), BA (Education Studies), Diploma in
Clinical Nurse Education, RGN, RMN, RCNT, RNT
Director of Nursing, Westminster Healthcare, London

Maria Scurfield RMN, DPNS, BSc (Hons)(Nursing Science)
Clinical Nurse Manager, Wearside Trust

David Sines PhD, BSc (Hons), RMN, RHMN, RNT, PGCTHE, FRCN
Professor of Community Health Care/Head of School of Health
Sciences, University of Ulster

Lesley Surman MA, BA, RN, RNT, RCNT, OND
Lecturer in Nursing, University of Manchester, School of Nursing,
Midwifery and Health Visiting

Lesley Wade
Lecturer in Nursing, University of Manchester, School of Nursing,
Midwifery and Health Visiting

Mike Wafer RGN, RNMH, BSc (Hons), MSc (Nursing)
Quality Advisor, Tameside and Glossop Community Trust

Stephen G. Wright RGN, RCNT, Dip N, RNT, DANS, MSc (Nursing),
FRCN, MHSN
Visiting Professor, School of Nursing, St Martin's College, University of
Lancaster; Director of the European Nursing Development Agency
(TENDA)

Andrew Yates BA (Hons), RMN, DipN (London), RNT
Lecturer/Clinical Nurse Specialist, University of Manchester/Tameside
and Glossop C & PS NHS Trust

Abebaw Yohannes MSc
Lecturer, School of Physiotherapy, Manchester Royal Infirmary, Central
Manchester NHS Trust

Preface

Over the past ten years people have become much more aware of the opportunities available to them once retired from full-time work. They know that they are living longer, that many have a disposable income, that there is social service and voluntary organisation support available to improve their standard of living and that, in short, they have as much right to access services and live life to the full as younger members of our society. This book aims to help them do just that.

The chapters are written by expert professionals who are working day by day with older people, helping them to continue to live in their own homes, following their own lifestyle and enjoying what each week brings. They are about how health care professionals can help the older person maintain a high quality of personal living, how adaptation to changed circumstances can be achieved, and how support can be accessed. They are about providing care unobtrusively – not as a care giver particularly, but as a colleague who can help, assist and support.

The book is unique, not only in taking this perspective but also in the breadth of information it contains. Much has been written about older people, but less about those with a learning disability or mental health disorder to which they have long adapted and with which they need community support. In June 1996 the government issued *Primary Care: the Future* (Department of Health, 1996), which encouraged those working in the community to look towards continuity of care, co-ordination, partnership and people-centred activities through which choice is available and options offered. The authors are skilled with this approach to working, not only with each other but also with older people, whether living alone or in a group.

As I reach my mid-fifties I am very conscious that I want professional help, advice and support to be available as I age; what I don't want is to be treated as though old age is an illness and I am a patient.

Betty Kershaw

References

DoH (1996) *Choice and Opportunity: Primary Care – the Future*. HMSO: London.

New Labour because Britain deserves better (1997) Labour Party Manifesto, March 1997, London Central Office.

Steiner, A and Vaughan B (1996) *Intermediate Care*. King's Fund Publishing, London.

Introduction

Stephen G. Wright

Old age ain't no place for cissies.
(attr. Bette Davies)

Bette Davies had a reputation for being a tough minded film star, and was reputed to have become even more so in her old age. If we scan the horizon of those who are old today and those who will be old when the new millennium dawns, we find mixed views of progress, opportunity, danger and deprivation. Being old still demands considerable toughness and resilience: it is often not a place for the faint hearted. As the chapters in this book illustrate, old age can be a time of great joy and fulfilment – but it can also be one of great suffering and distress, especially for those whose health fails, those without family or community support, those whose income is low, those whose education and housing are poor, those from working class or ethnic minority backgrounds and those who are disabled or dying. Our culture still advantages in almost all respects the white, male, middle class and youthful whose first language is English.

Our continued worship at the altar of youth, money and masculinity means that those who possess none of these qualities may find themselves up against all manner of discrimination and disadvantage. No-one escapes. To a greater or lesser extent anyone who reaches old age (whenever this nebulous concept starts) can expect to meet some form of alienation from full participation in the world, whether it be prejudice or expectations of how old people are supposed to think, feel and behave.

Witness the media hype a few years ago when a nurse disguised herself as an old woman and merely tried to go about town to do her shopping. She detailed a catalogue of abuse, being ignored, sworn at, pushed aside and generally made to feel useless, foolish and unwanted in the great majority of her social encounters. Of course, much of the media reported this with horror and saw it as a sign of the times – of moral decay – that the old should be treated thus. Conveniently and hypocritically, it forgot about its own part in creating a climate where old age is viewed as an almost exclusively negative phenomenon. To any old person this was not new. Many generations have witnessed the consequences of being old and at the bottom of the social pecking order. Those who escape these pressures are relatively few – usually the better off and better educated, as Phillipson's (1982) thesis on capitalism and the construction of old age has illustrated.

As the issue of the 'problem' of an ageing population receives ever greater attention, professionals like nurses are going to have to review their approaches and practices. This book seeks to address much of this updated thinking arising from nursing. Others, meanwhile, are 'deconstructing' the seemingly pervasive image of old age being a negative phenomenon. Ram Dass (1995), a well known spiritual leader in the USA, has turned to aspects of his own ageing in much of his current teaching and is preparing a book on the theme. He has argued that one positive aspect of 'slowing down' physically and growing old means that we can concentrate more on that 'inner journey', and that we should perhaps help people to prepare for this through teaching meditation techniques, for example. Saxby (1983) has written movingly of the opportunities for transforming relationships between the old and the young. Chopra's recent (1993) thesis opens up whole new territories for thinking, and research into the process of ageing that transcends many of the limitations of the currently dominant biological models.

The myth that somehow in the past older people had a better deal is just that – a myth. It seems that the old person's status and participation in the world has always been determined just as much by the expectations and prejudices exhibited today. If old age was venerated at all, it was probably because so few people ever reached it. Now, as more people than ever before can look forward to three score years and ten, or maybe twenty, thirty or forty, what is happening? Almost every report, account or story of the ageing population represents it as a problem. Old people are frequently referred to as burdens on society – *they* have become the problem, rather than the values of the society they inhabit.

Such values percolate our every action, our language, our political decisions. In writing this I am falling into the same trap myself: in describing the phenomenon of ageing I inevitably objectify it, referring to it as a thing 'out there' to be discussed and commented upon. Older people are not *they* but *we*; ageing is *in here* not *out there*. Our tendency to categorise and stereotype to help to reduce a concept to manageable proportions may help us to identify and solve problems. However, it also leads us to distance ourselves from the phenomenon, to set it apart as if it were something that happens to others and not to ourselves. We come to see older people, as Elder (1977) so succinctly described in her experiences, as aliens among us.

This would be comical if it were not so dangerous. Our capacity to distance ourselves from that which is different (and especially, as in the case of ageing, being associated with deep seated fears in our culture) and to create a sense of 'otherness' allows us at best to rationalise our prejudices under the guise that 'they' are not the same as us. When we cease to see other people as connected to or just the same as ourselves, and see them instead as stereotypical groups with given feelings and behaviours, we believe we can safely put them away from us. We cease to identify with them as individuals; rather, they become objects 'out there' – at best deserving of our pity and help, and at worst to be removed from our sight or treated as less than human. The nightmares of concentration camps, be they the infamous ones of World War II or the more recent ones in Bosnia, and of the litany of human oppression down through the ages have roots identical to those of the catalogue of misery which continues to be inflicted upon the old. When we no longer see another person as a human being with thoughts and feelings and a history and value like ourselves, we create the context for all manner of abuse. We can do anything to 'them' because 'they' are not the same as 'us'; 'they' become less human. There continue to be dark corners of nursing where such inhuman values are acted out. Not all these are about obvious physical or mental maltreatment. More often they seem to fall into the category of the 'slow drip' of inhumanity that 'wears down' (de Beauvoir, 1972) the old person's dignity and self respect bit by bit – the denial of little freedoms such as what to wear, what to drink or where to go. Sarton's (1967) touching story also illuminates another dimension: how the carer fails to get inside the older person's world (perhaps because it would frighten them too much with their own fears about ageing and mortality). In one scene she writes of how her nurse, Harriet, hides behind a series of clichés and glib phrases to avoid the anxiety of encountering the real feelings and demands of an old lady:

> Nothing can really be done to help us on the downward path, so mentioning the horrors of growing old alone becomes a terrible burden. There seem to be only a few responses possible. One is the dreadful false comfort of the cliché – 'it can't be as bad as all that' or 'things will surely be better tomorrow, dear'.

> I suffer excruciatingly from endearments that are casual or perfunctory, because I am so starved for real deep feelings, for love itself, I suppose. But the crucial response to a *crie de coeur* is not to believe or to pretend that it is a lie.

> This is Harriet's weapon – 'you must imagine that you can't sleep. I heard you snoring at four this morning'.

> There is also the cajoling response, the one that treats the old person as an infant, the 'now, now, quiet down' sort of thing. 'I'll bring you some tea.' So, the person is lying there in distress but a cup of tea solves everything.

> One could only be answered differently by true caring and that, I suspect, would show itself in silence, by the quality of listening or some shy gesture of love.

Old age is really a disguise that no-one but the old see through. I feel exactly as I always did, as young inside as when I was 21, but the outward shell conceals the real me, sometimes even from itself, and betrays that person deep down inside under wrinkles and liver spots, and all the horrors of decay. I feel things more intensely than I used to, not less. But I am afraid of appearing ridiculous. People will expect serenity of the old. That is the stereotype, the mask you are expected to put on. But how many old people really are serene?

The professional and general media carry endless reports of failings in care when old people come into the hands of professional carers. Sometimes it seems as if the problem is solved as the guilty people are punished or the inadequate unit is reorganised, but it only reappears in another setting – different place, different people, same problem.

Of course, the professions' responses when their weaknesses are exposed is to affirm that such incidents are in the minority, that most carers are conscientious and are always giving of their best to the patients, clients or residents. There is some truth in this, and we do need to keep matters in perspective. Nurses in particular have been at the leading edge of the development of nursing practice in relation to older people – so much so that many nurses in the specialty have matured beyond the need to feel defensive about their work, which was once relegated to the bottom of the status pile in nursing and dismissed as a low-tech Cinderella service. It is not so long since I worked in a nursing development unit (NDU) whose work was well publicised from the middle 1980s. I recall being treated a few years before to words of wisdom from one senior colleague who regarded 'geriatric' nursing as suitable only for those who had 'not passed their finals first time', were 'kind and caring but not very bright', had been disciplined for various reasons and were therefore 'no longer suitable for the acute wards' or who quite simply 'had weak brains but strong backs'. I remember well my fury at the time – enough to retreat to my ward and record the conversation for posterity! My colleagues and I vowed that we would make that person eat those words, and we did, as our unit became well known and took its place at the cutting edge of developing the nursing care of older people in particular and nursing in general. The Tameside NDU joined the growing band of units and individuals, increasing incrementally as the years went by, who were transforming both the image and the practice of the specialty. There is now greater recognition of its value and complexity. High-tech care is involved as well, but the care of older people remains essentially 'high-touch' in terms of the nature of the nurse–patient relationship, requiring an intimacy and complexity of thought and action every bit as demanding as other nursing specialties. There is less need, perhaps, to feel defensive or to justify the special nature of nursing older people – in that sense it seems to have come of age. Although there are still outmoded values and perceptions lurking in some corners of nursing, for the most part the nursing of older people now stands on an equal footing with other branches of nursing.

This change in perceptions and practices has been spurred on by many factors, not least the growing numbers of older people. No longer consigned almost exclusively to the 'geriatric wards' of the old work-houses, the over-60s now form the bulk of the case loads in almost every nursing setting in both hospital and community. It seems that everyone is a nurse for the older person now! So more nurses have come to realise that this part of nursing is not so simple or 'basic' after all. However, this also makes it imperative that the innovations in practices fostered in the specialty over the years must now be spread to every sector. Thus, nurses of older people now commonly find themselves acting in a consultancy capacity to other specialties. Meanwhile, a check through the high profile awards for nursing innovation sponsored by several journals and other organisations will reveal that, of the nurses in prominent leadership positions, and changes in practice such as self medication, primary nursing, NDUs, continence care and countless other aspects, great numbers have had their origins or received their greatest boost from the nursing of older patients. The conferences, debates and workshops on relevant themes from the specialty have swelled professional knowledge and debate, as has the enormous expansion of the available research and literature, to which this book is a significant contribution.

Thus there are many grounds for optimism, but we need to be wary of overindulging in self-congratulatory mirror gazing. The battle for compassionate creative caring in nursing is far from universally won and outside the profession the obstacles sometimes seem as insurmountable as ever. The deeply rooted undervaluing of the aged and ageing has knock-on effects other than the abuses mentioned earlier. It encourages the view that as the ageing population expands, and especially in times of perceived economic difficulties, the old are the problem and not the values and standards of the society they inhabit. For example, it is widely accepted that health and social care have unlimited demand, but that supply (i.e. money) is finite. Perhaps nurses, who have historically made great store of their intimate understanding of patients' needs and their commitment to work in partnership with them, could contribute to the questioning of this nostrum. The myth of 'infinite demand: finite resources' appears to be just that – a myth. There is no evidence that older people are increasingly demanding costly high-tech health care and medical intervention; in fact, it could be argued that the reverse is the case. In other words, we often reach a time which the ancients called *satietas vitae* – a fullness or sufficiency of life, characterised by a desire for a peaceful non-interventionist death as life draws to a close. Furthermore, presenting the image that older people are necessarily frail and demand-ing of support flies in the face of the evidence discussed later in this book. Only a minority of older people, less than 5 per cent, are in need of some kind of institutional care such as hospital, nursing or residential home (Hall, 1996). The rest, it seems, are quietly getting on with their lives with minimal medical or social intervention, and probably equally quietly resenting the general image portrayed of them as helpless and burden-some. Furthermore, Wyke's (1994) report indicates that we may not only be living longer by the year 2050, because of continued advances in health care which may make lifespans of 130 or 140 years the norm, but that such an old age will be a healthy and more vigorous one.

If we continue to perceive old age as negative and associated with inevitable decline, we will indeed continue to have anxieties about funding health care costs. However, if we let slip the mask of outmoded prejudice, the real challenges seem to be about rethinking our approach to the age of retirement, about how our working and leisure lives are planned, and so on.

Thus, the real issues for society about ageing are not so much about finite resources, but how we choose to make use of them and what we choose to see as priorities. Furthermore, such rethinking and reprioritis-ing demands that our society free itself of the mire of old notions and prejudices about ageing that keeps us stuck in unimaginative, outworn and unproductive solutions. Meanwhile, the siren voices that associate more old people with more costs to society appear to be holding sway and, worryingly, are feeding the calls to find solutions (the 'final solu-tion'?) which many may regard with alarm. While the debate continues to be presented in reductionist terms ('we have only so much money – do we provide a long-term bed for the 80-year-old or an intensive care bed for the child?'), it is little wonder that no more imaginative solutions can come forward. Meanwhile, older people are led increasingly to feel that they are a burden or 'in the way'. The inevitable consequence of this, and a scenario loved by those who would like quick fix solutions to cut costs, is that the old should be 'encouraged' to die. Vincent (1994) reports one example from the Netherlands where acts of euthanasia in certain circum-stances have been decriminalised. In this case, a doctor who 'confines himself to one act of euthanasia per month on the grounds that he finds it emotionally burdensome work, has been at pains to point out that old people who wish to die in order to relinquish their hospital beds to worthier patients should be treated as national heroes'. Such thinking provides an excuse for policy makers and those who hold the purse strings to avoid difficult resource allocation decisions and to avoid making the effort to look for more creative options. Furthermore, it conforms to stereotypical views of ageing and, in the use of the word 'worthier', betrays all the prejudices and value judgements about ageing and the old that ultimately lead to a social acceptance of killing as a serious option to deal with the 'problem' of ageing. We may be left wondering whether the awards made to the 'national heroes' in these circumstances will be made while they are alive or posthumously.

What part can nursing play? Each nurse who works with older people can play a part, and this may involve doing more than giving the best quality care to our patients or clients. We can, for example, challenge negative perceptions about ageing whenever and wherever we encounter them. We can become active, locally and nationally, at political and organisational levels, in all manner of settings from our employers to political parties to professional bodies, and lobby for the rights of those who are ageing (this means ourselves). We can participate in professional debates, dialogue, research and knowledge building that help to diminish ignorance (as this book seeks to do). We can help to create and participate in imaginative educational programmes that help those who seek to care for the ageing to move beyond empathy, which tries to see the world and another's suffering from the other's point of view, towards compassion, where we see that person's world not as separate from our own, but as one and the same (*com-passion* = feeling and being with). When we see ourselves not as separate from but as connected to other human beings in this way, perhaps we can truly begin to act compassionately for older people and bring real meaning to that much overused and glibly spoken phrase 'the nurse as the patient's advocate'. When we act with compassion, we act for ourselves because there is no 'other'. Sogyal Rinpoche (1992) writes from a Buddhist perspective and gives nurses much food for thought and action about caring for those who are old. He asks 'What is compassion?' and notes that 'it is not simply a sense of sympathy or caring for the person suffering, not simply a warmth of heart towards the person before you, or a sharp clarity of recognition of their needs and pain, it is also a sustained and practical determination to do whatever is possible and necessary to alleviate their suffering.' Nursing has always been more than being compassionate: it is also an action discipline, and there is much that nurses can do to advance the cause of the older person when we translate compassion into action.

To act compassionately means that we have to be inside the other person, connected to them so that they cease to be a 'they' but are part of 'we'. By listening to what older people have to say, by hearing their story, we can come to understand what it means to be old, for their story is our story too. Monitoring standards of care, as this book suggests, is one way we can do this, but there are countless others – such as facilitating patients' or residents' committees, supporting advocacy schemes or constructing in our working practices 'laws and conventions' (Blythe 1987) practices that are determined by the needs and wishes of the older person and not dominated by professional control or what we think of as best.

Each of us may be old someday, so there is an investment for us in making life better for those who are old now, for the time may come when 'we' are 'they'. Often the old are argued to 'keep thinking young'. Perhaps in the meantime it would profit us to 'keep thinking old'!

Some years ago Linda Thomas, a professional colleague and friend, introduced me to a poem which encapsulates some of the values and attitudes which this chapter has sought to discuss. At the time, Linda Thomas was adviser in the care of older people for the Royal College of Nursing. She is a fine example of compassion in action, and has done as much as anyone I know in her own quiet way to advance the cause of the old and those who care for them. I would like to dedicate my introduction to this book in gratitude to her, and conclude by reproducing that poem. It offers, perhaps, the opposite perspective from the 'Crabbit Old Woman' cited later in the book, and illuminates how each of us can challenge the stereotypes of ageing, which serve none of us well:

> When I am an old woman I shall wear purple
> with a red hat which doesn't go and doesn't suit me.
> And I shall spend my pension on brandy and summer gloves
> And satin sandals, and say we've no money for butter.
> I shall sit down on the pavement when I'm tired
> And gobble up samples in shops and press alarm bells
> And run my stick along the public railings
> And make up for the sobriety of my youth.
> I shall go out in my slippers in the rain
> And pick flowers in other people's gardens
> And learn to spit.
> You can wear terrible shirts and grow more fat
> And eat three pounds of sausages at a go
> or only bread and pickle for a week
> And hoard pens and pencils and beermats and things in boxes.
>
> But now we must have clothes that keep us dry
> And pay our rent and not swear in the street
> And set a good example for our children.
> We must have friends to dinner and read the papers.
>
> But maybe I ought to practice a little now?
> So people who know me are not too shocked and surprised
> When suddenly I am old, and start to wear purple.
>
> (Joseph, 1991)

References

de Beauvoir S (1972) *Old Age*. Penguin, Harmondsworth.
Blythe R (1987) *The View in Winter*. Penguin, Harmondsworth.
Chopra D (1993) *Ageless Body – Timeless Mind*. Harmony Press, New York.
Elder G (1977) *The Alienated – Growing Old Today*. Writers and Readers Publishing Co-operative, London.
Joseph J (1991) Warning. In Martz S (ed.) (1991) 'When I am an old woman I shall wear purple'. PMP, Watsonville.
Hall JK (1966) *Nursing: Ethics and Law*. WB Saunders, London.

Phillipson C (1982) *Capitalism and the Construction of Old Age*. Macmillan, London.

Ram Dass (1995) *Conscious Ageing*, a collection of tapes available from the Hanuman Foundation, New Mexico, USA. A book on the theme is currently in press.

Sarton M (1967) *As We are Now*. Women's Press, New York.

Saxby J (1983) Jane Saxby. In Jones B (ed.) *Three Lives*. NFCO, London.

Sogyal Rinpoche (1992) *The Tibetan Book of Living and Dying*. Ryder, London.

Vincent S (1994) *Exits. Guardian Weekend* Special Report, pp 6–10.

Wyke A (1994) The Future of Medicine – Peering into 2010. *The Economist* 330, suppl. 10/3.

1

The ageing process

Ken Barker

When you woke up this morning to commence your daily rituals and routine, as you got out of bed, did you consciously reflect on the ease or difficulty of the movement compared with yesterday, last week, five years ago? Did you gaze into your bedroom or bathroom mirror? For what? A stretch of the cheek here to tighten out those lines, a few fingers through the hair to reorientate those strands of grey? Is it time for the moisturising cream, the colour rinse? Has a partner or relative kindly pointed out the thinning here and there, the midriff enlargement, or the 'uncoolness' of your dress sense or your music taste?

Well of course you are older . . . but are you old? You know your age . . . but are you aged? Take a minute to identify what your images of ageing are and write them in the box below. Indicate with a P or N whether these are positive or negative reflections.

You could have included among your reflections greying, thinning hair, loss of skin elasticity, loss of energy, diminished mobility, bereavement, isolation, financial worries. Equally you could have considered maturity, accumulation of knowledge, the development of wisdom and problem solving ability, freedom to enjoy leisure and financial security. When reflecting on others, perhaps your patients and clients, did you include arthritis, atherosclerosis, high blood pressure, osteoporosis, prostatism, dementia, Alzheimer's disease and senility?

These features pose one of the largest problems in considering the ageing process. It is difficult to separate the effects of the background chronological process from the pathological effects of disease which may be superimposed on it. Thus, disease may overlay or change in some manner the entire biopsychosocial 'programme' of the individual.

'Ageing', according to Carter (1980), is associated in most people's minds with 'old age' – a concept that people in this country define by statutory retirement age. To many, ageing is attributed to changes seen in older people (a classification that varies with the age of the observer). Although this definition includes the multiple pathologies often found among older people, it also recognises that ageing biologically is a process along the continuum from conception to death (Figure 1.1). We can recognise this by studying the life cycles of other species. We can also acknowledge that the health of all living organisms is affected by environmental and other factors, whether intrinsic (internal) or extrinsic (external).

Conception	Childhood	Adulthood	Old age
Embryo	Growth and	Homeostasis	Deterioration/
Foetus	development		senescence

Figure 1.1 Lifespan continuum. (After Carter, 1980)

In the life of the embryo, visible changes occur with a rapidity that continues through the foetal stage and through childhood and adolescence. However, in adult life, many years have to pass before differences or changes can be detected. Yet the rate and effects of these changes are individualised. We all probably know someone aged 70 or 80 who looks fitter or younger than some 50-year-olds.

The age of an individual is obviously the amount of time a person has lived, and ageing therefore is the process of growing old – a chronological event. Quite often, though, it is measured in terms of the physical and psychological deficits, deteriorations or debilities acquired as our life progresses. Herbert (1992) asserts that we age at different rates due to inconsistencies in our biological systems' reserves. It is this that ensures individuality and makes it difficult for the observer to correlate a specific change within a species to a particular age.

Christiansen and Grzybowski (1993) offer clarification of two other terms used erroneously to describe ageing. In the box below, indicate your understanding of the words 'senescence' and 'senility'.

Senescence

Senility

Are these accurate descriptions of ageing? You may have accepted both into your concept of the ageing process, as both indicate progressive changes in a personal appearance or functional capacity as one grows old.

Christiansen and Grzybowski define *senescence* as the accumulation of harmful events and *senility* as the accumulation of the most harmful senescence events.

Senescent and senile changes are therefore measurable. They are also harmful in that they reduce the likelihood that the individual will be able to resist or recover from challenges caused by environmental or homeostatic imbalances. Older people's susceptibility to acute and chronic disease processes obviously affects their homeostasis.

However, Carter (1980) advised against the adjective (the label) 'senile', stating that, 'in practical terms it usually only implies that the person being spoken about is older than the speaker!' Even the word 'old' has both positive and negative applications.

Consider the following:

- Advanced in years
- Having been long or relatively long in existence
- Worn out, out of date, superseded or abandoned
- Belonging to former times
- Long practised or experienced
- Having the characteristics of age
- Familiar or accustomed
- A general word of familiar or affectionate approbation or contempt.

These are all part of the definition of 'old' provided in *Chambers 20th Century Dictionary*.

Ageing can therefore be seen as a lifelong process, a feature of human existence (in fact of every living thing), not just occurring in older people.

Table 1.1 The UK population: proportions by age

Year	Total population (millions)	Percentage by age				
		<16	16–39	40–64	65–79	80+
1951	50.3	—	—	31.6	9.5	1.4
1961	52.8	24.8	31.4	32.0	9.8	1.9
1971	55.9	25.6	31.3	29.2	10.9	2.3
1981	56.4	22.2	34.9	27.8	12.2	2.8
1991	57.6	20.3	35.2	28.7	12.0	3.7
Projections						
2001	59.2	21.3	32.6	30.5	11.4	4.2
2011	60.0	20.1	30.0	33.7	11.7	4.5
2021	60.7	19.5	30.5	31.9	13.6	4.5

(Adapted from OPCS (1993) Table 1.3, p 14)

However, changes that occur may leave the individual vulnerable to internal homeostatic imbalances or to environmental insult, which may be harmful. There is increased likelihood of these factors occurring in later life because of natural age related changes in body system functioning. Yet the affects of ageing have to be considered separately for each individual, especially as logic tells us that the longer one lives the more likely it is that health may be affected by extrinsic factors too.

Look at Table 1.1. Identify the trends affecting the elderly population and suggest reasons for them.

Trend 1

Rationale

Trend

Rationale

You should have identified two major themes: firstly, that the proportion of the population aged 65–79 years increased steadily from 1951 to 1981. Over the last ten years there has been a slight reduction, and numbers will continue to fall – but only over the next 20 years, when a further rise is anticipated. Over the same period, the number of persons in the most elderly division, those over 80, rises until 2011. The projection is that the population of the UK will continue to rise and that an increasing proportion will be elderly and very elderly. Other figures (OPCS, 1993) remind us that life expectancy is increasing.

Over the period covered in the table, the number of 16-year-olds and under has been falling and will recover only slightly in the early part of the next century.

In exploring reasons for the changes you may have considered the fall in birth rate (which explains the reduction in the younger age groups) or improvements in housing, sanitation and nutrition, the eradication of many previously fatal infective diseases, and better medical and surgical intervention resulting in the control of many illnesses. Nursing and social work have played a major part in the changes. And we must not forget the impact on life expectancy of the two world wars.

In fact, the OPCS Census of 1993 indicates a reduction in mortality over the last 40 years from injuries and poisoning, respiratory diseases, circulatory diseases (still the greatest killer), infectious diseases and all other diseases with the exception of cancer. The increase in cancer deaths is a result partly of better diagnosis of the disease with improved technology and therefore the inclusion of this diagnosis more readily on death certificates. The incidence of cancers also increases generally with age and therefore we will see more in our increased numbers of older people. Yet, despite this, the life expectancy of older people of all ages has increased over the last 90 years and projections are that it will continue to do so.

Briefly comment on the trends indicated by the figures in Table 1.2.

Trends

The life expectancy of a newborn child was expected to increase from 45.5 years for males and 49 years for females in 1901 to 74 and 79.5 years respectively in 1996. Thus, for every year a person lives, their life

Table 1.2 The number of further years a person might expect to live, by age and gender: trends from 1901 and a projection to 2001

	At birth		At 1 year		At 10 years		At 20 years		At 40 years		At 60 years		At 80 + years	
Year	M	F	M	F	M	F	M	F	M	F	M	F	M	F
1901	45.5	49.0	53.6	55.8	50.4	52.7	41.7	44.1	26.1	28.3	13.3	14.6	4.9	5.3
1931	58.4	62.4	62.1	65.3	55.6	58.6	46.7	49.6	29.5	32.4	14.4	16.4	4.9	5.4
1961	67.9	73.8	68.6	74.2	60.0	65.6	50.4	55.7	31.5	36.5	15.0	19.0	5.2	6.3
1991	73.2	78.6	72.8	78.1	64.0	69.3	54.3	59.4	35.3	39.9	17.8	21.8	6.5	8.1
1996	74.0	79.5	73.5	78.9	64.7	70.1	54.9	60.2	35.8	40.6	18.2	22.4	6.7	8.6
2001	74.5	79.9	74.0	79.3	65.2	70.5	55.4	60.6	36.2	41.0	18.7	22.7	7.0	8.8

(Adapted from OPCS (1995))

expectancy becomes greater, with overall increases since 1901. Consistently, the life expectancy for females is greater than that for males.

Data show that the population of pensionable age (men over 65 years and women over 60 years) is continuing to rise. As the age bandings within the population change their dimensions and interrelationships, there are bound to be wider societal implications. The public sector services, especially health and social care provision, will see demand increase. Between 1979/80 and 1989/90, total health expenditure in England and Wales on health services for older people increased by 43 per cent (and for personal social services 48 per cent), with an estimated £6700 million spent on hospital and community health services in 1990/91, for those of pensionable age – which represented 45 per cent of total spending on all age groups. (the Government's expenditure plans 1992/3–1993/94, cited in Tinker *et al.*, 1994).

In parallel with these trends, Christiansen and Grzybowski (1993) inform us that the World Health Organization (WHO) have data suggesting that a new phenomenon has arisen in all the industrialised countries of the world: that of a society which is 'dominated . . . by the concerns and needs of an aged or ageing population'.

The WHO defines age thus:

- Elderly: 60–75 years
- Old: 76–90 years
- Very old: 90 + years

The ambiguity of many of the terms used to categorise or describe the elderly may give rise to ageism – which is a stereotyping attitude and therefore is no better than a form of contempt, because the ageist individual visualises old people as a uniform group usually decrepit and 'senile' – in the derogatory sense. This attitude encompasses a homogenised group of passive and sexless individuals incapable of self care.

Often *Images of Ageing* demonstrate the attitudes and observations of the casual on-looker and show great variability in the expression of physical and cognitive abilities. Many would-be philosophers also apply a quality to their 'prose' that reflects the value of age, or the aged, to society. It is all too easy to let value slip into tolerance.

A great deal of the ageing process is likely to pass us by if not for the 'kind' observations of others. If the majority of people consider changes in appearance to be signs of ageing, why do we look for them? The society to which the ageing population belongs is providing an increased commitment, but older people have contributed in the past to the creation and stability of that society. Why should it now create pressures which are fashion-enforced and activity restricting? Consider the following:

- Age restrictions on employment (especially that requiring training or education) imposed by a mandatory retirement policy
- The pressure of advertising aimed at younger stylish or 'attractive' age groups: only recently has it been recognised that both the older person and the 'fatter' one like to dress attractively
- Media images that present attractiveness as the norm and create subconscious coercion to conform – such as those associated with expensive cosmetics, emollients and regenerating creams (advertised by big business as carrying water back into the ageing skin) and with cures for baldness
- Social attitudes that perpetuate the myth that old age is a helpless condition, that the elderly are of no social use, are a burden, or have nothing to offer and therefore are given no valuable role.

Yet do the majority of us not wish for a ripe old age? If so, we can be reassured by a BBC report (January 1997 CEEFAX) that scientists at the University of Manchester estimate that current technology and improvements in medical intervention will soon give us a life expectancy of 200 plus. Among all these pressures it is imperative that we all have regard for all the experiences and stimuli that have shaped older people through their lives. It is only by taking this holistic approach that we may see through the 'static', through the negatives, and give the value we would all hope to receive. Or do we expect the same as *we* age?

The Portuguese have a proverb: If you wish good advice consult an old man. How much more valued would older people be if we all followed that advice.

But there is more still. It is very easy to see the person in front of you now, hale and hearty or ailing and dependent, and to look no further. A poignant reminder can be found in the following poem, a life account written by an elderly resident of a nursing home in Ireland. This poem was shown to me when I began nurse training in 1976 and is still appearing in texts concerning the care of the elderly and being shared with students today. Take a few minutes to read it. Reflect on its significance to your past experiences with older people and consider the biopsychosocial factors of her life and upon which she is reflecting.

Kate

What do you see nurses
   What do you see?
What are you thinking when you
   are looking at me
A crabbit old woman
   not very wise,
Uncertain of habit
   with far-away eyes.
Who dribbles her food
   and makes no reply,
When you say in a loud voice
   'I do wish you'd try'
Who seems not to notice
   the things that you do,
And forever is losing
   a stocking or shoe,
Who unresisting or not
   lets you do as you will
With bathing and feeding
   the long day to fill,
Is that what you're thinking,
   is that what you see?
Then open your eyes nurse,
   You're not looking at me.
I'll tell you who I am
   as I sit here so still,
As I use at your bidding
   as I eat at your will.
I'm a small child of ten
   with a father and mother,
Brothers and sisters, who
   love one another,
A young girl of sixteen
   with wings on her feet,
Dreaming that soon now
   a lover she'll meet:
A bride soon at twenty,
   my heart gives a leap,
Remembering the vows
   that I promised to keep:
At twenty-five now
   I have young of my own
Who need me to build
   a secure happy home.

A young woman of thirty
   my young now grow fast,
Bound to each other
   with ties that should last:
At forty my young ones
   now grown will soon be gone,
But my man stays beside me
   to see I don't mourn:
At fifty once more
   babies play around my knee,
Again we know children
   my loved one and me.
Dark days are upon me,
   my husband is dead,
I look to the future
   I shudder with dread,
For my young are all busy
   rearing young of their own,
And I think of the years
   and the love I have known.
I'm an old woman now
   and nature is cruel,
'Tis her jest to make old age
   look like a fool.
The body it crumbles,
   grace and vigour depart,
There now is a stone
   Where I once had a heart:
But inside this old carcase
   a young woman still dwells,
And now and again
   my battered heart swells,
I remember the joys,
   I remember the pain,
And I'm loving and living
   life over again.
I think of the years
   all too few – gone too fast,
And accept the stark fact
   that nothing can last
So open your eyes nurses,
   Open and see,
Not a crabbit old woman,
   look closer – see ME
   (quoted in Carver and Liddiard, 1978).

It should be remembered that the majority of people over 65 are able to lead entirely independent lives: 50 per cent of all people over 65 and 33 per cent of over-85s report no disability at all (Tinker *et al.*, 1994).

Why do we age?

Throughout the years much has been written about ageing and the ageing process in literature, philosophy and scientific literature, and it is only by taking a scientific approach that we can really address *why* we age by understanding *how* we age.

Look around you, and within the wider environment think how you recognise ageing in such things as cars, bridges, elastic bands and food. Obviously, wear and tear, perishing, metal fatigue, rusting (oxidation), rancidity, desiccation and decay all play their parts. Humans can be measured against some of these changes because we are subjected to the same environmental conditions. We are, after all, made up of foodstuffs ('We are what we eat'), and we have molecules in common with some of these substances.

But there are other perspectives that colour our view of ageing.

You have probably heard that our allotted span is 'three score years and ten', . . . '70 years: or 80 years if we are strong' (Psalms 90: 10), but this is about length of life rather than ageing. In general literature the theme has been developed:

> God the Lord wishes to determine the life of his creatures and to the ass, the dog, the ape and lastly the man he allots 30 years each. But for the animals this is too much and God has compassion upon them and gives the ass only 18 years, the dog 12 years and the ape 10 years. Man with 30 years has too little and God has compassion upon him and gives him the 18 years and the 12 and the 10 years of the other animals. Hence for the first 30 years, man lives a human life; but then in succession come the burdened life of the ass, the snarling years of the dog and the foolish years of the ape – the laughing stock of the child. (Jakob Grimm, 1860, cited in Carter, 1980, p. 120)

The above, whilst comico-tragic, obviously reflects a viewpoint which may be considered vaguely scientific as it compares humans with other species. It also relates age with a quality or purpose of life. Does this view persist now? Remember that there is more than one way to deride the elderly. Very early postulates relate duration of life to an animal's period of growth, being a function directly of their eventual size (Aristotle 384–322 BC). It is interesting to note the recognition that youth laughs at old age.

Ageing? Why should we worry? Our life span is in the hands of God. However, if we are to believe Aristotle, it lies in the hands of nature. 'Nature does everything for the best.' An example to illustrate his point can be seen in the dehiscence of adult teeth in older generations. From

Aristotle's viewpoint, this would be logical: as you won't be eating for much longer because of the imminence of death, you don't need teeth. Cause or effect? A similar event occurs in nature, in African elephants. Throughout their lives they grind away their teeth. When they become unable to eat they starve to death.

From your reading and your own experience, you will know that humans do not have an allotted span, nor does it lie 'in the hands of nature'. However, Weismann (1882) asserted that it was senseless to have unlimited life, reasoning that tissues of the body that are deteriorating or wearing out just can't keep up with the demand to replace themselves. Obviously when a critical point is reached death would occur. Within a society this may be beneficial, preventing a drain on resources and indeed making way for the young. Weismann also wrote that, 'the worn out are not only valueless but indeed harmful as they take the place of the sound'. Within wider spheres of biology, the support for these assertions, which echo the sentiments of another philosopher (Epicurus, circa 400 BC), is limited to a few species of moth (Waddington, 1980, in Carter, 1980, p. 120).

It is easy to see where the expression 'to wear out' came from. Your own experience will have taught you that materials wear out at different rates, not least based on the properties of the individual substance. The modern view of nursing, which espouses holism and individualism, is perhaps the key to longevity in humans. From the moment of conception we have a genetic programme to initiate and drive our development, which produces an organism that is subjected to environmental pressures. These pressures vary from those that are subtle, such as the intrauterine blood supply, to others, like environmental pollution, which are much more obvious. Environmental and interpersonal interactions impact on the genetic programme in ways that are purely individualistic. Not even identical twins have exactly the same environmental and interpersonal interaction.

Jalavisto (in Ackerman, 1951, p. 321) demonstrated that longevity and life expectancy appear to be linked to maternal age, suggesting a genetic link, but emphasised that because of our individuality there is no guarantee that we will meet our full genetic potential. This is demonstrated when, for example, we consider a person who carries the genes for 'tallness' who fails to reach this potential because of illness, malnutrition or lack of parental affection and stimulation as a child.

Having now touched on historical theories, it is time to explore further.

To make sense of the biological theories that seek to explain the ageing process one needs to understand thoroughly the cell and its growth and functions. Take time out to:

1. Reflect on your knowledge of cell structure. Does Figure 1.2 look familiar?

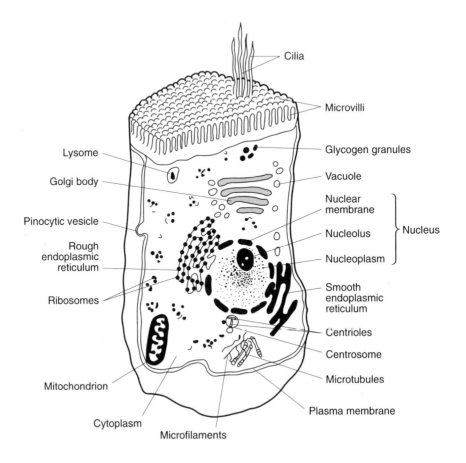

Figure 1.2 Structure of a typical cell. (With permission from Clancy and McVicar, 1995)

2. Identify the role or function of each of the labelled organelles and note the structure of the cell membrane (Figure 1.3).
3. Consider the importance of protein in cell structure and regulation.

Cells

The human organism, like all organisms, is composed of cells (see Figure 1.2) which are the basic living structural and functional unit (Tortura and Grabowski, 1993). The human body comprises 'trillions of cells and the substances between them' (Seeley, Stephens and Tate, 1992). All body cells originate from male and female gametes fusing and undergoing *mitotic* division from the zygote onwards. (Remember that *meiosis* occurs only in sexual cell division.)

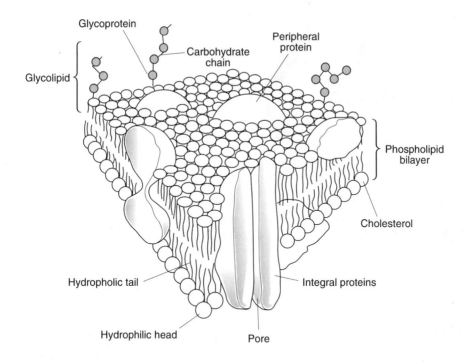

Figure 1.3 The fluid mosaic model of membrane structure. (With permission from Clancy and McVicar, 1995)

Mitosis is the cell division that produces daughter cells with the same genetic content: *diploid* cells produce *diploid* cells. Recall what happens in:

- Interphase
- Prophase
- Metaphase
- Anaphase.

Mitosis is only one brief part of the cell's life cycle (see Figure 1.4). For the remaining time there is a growth in size (both surface area and volume) during which it expresses the uniqueness of its deoxyribonucleic acid (DNA).

The cell cycle is only one part of the ageing process. Note that in biological organisation there are subcellular classes and ultimately molecular organisation (see Figure 1.5) and that ageing probably occurs at all levels. Cells proliferate from fertilisation extremely rapidly. Growth slows down as they become committed to specific functions within the body. The cellular life span of all of the body cells can conveniently be discussed under three main groupings:

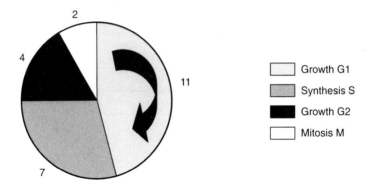

Figure 1.4 The cell cycle. In a typical adult lymphocyte, the G1 phase takes 11 hours, the S phase 7 hours, the G2 phase 4 hours and mitosis (the M phase) 2 hours, approximately. The cell cycle varies according to the cell's type and function.

- Cells that continue to proliferate throughout life, replacing dead or damaged tissues where the rate of production and rate of loss are balanced in homeostasis, e.g. skin, bone marrow and mucous membrane
- Cells that stop proliferation when sufficient numbers are achieved but which can resume division if necessary to replace damage, e.g. liver
- Cells that cease growth altogether when sufficient numbers are achieved and then reject their replicatory structures, e.g. muscle cells and neurons: loss due to damage or death of such a cell is irreversible (at present).

There is also a complex control system of genes (cellular growth promoters and inhibitors, tumour suppressors and oncogenes) that regulate the life cycle of cells by the protein expressions, and chemical reactions and interactions, occurring within the cytoplasm (Ludlow *et al.*, 1989). Genes are lengths of the DNA molecule which 'code' for the individual proteins. Figure 1.5 places cells in the context of the whole organism. Think about the importance of the genetic component: the human genotype is estimated at some 100 000 genes, which give us all our individual characteristics. Consider the effect on the organism as a whole of external (extrinsic) and internal (intrinsic) factors impinging on function and structure at all the levels in the chart. For example, within the last 50 years consider not only the effects of the atom bomb and nuclear reactor accidents on the survivors but how the altered physiology caused these effects to develop. It is worth noting that Kagan and Levi (1974) believe that we inherit predispositions to certain disease processes, and that these react with the environment to give us our unique response. This could explain why people age at different rates within the same 'allotted span'.

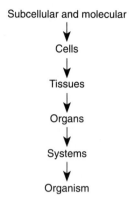

Subcellular and molecular

↓

Cells

↓

Tissues

↓

Organs

↓

Systems

↓

Organism

Figure 1.5 Levels of biological organisation.

Deoxyribonucleic acid (DNA) and ageing

This is a complex molecule, which carries the genetic blueprint of an individual's biological structure and regularities. It consists of two parallel 'backbones' of the phosphorylated sugar deoxyribose protruding out of which are the bases adenine (A), thymine (T), guanine (G) and cytosine (C). It is organised into a ladder-like structure, which is spiralled in a helter-skelter into the classic double helix (Figure 1.6) identified by Watson and Crick (1953). The rungs of the ladder consist of two complementary bases bonded in the middle with hydrogen bonds. The pairing of these bases is not random, but specific, and this specificity is required for the correct functioning of the molecule. Cytosine binds with guanine and vice versa: adenine binds with thymine and vice versa.

Looking at Figure 1.6(b), visualise, if you can, damage to one of the strands. Provided that the other strand is intact, because of the specificity of base pairing, the other strand can be repaired by enzymes which attach the correct complementary bases in the correct sequence.

During mitosis it is important that the daughter cells (the cells produced by the division) have the same genetic information as their progenitor. Internal processes then regulate the expression of this information into structure or function. (In mitosis, when the dividing cell is large enough and has duplicated all its chromosomes/genes, it cleaves into two daughter cells, each identical genetically to each other and to the original. Depending on how these cells differentiate – which genes are activated – they may function in exactly the same way – or differently.)

The DNA of the progenitor cell has to be replaced exactly. Imagine the whole structure of DNA as a large zip fastener with the binding parts being the hydrogen bonds between the base pairs forming the rungs of

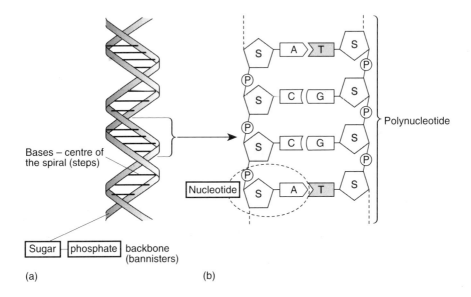

Figure 1.6 (a) The double helical structure of DNA. (b) Magnified view of DNA components: S, sugar (pentose); P, phosphate; C, T, A, G, bases – the pyrimidines cytosine and thymine, and purines adenine and guanine. (With permission from Clancy and McVicar, 1995)

the ladder. Enzymes split the band along the length of the molecule (which can be millions of bases long) at the hydrogen bond. Other enzymes then structure two reciprocal chains using the primary chains as templates.

You can see that, as the original DNA molecule 'opens', new strands are formed (one for each of the original backbones), enabling the DNA to replicate. One copy will go into each daughter cell.

DNA is the code that determines whether you develop into a human, a monkey, a frog or a fish. There are a lot of similarities in the DNA of these species, more than you would imagine, but this is logical as we all shared a common evolution.

How does DNA work? It is known that in each nucleated cell of the human body within the nucleus are 46 chromosomes, which contain in total about 100 000 genes – our genotype. Genes singly or in combination give us our traits or individual characteristics – single gene traits, or polygenic traits. e.g. eye colour, skin colour, height, ability to 'tongue roll'. These are some of the obvious visible ones. Less obvious are the structure of haemoglobin, enzymes for cellular regulation, growth promoter genes, growth inhibitor genes, chemical receptor genes, membrane ion channel genes, and many more.

All of these traits are characterised by specific proteins, which are involved either in the structure itself or in the regulation of that structure. The gene is a length of DNA that carries the code for a specific protein – which gives the characteristic to the body. Proteins are made up of chains of amino acids bonded together in an order which is specific for that protein: change the sequence of amino acids and you will alter the structure and may alter the function of that protein. Consider this with regard to the role of proteins in cell membranes, for example. Gross changes may alter the protein itself. The proteins are also folded characteristically so they have three-dimensional shapes as well as chemical formulae. It is known that the shape and the amino acid sequence are both important in how the protein functions. This concept is becoming increasingly implicated in the attempted explanation of prion diseases such as bovine spongiform encephalopathy (BSE) and Creutzfeld–Jakob disease (CJD) (Prusiner, 1991).

If DNA is the code book, genes are each individual sentences. The body 'reads' the DNA in sequences of three bases known as triplets or codons (Figure 1.7). It is the triplet that is the code for an amino acid: the sequence of triplets determines the order in which the amino acids are placed within the protein, via an intermediate chemical messenger RNA (mRNA).

UUU ⎫ phe	UCU ⎫	UAU ⎫ tyr	UGU ⎫ cys
UUC ⎭	UCC ⎪	UAC ⎭	UGC ⎭
UUA ⎫ leu	UCA ⎬ ser	UAA ⎫ 'stop'	UGA 'stop'
UUG ⎭	UCG ⎭	UAG ⎭	UGG trp
CUU ⎫	CCU ⎫	CAU ⎫ his	CGU ⎫
CUC ⎪ leu	CCC ⎪ pro	CAC ⎭	CGC ⎪ arg
CUA ⎬	CCA ⎬	CAA ⎫ gln	CGA ⎬
CUG ⎭	CCG ⎭	CAG ⎭	CGG ⎭
AUU ⎫	ACU ⎫	AAU ⎫ asn	AGU ⎫ ser
AUC ⎬ ile	ACC ⎪ thr	AAC ⎭	AGC ⎭
AUA ⎭	ACA ⎬	AAA ⎫ lys	AGA ⎫ arg
AUG met	ACG ⎭	AAG ⎭	AGG ⎭
GUU ⎫	GCU ⎫	GAU ⎫ asp	GGU ⎫
GUC ⎪ val	GCC ⎪ ala	GAC ⎭	GGC ⎪ gly
GUA ⎬	GCA ⎬	GAA ⎫ glu	GGA ⎬
GUG ⎭	GCG ⎭	GAG ⎭	GGG ⎭

ala, alanine; arg, arginine; asn, asparagine; asp, aspartic acid; cys, cystein; gln, glutamine; glu, glutamic acid; gly, glycine; his, histidine; ile, isoleucine; leu, leucine; lys, lysine; met, methionine; phe, phenylalanine; pro, proline; ser, serine; thr, threonine; trp, tryptophan; tyr, tyrosine; val, valine.

Figure 1.7 The mRNA codons for amino acids (mRNA cannot 'hold' Thymine and substitutes it for uracil = u).

Proteins are made in the ribosomes, outside the nucleus. DNA cannot pass out of the nucleus so the code has to be copied (in a process called *transcription*) on to a molecule that can, i.e. messenger RNA. Once mRNA is on the ribosome, *translation* of its codons occurs by transfer RNA bringing the correct amino acid to deposit in the correct place on the developing protein chain.

Imagine the number of cell divisions that occur in a lifetime. Is DNA going to be copied exactly each time? Remember that a change in DNA structure from the original is known as *mutation*. From conception, the developing organism is subjected to external influences. We know that the smaller the number of cells, potentially the greater the impact these have on mitotic replication of DNA or the transcription process into protein. The mutation will be carried from its time of origin into all subsequent divisions. This is clearly demonstrated if we remember the impact of cigarette smoking during pregnancy on the birth weight and subsequent health of the baby.

How many environmental mutagenic effects will we experience throughout our lives? Will they damage our sexual cells and affect our offspring? Or will they have a positive effect? Will they act singly or, over months or years, combine to cause their effects?

Remember, too, that structurally we are made up of simple and complex chemicals. What reactions occur as our chemicals come into contact with other chemicals? Even such things as common as the oxidation of foodstuffs mentioned earlier may affect the fats and proteins of which we are made – remember membrane structure? Let us attempt to illustrate the concept. Remember that each triplet code identifies a specific amino acid in a position in a protein. Consider a chain of DNA with a 'frame deletion' (perhaps because of radiation damage).

Original sequence:

AAT	GCC	GAA	CTT	ATG	CAG
TTA	CGG	CTT	GAA	TAC	GTC

Sequence after damage, i.e. deletion of A and T second and third bases of the first triplet:

AGC	CGA	ACT	TAT	GCA	G—
TCG	GCT	TGA	ATA	CGT	C—

The first triplet after the damage will become:

AGC
TCG

which is a different code and may result in different amino acids being substituted.

Because of the knock-on effect of this deletion, a different DNA code has been produced by the mutational effects of whatever caused the change. The random occasional changes or errors in replication that occur during our lives (error prone replications) may accumulate to cause protein alteration, whereas a single error may be inconsequential on its own. Reflect on your experience of dealing with patients suffering from cancer – we can use radiation to shrink or obliterate tumours, but at what risk? Radiation is a known mutagen and can sufficiently alter the DNA of growth regulator genes to disregulate the cell cycle. We are exposed to background cosmic radiation every minute of our lives, but we all have individual exposure rates because of our other activities and so the effects too are therefore individual.

It may be an accumulation of error prone replication throughout our life, or cumulative chemical combination as we produce and excrete wastes, or the absorption of pollutants in food or from the environment that changes our DNA, causing the changes in our protein structures that we see as ageing. Or it may be a hitherto unidentified process or processes working through different mechanisms and at different organisational levels that ages us. The changes may be entirely chemical.

The impact of DNA technology has tended to point to DNA as the seat of ageing. Several researchers have associated gross chromosomal changes, including apparent whole chromosomal gain or loss, with the ageing process. McKenna (1982) identified that Jacobs *et al.* (1963) worked with specific chromosomes confirming this; Schneider (1979) confirmed work by Pierre (1974) showing that in males the Y chromosome is most commonly missing and that Fitzgerald *et al.* (1975) identified that in females it was an X chromosome most commonly missing. McKenna also suggests that these may be the least deleterious chromosomes to lose. Females have two X chromosomes per cell, one of which is usually inactivated, and the Y chromosome contains little genetic information and is therefore least likely to affect the cell by its loss. However, cells with incorrect chromosomal numbers may affect the manufacture of all proteins and therefore lose their identity to immune surveillance. This produces a greater chance of producing autoimmunity, in which the body reacts to destroy the changed cell. So is this the cause of ageing or an effect seen by the ageing process? The question is still unanswered. It is known that genetics is involved somehow, as Karlman and Sander (1949) and, in a more comprehensive study, Jalavisto (in Ackerman, 1951, p. 321) have demonstrated that longevity is inherited. In general, the longevity of a father influences that of his sons whereas that of the mother influences the lifespan of both her sons and her daughters. It is also known that females live longer than males, – which is strongly suggestive of genetic involvement.

Hayflick and Moorhead (1961) identified that, in the laboratory, cells appear to have a limited replicative capacity. They found that fibroblasts undergo only 40–50 doublings before ceasing division. The implications of this would be a capability for growth and/or tissue replacement which had a finite duration, culminating in a situation of tissue degeneration as worn out or damaged tissue was not replaced – a state of altered homeostasis.

These findings parallel closely the earlier philosophical theories of 'allotted span' and 'wear and tear', but are not exclusive. However, as Clancy and McVicar (1995) point out, this capacity for division is apparently not achieved in vivo, in normally aged individuals or in those who have accelerated ageing (progeria). It does suggest, however, an intracellular regulation.

It is known that a complex arrangement of growth inhibitor and promoter genes (involving tumour suppressor genes and oncogenes), which interact with a whole range of intracellular chemicals, e.g. phosphates, regulate the cell cycle (Ludlow *et al.*, 1989; Mittnacht and Weinberg, 1991; Weinberg, 1992). It is also known that these are genetically determined (hence coded) in DNA. It is a logical conclusion that, if cycle regulator genes influence cellular ageing, they are subject to mutation or chemical reactions that will affect the regeneration process and have organism-level effects.

The regulator genes of a cell cycle are working in inhibitory/activating patterns probably based on internal feedback systems over short cyclic phases. But consider the inherited gene that results in Huntington's disease. It spends a large part of the individual's life in a latent or silent state, suggesting that gene latency could be protracted. This raises the question of what other genes remain within our genome in such a latent state.

Are we working to some wider genetic programme involving feedback regulators not yet identified? Many researchers have looked, and some still do, for a central timing mechanism: a 'biological clock', which by some mechanism influences our chronological development. It is accepted that the human species is subject to a number of biorhythms, which drive functions that have phasic cycles (Moore Ede *et al.*, 1982), but evidence for a central ageing clock is not conclusive. If such a clock is present, logic would dictate that it is either nervous or hormonal as these are the key body regulators.

Perhaps not all cells are capable of internal self regulation and paracrine communication, and so intracellular mechanisms retain their popularity. What better site than DNA? However, this is only one theory: there are many others.

Biological theories of ageing

Disposable soma theory

Kyriazis (1994) reviews this theory as being nature's way to protect the language of life (DNA) by preserving it within a body (soma). Energy is expended to preserve the carrier until sexual maturity and passage of

DNA into a new individual, whereafter the body is no longer necessary and repair is arrested.

Somatic mutation theory

Sziliard (1959, cited in Schneider, 1987) seeks to explain ageing in terms of mutations in body cells. The mutation is often caused by failure of cellular mechanisms to repair damaged DNA, or even failure of DNA synthesis. New 'messages' alter cell function or structure.

Error prone catastrophe theory

Originally the hypothesis (Orgel, 1970; Burnet, 1980) was that errors in the enzymes involved in copying and translating DNA, and thus in their own manufacture, cause increases in base placement errors, i.e. codons are not expressed, copied or translated accurately. Eventually the cells disregulate and die.

Two areas of potential error are DNA transcription and translation, and protein synthesis. Orgel's (1970) modification involved the hypothesis that non-dividing cells do not mutate if protein synthesis occurs without error. By implication this means that, if errors occur, non-dividing cells also change. The impetus for this alteration is driven by the observation that some cellular proteins do change in the elderly, but not all. More recent work by Dice and Goff (1987) suggests that these changes are post-translational changes, i.e. they are not associated with transcription or translation.

It may be that aged cells cannot break down aged proteins or produce more, or both.

Cross-linking or collagen theory

Collagen is the most abundant protein in the body at 25 per cent – 33 per cent of total protein and is the major protein constituent of connective tissue (Stryer, 1988). To function effectively it has to be synthesised and deposited correctly. Consequently these are two areas that may be affected by age (Bjorkstan, 1968). Normal collagen forms bonds between the fibres naturally as we develop and age. Unfortunately, the number of cross-linkages that occur by the time we are elderly makes the collagen more crystalline and progressively inactivates it.

Waste products, e.g. highly reactive free radicals and aldehydes from intracellular metabolism, may react with the collagen (or even elastin) and hasten the changes in its structure and function. The collagen thus becomes more rigid and less elastic and may provide the base for calcification.

Waste product accumulation theory

This hypothesis (Carrell and Ebeling, 1923, cited in Schneider, 1987; Sohal, 1981; Sellcoe, 1992) is that cellular ageing accumulates waste products of metabolism inside cell vacuoles, which gradually fill up the available space and limit movement of substances through the cell, affecting its function.

Such products have been identified in specific areas, e.g. neurons accumulate lipofuscin and β-amyloid, but no conclusive evidence exists that they are harmful.

Free radical theory

Harman (1956) suggests that toxic products of oxygen metabolism accumulate within the cell or tissue fluids. These free radicals are molecules or atoms with spare bonding capability. They are highly reactive and combine with intracellular DNA or protein and fat molecules, disrupting cell structure and causing problems with information storage or retrieval and both enzyme and membrane function. If ion channel proteins are involved, the permeability of the membrane is altered and then the cell's stability, potential for nourishment and excretory capacity are affected.

Rate of living theory

This hypothesis (Pearl, 1928; Carlson *et al.*, 1957, both cited in Schneider, 1987) suggests that ageing is caused by an increased rate of damage to cells and tissues associated with the increased metabolism of growth and development and with daily activity. The damage ultimately affects repair mechanisms and thus persists. The hypothesis is not popular at present.

Wear and tear theory

This theory (Pearl, 1924, cited in Schneider, 1987) is very similar to some already suggested. It, too, attributes ageing to an accumulation of the products of metabolism as we use our body structures on a daily basis.

Endocrine theory

This is a popular theory (Karenchevsky and Jones, 1947, in Schneider, 1987) that ties in with the idea that ageing, like most body functions, is regulated by a major control system. It also incorporates the premise that humans in general live long enough to reproduce and rear young, and are then redundant. This is an evolutionary viewpoint.

If we examine especially the reproductive capability of women, many ageing changes start to become visible in the third decade of life and proceed towards and culminate in the menopause, whereafter they accelerate.

Kyriazis (1994) reminds us that the hormones which give us our reproductive capability protect the body in a wider sense, e.g. the cardioprotective effects of HRT. Growth hormone production is reduced as we age. (Remember that, following the fusion of our bone epiphyseal plates, growth hormone is responsible for tissue repair and regeneration.) Other pituitary hormones, which affect a multiplicity of body functions through their effects on other tissues, are claimed to decrease in efficiency. The disregulation may be influenced by the body clocks identified earlier, through intracellular mechanisms or through the action of the pineal hormone melatonin.

Immunological theory

Walform (1969, cited in Schneider, 1987) and Hartwig (1992) suggest that ageing is associated with a declining efficiency of the immune system, but Herbert (1992) asserts that this is evidence for increased pathology with age rather than for ageing itself.

Responsiveness of both the cell mediated and the humoral immunity systems declines with age, and we see obvious involution and atrophy of immune tissues, e.g. spleen, thymus, lymph nodes and bone marrow. Hartwig (1992) suggests failure or inefficiency of T lymphocyte modulation of immunity as the culprit.

As cell proteins change with age, especially on the cell surface, auto-antibody production increases, with the body beginning to react against itself – thus reducing efficient cell numbers. Tissue 'surveillance' decreases, giving rise to a greater incidence of neoplastic changes, which persist, thus increasing the incidence of malignancy. Humoral immunity and reduction in second line defensive proteins reduces resistance to infection.

It can be seen that several theories overlap and thus, rather than having one single cause, the ageing process is likely to be multifactorial (Kagan and Levi, 1974).

Non-biological factors

Let us not forget that humans, as social beings, are affected by their surroundings and both their own activities and the activities of others. As sentient beings, we develop values and attitudes to our place in society and to society in general. The longer we live, the greater the impact social and psychological factors may have on us. Certainly there is usually the time to be affected. How must it feel to see societal values change from your own, to have your values considered old fashioned? How must it feel to see the people around you, your friends or your partner, die?

Acquiescent functionalism attributes problems within an elderly population to the difficulties in adjusting to growing old ('The mind is willing but the body weak').

Structured dependency maintains that the dependency of old age is a social construction and relates to old age by virtue of class, occupation and wider gender issues, which society reinforces.

Conclusion

True ageing changes are intrinsic; they are a feature of chronological development. As one ages, the balance of the body alters – some tissues deteriorate. As compensation by other systems and tissues is attempted tissue deterioration may predispose, with external factors, to multiple pathology. The polypharmaceutical correction of this may further affect the balance.

To the observer, the difficulty exists in determining the true ageing processes, and there are many theories seeking to explain these and to separate them from a natural wasting of body reserves through lack of use or inability to use them, or from pathologies which are seen more frequently in the aged.

It is better not to stereotype people, as individuality in both lifestyle and physiological reserves plus individuality of the ageing processes means that the aged are *not* a homogenised group of society. Individualism and holism are the keys to successful intervention, and must be paramount in any assessment process. As Doctor Hana Hermanova (*World Health*, November/December 1991, cited in Herbert, 1992) has said:

> Old age is not a disease and cannot be prevented. The occurrence of chronic degenerative diseases in old people can however be diminished, though not by means of curative medicine alone: middle aged people should be the target for health promotion with a view to preventing disability in old age.

Effects of ageing within the systems: a summary

It is difficult to categorise the effects of ageing, as most body systems demonstrate a reserve functional capacity which varies with the individual. Limitations in system function depend on the extent of the reserve and the rate of its loss.

Skeleton

This can be divided into axial and appendicular components, which are described in terms of microscopic structure, shape and size. Their growth and development depend on a combination of genetics and correct diet – containing protein, vitamins (especially vitamin D) and minerals. The mineralisation is hormonally regulated but, throughout life, activity that stresses the skeleton influences how the mineral is deposited, and consequently strength. Bones should have clearly defined margins, but in older adulthood they change shape and, because of altered mineralisation, also change texture. The clear lines on radiographs diminish, and the bone has a 'shaggy' appearance. Bone deposition and reabsorption disregulates, bone can start to be laid down at the edges of articulatory surfaces (*Lipping*), and this may affect joint movement by limiting the range of articulation. Movement may become less fluid, require more effort and cause pain.

Increasing age sees an individualised increase in bone reabsorption, which causes the bone to lose diameter and density. Especially in females the rate of reabsorption is said to be influenced by the mineral reserve, built up by activity throughout adolescence and into young adulthood. We see:

- Reduction in size
- Increasing porosity (more so in women who do not receive post-menopausal hormonal supplements)
- Less stress tolerance, which at its most extreme may result in a more easily fractured bone or spontaneous fracture (Payton and Poland, 1983).

The spine may develop curvature anteriorly because of reduced bone size and unequal wasting of spine muscles (kyphosis or 'dowager's hump').

Joints

Some people show changes in the structure of the synovial fluid component, which affects joint lubrication and nourishment of articulatory cartilage. This may subsequently degenerate, leading to the collapse of the joint or to growth of bony projections through it into the joint. The plane of movement may also be altered by unequal changes in the skeletal muscles that control it.

The slightly movable joints created by the intravertebral disc narrow as the disc atrophies, which contributes to diminished size and stooping. Nervous tissue degeneration will also affect muscle control.

Muscles

We reach our maximum strength between the ages 25 and 30, and then most individuals experience a diminishing speed, stamina and power. There is a reduction in all fibre types within skeletal muscle. These are replaced by connective tissue, which causes the above effects.

Activity plays an important preservative function. Exercise can improve disused muscle function, increasing both contractive proteins and innervation. This process maximises at approximately 50 years, to be followed by steady deterioration (Dublin, 1992).

Integument

A main integumentory component is the protein collagen, which alters in chemical composition with age, causing it to adhere to or form links between its fibres.

The skin becomes dry, thin and inelastic. There is a reduction in dermal and subcutaneous tissue fluid, causing a loss of turgor which leads to sagging as the number of skin folds increases. Pigmentation changes occur (liver spots) and more naevi are seen.

More air in the shafts of the hair causes greying, and there is a tendency to thinning in both number and texture of hairs (Whitehouse, 1992). There are strong genetic links here.

The keratinisation of nails becomes overdeveloped. This alters their growth characteristics: they become rigid, thick and horn-like in texture. If not cared for properly, they will ingrow.

Urinary system

Kidney

Between the ages of 30 and 75 years, there is a decrease in the functional units, the nephrons, by about 50 per cent. There is reduced blood flow to the kidney, causing a reduction in excretory capacity and ability to diurese. There is a potential to retain more urea but, as the dietary intake may be reduced, urine composition may not alter very much.

Bladder

The bladder and its neural controls are affected. The bladder muscle exhibits diminished tone. The number of receptors on the muscle reduces with age, with a resultant reduced stretch–relaxation response. A slower ascending nerve fibre relay results in reduced voluntary control because the internal sphincter opens involuntarily on spinal reflex. As the bladder capacity diminishes it will reach its threshold volume earlier and initiate the stretch reflex, opening the internal sphincter. This will cause pressure on the external sphincter – the pelvic floor (skeletal muscle) – where voluntary control via slower ascending and descending fibres may be diminished or delayed. This results in voiding problems.

In men, benign senile hypertrophy of the prostate may result in bladder neck obstruction. Progressive deterioration in stream, capacity and control may culminate in retention of urine.

Respiratory system

This is affected by changes in the thoracic structures, nervous control and spinal structure. With calcification of the costal cartilages, the ribs fix more firmly to the sternum and the chest becomes less flexible. Its ability to expand and contract is restricted further by atrophy or wasting of the intercostal muscles and diaphragm. These combine to create a reduced ventilatory capacity, which may lead to poor aeration of the lung bases especially. There is a reduced tolerance to this because of air passage narrowing and reduced central sensitivity of chemoreceptors to carbon dioxide levels.

Cardiovascular system

Degenerative diseases of the heart and blood vessels feature among the most common and serious effects of ageing. Arteries show increased fatty deposits, especially of high density lipoproteins (HDLs) as the body fat to body muscle ratio increases.

Atheroma may develop as a result of the effects of glucose on cell wall proteins.

Mineralisation of elastin in vessel walls by calcium causes a decreased ability to stretch and recoil, thus increasing diastolic pressure. The effects depend on the extent and the vessels involved: the more calcified and inelastic they become, the greater the risk of atherosclerosis.

Pathological disorders that result include coronary heart disease, ischaemic heart disease, hypertension, cerebrovascular accidents and heart failure (Frantz and Ferrell Torry, 1993).

The blood composition and volume are relatively unaffected by age apart from a decrease in the number of circulating lymphocytes.

Special senses

The eye

Most people are far sighted by age of 65 years, but this is not the typical long sight (*hypermetropia*) due to the shape of the eye. With age the lenses harden, thus losing elasticity and their ability to focus 'down'. This is known as *presbyopia*. It starts to develop around the age of 40–45 years, when the people affected may require bifocal or varifocal glasses.

Lens proteins alter with age and interrupt the passage of light through the lens as it becomes increasingly opaque. Severe opacities are known as *cataracts*.

The most serious eye problem in the elderly is *glaucoma*, caused by an increase in anterior chamber fluid pressures as movements of the natural intraocular fluid (aqueous humour) are disturbed. This may lead to blindness if not corrected, owing to a rise in intraocular pressure causing nerve damage.

The ear

There is a loss of hairs on the organ of Corti in the cochlea. This changes perception of some frequencies of sound (which frequencies are affected will be determined by what parts of the cochlea are involved). In the middle ear the ossicles, which are connected by synovial joints, become less mobile, and the muscles that move them lose tone. Thus, the transmission of sound and its conversion to electrical impulses for conduction to the brain are impaired. These two effects cause a diminished perception of sound pitch and amplitude, i.e. the person can't hear soft noises as well as they could. Hairs are also lost from the vestibular apparatus which controls equilibrium or balance in addition to neural atrophy. This may result in loss of balance producing a characteristic widening of the elderly person's stance to counter this and a tendency to hold their arms away from their body.

Taste

There is a loss of taste buds on the tongue due to progressive scarring, and this occurs from the age of 30 onwards. There is also atrophy and demyelination of the sensory relay nerve fibres, which degenerate. The effect is loss of taste perception, which affects salivation and mouth cleanliness and may affect appetite. Only 30 per cent – 40 per cent of the taste buds a person has at the age of 40 are still functioning at the age of 75.

Touch

This declines with age, especially in the palms and other hairless areas. Specific receptor types (Pacinian and Meissners) reduce in number, altering response to graded pressure. With peripheral neural atrophy, or in the cord or cerebral cortex, this produces a diminished ability to recognise the part of the body being touched.

Reproductive systems

Most men and women remain sexually active in their later years (despite social views otherwise), but mechanisms of response change as fertility declines in both genders. Erection is more difficult to achieve and maintain in the male, and the urgency for sex may decline in both partners. Relationship and companionship may take priority over intercourse. Reduced oestrogen levels in the female cause the vaginal epithelium to keratinise, and its lubrication is greatly diminished. This may make intercourse difficult, stressful and sometimes painful. The oestrogen related menopause may occur at any time from 40 to 60 years of age.

Oestrogen is a protective hormone in that it inhibits the osteoclastic reabsorption of bone. This process loses its inhibition after the menopause and, depending on the woman's mineral reserve, may lead to osteoporosis. The loss of oestrogen may lead to redistribution of body fat, water and facial hair.

Physical relationships may be further hampered by reduced articulation of the large joints (hips and knees).

Nervous system

Throughout adulthood there is a steady loss of cerebral cortical neurons, which leads to diminished sensory motor and associative control. (Between the ages of 30 and 70 years, the average brain weight decreases by 44% and nerve conduction velocity by 10%.) Although memory may be affected, especially short term, the changes are very individual and only a minority cause dementia. Peripheral neurons exhibit diminished receptor sensitivity. Their number and the conduction velocity of the action potential are reduced. There is a delayed reaction time, and reflexes may be slower. Perception reflexes and responses may also be delayed. The balance of the various neurotransmitter 'cocktails' is affected by altered neurotransmitter production and receptor population changes. Altered dopamine levels and receptor interaction may affect mood and co-ordination, as happens in Parkinson's disease. Altered acetylcholine levels have been implicated in Alzheimer's disease.

Within the brain, some people show a deposition of amyloid (an inflammatory response protein), which may cause the neuronal transport filaments to block or tangle, interfering with cell nutrition. These processes have also been implicated in Alzheimer's disease.

References

Ackerman U (1951) *Essentials of Human Physiology.* Mosby, New York.

Bjorkstan J (1968) The crosslinkage theory of ageing. *Journal of the American Geriatric Society* **16**, 408-27.

Burnet FM (1980) *Endurance of Life: The Implications of Genetics for Human Life.* Cambridge University Press, Cambridge.

Carter N (1980) *Development, Growth and Ageing.* Croom Helm, London.

Carver V and Liddiard P (eds) (1978) *An Ageing Population.* Hodder and Stoughton/Oxford University Press, London.

Christiansen JL and Grzybowski JM (1993) *Biology of Ageing.* Mosby, Missouri.

Clancy J and McVicar A (1995) *Physiology and Anatomy: A Homeostatic Approach.* Edward Arnold, London.

Dice JF and Goff SA (1987) Molecular determinants of protein half-life. *Eucara, FASEBJ,* November 1 (5), 349-57.

Dublin S (1992) The physiological changes of ageing. *Orthopaedic Nursing* 11, 45–50.

Frantz RA and Ferrell Torry A (1993) Physical impairments in the elderly population. *Advances in Clinical Nursing Research* 28, 363–70.

Harman D (1956) Ageing: a theory based on free radical and radiation chemistry. *Journal of Gerontology* 11, 298–300.

Hartwig M (1992) Immune control of mammalian ageing, a T cell model. *Mechanisms of Ageing and Development* 63, 207.

Hayflick L and Moorhead PS (1961) The serial subcultivation of human cell strains. *Experimental Cell Research* 25, 585–621.

Herbert R (1992) The normal ageing process reviewed. *International Nursing Review* 39, 93–6.

Kagan AR and Levi L (1974) Health and environment. Psychosocial stimuli – a review. *Social Science and Medicine* 8, 225–41.

Kyriazis M (1994) Age and reason. *Nursing Times* 90, 61–3.

Ludlow JW, DeCaprio JA, Huang CM, Lee WH, Paucha E and Livingstone DM (1989) *SV 40 lart T* antigen binds preferentially to an under phosphorylated member of the retinoblastoma susceptibility gene product family. *CELL* 56, 57–65.

McKenna PG (1982) Down the line. *Nursing Mirror,* 21st July, 26–9.

Mittnacht S and Weinberg RA (1991) G1/S phosphorylation of the retinoblastoma protein is associated with an altered affinity for the nuclear compartment. *CELL* 65, 381–93.

Moore-Ede MC, Sulzmann FM and Fuller CA (1982) *The Clocks that Time Us.* A Commonwealth Fund book, Harvard University Press, Cambridge MA.

OPCS Office of Population Censuses and Surveys (1993) *The 1991 Census of Persons Aged 60 and Over, Great Britain.* HMSO, London.

Orgel LE (1970) The maintenance of the accuracy of protein synthesis and its relevance to aging: a correction. *Proceedings of the National Academy of Science (USA)* 67, 1476–9.

Payton OD and Poland JL (1983) Ageing process. *Physical Therapy* 63, 41–7.

Prusiner SB (1991) The molecular biology of prion disease. *Science* 252, 1515–22.

Schneider EL (1987) Theories of ageing: a perspective. In Warner HH, Butler RN, Sprott RL and Schneider EL (eds) *Modern Biological Theories of Ageing.* Raven Press: New York.

Seeley RR, Stephens TD and Tate P (1992) *Anatomy and Physiology – International Edition.* Mosby, New York.

Sellicoe DJ (1992) Ageing brain, ageing mind. *Scientific American* **267**, 134–43.

Sohal RS (ed.) (1981) *Age Pigments.* Elsevier Press, Amsterdam.

Stryer L (1988) *Biochemistry,* 3rd edn. WH Freeman & Co., New York.

Tinker A, McCreadie C, Wright F and Salvage AV (1994) *The Care of Frail Elderly People in the United Kingdom.* HMSO, London.

Tortura GJ and Grabowski SR (1993) *Principles of Anatomy and Physiology,* 7th edn. HarperCollins, New York.

Watson JD and Crick FHC (1953) Molecular structure of nucleic acid: a structure for deoxyribose nucleic acid. *Nature* 171, 737–8.

Weinberg RA (1992) The retinoblastoma gene and gene product. *Cancer Surveys* 12, *Tumour Suppressor Genes, the Cell Cycle and Cancer,* pp 45–7.

Whitehouse MJ (1992) The physiology of ageing. *Journal of Intravenous Nursing* 15 (suppl) S7–S13.

2

Promoting quality of life: the development of specialist practice

Jim Marr

In the last 20 years, nursing care of older people has undergone dramatic changes for the better, and there has been a distinct focus on maintaining and improving their quality of life. This chapter presents a historical outline to lay the foundations for some of the more specific sections of the book.

Epidemiology and demographic changes

As a result of the cumulative achievements of health care and the social and economic progress of the twentieth century, a greater proportion of the British population now reaches the age of retirement than ever before. Most people now expect a long and healthy retirement, free of major illness and disability. Most people expect, and desire, to stay in their own homes for as long as possible and to live as independent a lifestyle as they can. However, not all older people achieve this because of the many chronic and disabling conditions that become more common in later life. These are not an inevitable consequence of ageing, but it is acknowledged that conditions such as dementia, stroke and osteoarthritis, as well as other cardiovascular and respiratory disorders, have an increased incidence and prevalence in later old age (over 75 years). Many of these conditions require complex medical treatment and active inpatient or outpatient rehabilitation programmes, and these services become the basis of community or institutional care. Older people, therefore, are major consumers of health and social care. Since the mid-1980s, this issue has been brought into sharper focus by government policies that attempt to address the increasing 'burden' of the ageing population of the UK and the ability of the nation to finance this increasing level of care services. This shift in perception to one in which older people have become a burden has been identified by Phillipson and Walker (1986) as the 'social construction of old age'.

Nursing care

Within the field of nursing, major advances have been made in the care of older people in the last twenty years or so, and a specialty has developed which is founded on an increasing knowledge of the ageing process and a rise in gerontological studies. Much of this improvement is due to the work in nursing development units, which have pushed forward the practice of nursing, and established a process of change that has empowered nursing on a wider sphere across most specialties. This phenomenon has been described by Salvage (1990) as 'new nursing' and focuses on the management of change, creative practice and patient-centred care.

This new nursing was born out of the changes taking place within clinical nursing of older people, and the early nursing development units (NDUs) arose out of this specialty.

Historical perspectives

Twenty years ago, nursing practice was based on management and medical models with nurses making very little contribution to decision making. Nursing was seen as subservient to medicine, and care was very much based on routines and task allocation. An autocratic authoritarian philosophy was evident, with clinical practice founded on tradition and ritual (Walsh and Ford, 1989). Nurse education focused on learning how to set up trolleys and trays and on memorising lists of signs and symptoms of common diseases. Nursing documentation was based on doctors' orders and written in a shorthand of local abbreviations that made little sense to others. Care was recorded briefly in the nursing kardex with little consideration of individual needs. 'Care rounds' were performed on an assembly line basis, and tasks were identified in a hierarchy and allocated according to the seniority of the nurse, with technical skills being given the greatest importance. The more subtle care skills, such as comforting, communicating and supporting, were given little attention and appeared only on an *ad hoc* basis when all other work was completed. Although a body of nursing theory had begun to emerge in the USA, nursing practice in the UK was still based on keeping busy.

This ritualised practice was particularly evident in 'geriatric' areas, where older people were processed in a warehouse fashion in an attempt to delay death as long as possible. A typical geriatric ward would have housed thirty or more older people in an open Nightingale layout, and their day would be spent sitting beside their bed – often spending all day in their nightclothes. Meals would be taken from the bed table and routine toileting rounds performed with commodes and urinals. By late afternoon, most would be put back to bed, and night staff would continue this existence of turning, toileting and changing.

Nursing developments

In the early 1980s evidence of change had begun to emerge as nurses tried to assert themselves and seek higher status within the health care team. Bachelor (1980) identifies a number of factors that brought this about: the changing status of women in society, the higher status of nurses reflected in salary increases, the enhanced quality of entrants to nurse training, the women's liberation movement, the introduction of new management structures in nursing, the improvement in quality of nurse education, the increased number of men in senior positions and the rise in trade union involvement by nurses.

Also at this time the 'nursing process' (Yura and Walsh, 1973), a problem-solving approach to nursing, was introduced in the UK. This articulated for nurses a systematic approach to care, which focused on the individual needs of each person and encouraged a decision-making autonomous approach, much to the distress of many in the medical profession who saw it as undermining their authority.

The emergence of nursing models (such as Roper, Logan and Tierney's (1985) 'activities of living') gave nursing a further impetus.

Nursing development units

Influenced by nursing developments in the USA, Oxfordshire Health Authority set up an NDU in a small community hospital at Burford in an attempt to explore new approaches to the delivery of nursing care (Pearson, 1988). Following an intensive programme of staff development, a system of primary nursing was set up with individual nurses acting as key workers with 24 hour accountability for their patients. Nurses worked in partnership, giving informed choice in care that was patient centred and individualised rather than task orientated. The innovative work at Burford was regularly featured in national nursing journals, and research conducted within the unit, on older people with fractured femurs, showed that the higher quality of nursing they received increased their life satisfaction. Although the survey was small, it aroused interest and support from around the UK and, with that, encouraged the Burford unit to expand its services to incorporate community nursing. This first NDU established the principles of practice, research, management and education, all based in a clinically orientated unit. From this experience, the Oxford Nursing Development Unit was founded, with sixteen nursing beds specifically for patients who needed intensive nursing (Salvage and Wright, 1995).

In 1985 Tameside Nursing Development Unit was founded in Tameside General Hospital, Ashton-under-Lyne. This unit was based within the services for older people, and a change process was established throughout acute, rehabilitation and day hospital services whereby patient care was empowered through primary nursing, standard setting and the involvement of patients in the planning and management of their own care. The work at Tameside was widely publicised by its leader, Steve Wright, and this helped to influence and promote the NDU concept within the UK (Wright, 1989). Thus nursing in the UK was being very much led by the innovative work in old age services.

In 1988 the King's Fund Centre Nursing Development Programme was established to pursue clinical nursing development by piloting more NDUs and setting up a national NDU network. In 1991 the government allocated £3 million to established further NDUs in a programme managed by the King's Fund. By 1993, Barbara Vaughan, the new director of the King's Fund Programme, was overseeing the work of over 70 active NDUs within the country – many of which were involved in services for older people. This innovative work and its published literature inspired nurses around the country, and the nursing care of older people became firmly established as a specialty in its own right. From this work, quality of care for older people and nurses' clinical knowledge and skills had dramatically improved.

'High-tech' and 'high-touch' care

As nursing care of older people began to emerge as a specialty in its own right, the nurse's role developed to attempt to meet their special needs. Initially, much discussion took place in NDUs about the expansion or extension of the nurse's role as nurses learned new skills and took on new responsibilities. The expansion/extension debate was eventually addressed by the UKCC (1992) in their publication *The Scope of Professional Practice*. This gave nursing staff a freedom to develop further specialist skills and roles.

The quality of care of older people was further enhanced by discussion and debate on high-touch or high-tech care. As nurses reviewed and re-examined their role and the importance of their care skills, the therapeutic use of touch was a subject that appeared often in the nursing press. Issues around procedural touch (the touch involved in the technical procedures of nursing) and non-procedural touch (that used as a method of communication or comfort) were debated (Pearson, 1988). Nurses working with older people took on new procedural skills such as venepuncture, cardiac monitoring and subcutaneous infusions, but at the same time extended their care (or high-touch) skills into the realm of complementary therapies using massage, aromatherapy and relaxation techniques. Thus the quality of care provided for older people improved and the autonomy and specialist practice of nursing staff was developed and came into its own.

Management of care

As specialist clinical skills developed, traditional nursing roles and regulations were also challenged. Open visiting was supported, and relatives were encouraged to become partners in care. Overnight accommodation and facilities for refreshments were made available so that the older person could remain involved with, and be supported by, friends and family. Flexibility and choice in care became the norm as a consumer-orientated philosophy developed. Care and treatment regimens were explained fully, with true informed consent being sought. Care plans were formulated, and these were located at the individual's bedside and became true working documents. The older person was encouraged to read them and question nursing staff about their care and to contribute to the review process as they wished, adding comments and evaluating their progress. A patient-centred rather than a worker-centred philosophy emerged, with acceptable standards of care being formulated (RCN, 1991), agreed and regularly measured and evaluated. An open system of complaints and suggestions was also encouraged as the older people and their families were empowered within the health care system.

Primary nursing (Manthey *et al.*, 1970), where each registered nurse carries a case load of six to eight patients and is responsible on a 24 hour, seven days a week basis, became the preferred method of care delivery. Further publications such as *The Patient's Charter* (Department of Health, 1992) and *A Vision for the Future* (Department of Health, 1993) enabled and empowered nurses and those in their care to continue to develop quality standards.

Community care

While care for older people was undergoing major change in hospital services, government policy had been effecting major change within the community. *Growing Older* (DHSS, 1981) paved the way for the changes:

> Whatever level of public expenditure proves practicable, and however it is distributed, the primary sources of support and care for elderly people are informal and voluntary. These spring from the personal ties of kinship, friendship and neighbourhood. They are irreplaceable. It is the role of public authorities to sustain and, where necessary, to develop – but never to displace – such support and care. Care in the community must increasingly mean care by the community.

The origin of the term 'community care' remains obscure. However, it is not a new policy objective in the field of mental illness as there had, for a number of years, been a move to prevent and decrease institutional care and the institutionalisation of people with mental health needs.

In the 1960s, now famous literature such as Goffman's (1961) book on Asylums and *Sans Everything* by Barbara Robb (1968) began to highlight the unsuitability of large institutions and the depersonalisation, deprivation and neglect that patients were subjected to. Although the term 'community care' first meant de-institutionalisation, in later years this emphasis changed to include a degree of support that should be given or provided outside the institution. An exact definition of 'community', however, is difficult to find. In the Seebohm Report on Local Authority and Social Services (Home Office, 1968, p. 147) it is defined thus:

> The notion of a community implies the existence of a network of reciprocal social relationships which among other things ensure mutual aid and give those who experience it a sense of well-being.

Initially, the idea of community care was to reduce the number of hospital places, but over the years the notion has been elaborated by successful legislation, most notably published by the Department of Health in the 1980s – *Caring for People* (1989) and *Working for Patients* (1989). No-one would disagree with policies to reduce institutionalisation in support of a more normal lifestyle out of hospital, but the policy makers have been accused of having a hidden agenda in these decisions.

It may be argued that these policies are based on rising numbers of older people and 'dependent' individuals, and the cost implications thereof. Care in the community has been seen as a cheaper option to the costly provision of hospital beds. However, the notion of 'community' must include the provision of a whole range of services that enable people to choose to remain in their own home with dignity and independence for as long as possible.

Since the introduction of the Welfare State in the UK, there has been a move away from providing care in residential settings to providing it at home. As mentioned, much of this has been in the belief that care in the home is the cheaper option to the maintenance of large institutions, many of which date back to Victorian times and are therefore expensive to maintain and keep up. In support of this, there has been a move to transfer resources to the community, but the level of these resources has been a main cause of concern. Criticism has been made about under-funding and under-resourcing, particularly with the large number of people requiring these services.

During the 1970s, the economic difficulties experienced in the UK began subtly to change the term 'community care'. Increasingly, a clear distinction has been drawn between care in the community and care by the community. Victor (1987, p. 288) explains this change:

> Care in the community is best defined as the provision of care by the placing of professionals and specialist personnel in the community to provide services to clients in their own home. Care by the community stresses the provision of care by the lay/non specialists on a voluntary or semi-organised basis.

It is interesting to note how this subtle change from 'care in' to 'care by' the community has let the government off the hook, with major implications for service provision and the funding of these services. 'Care in the community' suggests a formal framework of professional help, funded by health and social services, whereas 'care by the community' suggests the informal network of friends and family. Cost differences could therefore be enormous, with a shift of responsibility for help and support from central and local government to the family. Although no formal procedures exist to enforce families to care, social obligations and expectations put pressure on some family members to care for those in need. The unavailability of statutory services further adds to this pressure.

Two models of community care are therefore evident:

- The community using its own resources via informal and voluntary support
- The community resources being supplemented from external sources mainly provided via national government.

More and more, however, statutory services for older people are being seen as a last resort measure with the emphasis mainly being placed on family and the informal sector.

Caring for, and about, older people

Many people with disability, striving to maintain their independence, reject the concept of care, claiming that it implies a passive role in which they are reliant on dominant able-bodied people. A favoured term is 'support' or 'assistance', as some degree of control and choice is then involved.

Much has been written about the concepts of 'caring for' and 'caring about' (Ungerson, 1983). Caring *for* someone suggests the practical tasks and skills involved in day to day support, whereas caring *about* suggests the wider aspects of rights and advocacy. With regard to community care, the 'caring for' is expected to be done while the 'caring about' aspects are not reflected in government policies, which appear continually to underfund and undervalue the services required by older people.

The responsibilities for caring usually falls to women, and thus caring is regarded as a woman's issue. More women than men are carers and more women (mostly older women) than men are cared for (Bernard and Meade, 1993).

How much care is required?

The ageing of the British population has been well documented. In the 1980s an alarmist phrase, 'the demographic timebomb', was used and abused by politicians as shorthand for the complex pattern of demographic trends. This was seen by some to be a misleading phrase which was of little use. However, Henwood (1992, p. 7) disagrees:

> It accurately conveys the sense of urgency and panic which has surrounded the increasing awareness of the ageing population alongside the decline of other age groups (notably young people aged 17–24) and wider changes in family trends.

Although the proportion of the population aged 65 and over has been growing since the turn of the century, it is only in the past 20 years or so that these numbers have been recognised as an important policy issue, with the real growth occurring in the oldest old, who are more likely to be dependent and the major consumers of services. Although there is not necessarily an expectation that increased old age brings frailty, the proportion of the population with some degree of disability rises markedly over the age of 75 and there is dramatic increase over the age of 85. The 1985 General Household Survey found that approximately 2 per cent of the older population (159 000) were bedfast and 8 per cent (670 000) were housebound; 3.6 per cent of all older people (301 000) were unable to go up or down stairs unaided, and 7.3 per cent (611 000) were unable to bathe themselves. These figures reflect a considerable level of disability and dependency among older people and therefore a considerable demand on services.

Projected figures are uncertain as it is possible that future generations of elderly people will be fitter. However, increased numbers of very old people (over 85) give some insight into the possible demands of the future.

Who cares?

Because caring is regarded very much as a women's issue, there is an implicit expectation in the policies of community care that women will still be available to, or choose to, provide care. Many of these policies also base themselves on a romantic idealistic view of 'family life' based on the nuclear family living close to older relatives. Within this family is an able-bodied woman who is supported by her husband and who is therefore free to provide care and support to the older person. This notion is now out of date, as the traditional community has changed with the break-up of the extended family and the expectations of married women to continue in employment. The reduction in family size and increased incidence of divorce and remarriage further complicate this idea and raise questions about the wisdom of policy makers. In her work on family obligations and social change, Finch (1989) notes that family relationships do not operate on the basis of ready-made rules of morality. The 'sense of obligation' to care is not reliable and, in many relationships, never materialises. It would be foolish to ignore the limitations of the family and the fact that many older people do not have relatives. Family support for them is impossible.

There is also no adequate framework of benefits and services to enable men and women to make rational choices about the balance between work and home responsibilities. Apart from the financial cost of caring, the most significant cost is the emotional and physical strain involved. Caring for a relative in their own or the family home is tiring and disruptive to family life. Family and marital stress is common, as is a disruption to social life. Other members of the family may distance themselves so that the main burden of care falls to one individual. Often the strain involved in this reaches crisis point. The cost of care is thus not to be minimised. No allowance is made for the lost opportunity or the reduced possibility of career development. The extra finances involved in the caring role are also exaggerated by the ability to earn only a part-time wage or retain only a lower position because of reduced time commitment to work. Although the cost to and the position of women are recognised by government, the role of public services is still seen to be an enabling one, helping people to care for themselves and their families by providing a framework of support (DHSS, 1981).

The superiority of family care cannot be assumed. The unequal gender responsibilities involved, plus the negative relationships that exist within families, do not lend support to the idealised notions of community care. The ability of the wider community to offer or provide support is also flawed, as voluntary services are restricted because of lack of available human resources, and rising crime figures encourage people to be less trustful of others and so to keep themselves to themselves. Notions of helpful neighbours, milkmen, postmen and children running errands are founded in the past.

Reasons for change

In its early stages, community care was defined in negative terms as the opposite of institutional care. Although there appear to be clear reasons for a move away from institutional care, the notion of community care was unfortunately a romantic image, conjuring up notions of the camaraderie apparent during the Blitz. This image has prevailed and may be responsible for the lack of specific objectives surrounding its policies and the fact that no specific definitions have been given about what exactly community care is.

The move away from institutional care was evident initially in the field of child care and mental incapacity, and few could argue for the physical, social and emotional deprivation that institutional care encouraged. As new drugs were discovered to combat the behavioural problems manifested in mental illness it became apparent that hospitalisation might not be necessary in the long term and that support could be given to maintain people in the community. Thus the notion of community care was possible because of advances in treatment regimens, such as new drugs. The majority of older people have always been cared for in the community, and the emergence of the specialist medical and psychiatric services since the 1970s has promoted the idea that long-term residential care should always be seen as a last resort.

In 1981 the definition of community care for older people took a significant turn with the publication by the DHSS of the White Paper *Growing Older*. The responsibility for their care was clearly stated to lie with the community, as this was claimed to be the most appropriate model. At this time the Conservative government was involved in scaling down government intervention and responsibilities, promoting instead private enterprise and individualism. This reduced reliance on statutory services and encouraged responsibility of the individual or the family to support and provide for themselves. Although this echoed Margaret Thatcher's policies of returning to Victorian values, it also supported the policy of a reduction in public expenditure as the demographic trends began to highlight the supposed inability of the country to support the increasing number of older people. Between 1951 and 1988, the proportion of the total expenditure attributable to the over-65 age groups leapt from 20 per cent to 49 per cent and the per capita spending on the over-75s rose from just over twice the average to almost five times the average (National Association of Health Authorities, 1989).

Few would not agree that the quality of life should be better for an older person living in their own home and that it is the right of the individual to remain in their home whenever possible. However, there was, and always will be, a need for some very severely dependent older people to receive continued care over a 24 hour period for reasons of physical or mental frailty or dependency. Although the cost of institutional care is high, there is no evidence that the intensive care required by some older people to live in the community is a cheaper option. A level of professional or formal care will always be required, especially for tasks of a more intimate and personal kind. There is a difference between friends and/or neighbours collecting shopping for an elderly person and dropping in to put them on the toilet. In support of this, there is evidence to suggest that elderly people prefer to rely on state services and formal cares than on their children (Arber and Ginn, 1991). Although consumer choice is said to be a fundamental principle of community care reforms, the fact that older people would choose formal rather than informal care has been ignored.

The reliance on care by the family also presumes that they are close by and can easily 'pop in'. However, the search for employment now encourages people to move to obtain work and so they may be less available. Frequency of visiting will depend very much on geography and on distance. In the 1950s, 40 per cent of older people lived with a child, but by 1990 this figure had dropped to only 5 per cent.

Reciprocity and empowerment

Much of the basis of community care has been motivated by costs and perceived expenditure, supporting the notion of the political economy theory of ageing (Phillipson and Walker, 1986). Sadly, this does not take into account the very real contribution made to society by older people, perceiving them only as consumers and not as contributors. The years after retirement offer opportunities for new experiences, growth, self realisation and reflection. It is important to remember that most older people continue to live active and constructive lives and many have made, and continue to make, notable contributions to society. Unless their reciprocity is acknowledged they are unlikely to be considered as equal members of society. Tinker (1991) warns that this is foolish and short-sighted. It also encourages the myth that no-one relies on them and they are therefore of little use.

Choice and flexibility of service provision are also said to be fundamental to community care. Care managers are encouraged to be creative in their use of resources. It may be argued that reliance on the state for income and health or personal care allows more autonomy than reliance on household members (Arber and Ginn, 1991). However, complete autonomy can be gained only with devolvement of the budget to the individual to allow them complete choice and flexibility. A decent level of personal spending power would allow access to the open market, promoting individualism and encouraging market forces. Individual liberty, competition, choice and flexibility would then be encouraged. It is difficult, however, to empower older people, and the idea of them being able to barter on an open market to maintain some degree of life quality is ridiculous and an alien concept to them. Forcing disabled and frail older people into this kind of arena would only increase their vulnerability and dependence. Those with mental health problems resulting in cognitive impairment would surely be losers again, unless carers or advocates were appointed to act on their behalf. Once more, family, friends and neighbours would need to be drawn into the support network – this time to use skills of finance, bargaining and retail.

Nursing home care

An independent report (Wagner, 1988) was commissioned by the government to study the provision of residential care by the statutory, independent and voluntary sectors. This study attempted to confront the idea of residential care being a realistic option for those requiring increased levels of care. Some of the recommendations of the report were later included in the NHS and Community Care Act (1990), which prompted a review for more appropriate domiciliary services and community care. It also called for the promotion of care homes in the independent sector. Initially, many of the privately run nursing homes received bad publicity as entrepreneurs sought to achieve a quick and large return on their investments. Large multistorey houses were bought and converted to make totally unsuitable environments for older people whose quality of life suffered as a consequence.

Desirable characteristics of homes, according to the Wagner report (1988), were for:

- *Privacy* – so that residents could be left undisturbed and free from intrusion

- *Dignity* – respecting the uniqueness of individuals and their personal needs
- *Independence* – a willingness to accept a level of risk without intervention
- *Choice* – the opportunity to select from a range of options
- *Rights* – maintaining the entitlement of citizenship
- *Fulfilment* – the realisation of personal aspirations and abilities.

These characteristics are still supported today and form the basis of the regulation and inspection of homes under the Registered Homes Act (1984).

Despite the early negative perceptions of nursing homes, many consider them to be the best option for older people with mental health problems. The advantages cited include the provision of safety and supervision, comfort and physical care, not having to worry about finances, and the reduction of loneliness (Wade, 1994). The involvement of large corporate organisations such as Westminster Healthcare have brought credibility and high standards of care for older people in purpose-built accommodation designed to meet their specific needs.

Conclusion

The health care of older people has improved dramatically over the last two decades both in hospital and in the community. However, there is still a long way to go. Each day in the press, we read of rationing of services – often based on ageist policies where older people's needs are viewed as secondary to those of younger people. The debate continues about payments for care, with an ongoing argument about what is health care and what is social care – because health care was always promised to be free at the point of delivery, whereas social care was not. Recently, the government announced an unpopular insurance scheme to enable people to begin to make plans for care costs in their old age.

In this political climate, therefore, it is becoming more and more important that nurses are able to articulate the specialist knowledge and skills which they use to care for older people. More than ever before, the spotlight is on us, as the care of older people moves into the next millennium.

References

Arber S and Ginn J (1991) *Gender and Later Life*. Sage, London.
Bachelor I (1980) *The Multi-disciplinary Clinical Team – A Working Paper*. King's Fund, London.
Bernard M and Meade K (1993) *Women Come of Age*. Edward Arnold, London.

Department of Health (1989) *Working for Patients*. HMSO, London.
Department of Health (1989) *Caring for People*. HMSO, London.
Department of Health (1992) *The Patient's Charter*. HMSO, London.
Department of Health (1993) *A Vision for the Future*. HMSO, London.
DHSS (1981) *Growing Older*. HMSO, London.
Finch J (1989) *Family Obligations and Social Change*. Polity Press, Oxford.
Goffman E (1961) *Asylums*. Doubleday, New York.
Henwood M (1992) *Through a Glass Darkly: Community Care and Elderly People*. King's Fund, London.
Home Office (1968) *Report of the Committee on Local Authority and Allied Personal Social Services (Seebohm Report)*. HMSO, London.
Manthey M, Ciske K, Robertson P *et al.* (1970) Primary nursing. *Nursing Forum 9*, 64–83.
National Association of Health Authorities (1989) *Will You Still Love Me?* Society of Family Practitioner Committees, London.
Pearson A (1988) *Primary Nursing*. Croom Helm, London.
Phillipson C and Walker A (1986) *Ageing and Social Policy*. Gower, Aldershot.
Robb B (1968) *Sans Everything: A Case to Answer*. Nelson, London.
Roper N, Logan WW and Tierney AJ (1985) *The Elements of Nursing*, 2nd edn. Churchill Livingstone, Edinburgh.
Royal College of Nursing (1991) *Standards of Care – Nursing and Older People*. Scutari, Harrow.
Salvage J (1990) The theory and practice of the new nursing. *Nursing Times 86*, 42–5.
Salvage J and Wright S (1995) *Nursing Development Units – A Force for Change*. Scutari, Harrow.
Tinker A (1991) *Elderly People in Modern Society*. Longman, Harlow.
UKCC (1992) *The Scope of Professional Practice*. UKCC, London.
Ungerson C (1983) *Why do women care?* In Finch J and Groves D (eds) *A Labour of Love*. Routledge and Kegan Paul, London.
Victor C (1987) *Old Age in Modern Society*. Chapman & Hall, London.
Wade B (1994) *The Changing Face of Community* Care. Daphne Heald Research Unit, London.
Wagner Report (1988) *Residential Care – A Positive Choice*. HMSO, London.
Walsh M and Ford P (1989) *Nursing Rituals*. Butterworth-Heinemann, Oxford.
Wright S (1989) *Changing Nursing Practice*. Edward Arnold, London.
Yura H and Walsh MB (1973) *The Nursing Process*. Appleton–Century–Crofts, New York.

3

Sensory deprivation
and the older person

Lesley Surman

This chapter is concerned with sensory loss in the older person. As nurses we meet older adults in the course of our everyday activities, be they as patients/clients, relatives, friends or significant others, or as the people we work with. It is advantageous for the nurse to be aware of the changes that can occur with the ageing process. This knowledge can help us in our everyday interactions with other people, facilitate harmonious relationships and promote independence and self esteem in ourselves and others.

We are all concerned, or afraid, to a greater or lesser extent with ageing (gerontophobia) (Thompson 1989). Here the common changes associated with the ageing senses are outlined. Case studies are offered for you to consider from a managerial, ethical or professional stance, and some will be referred to in later discussion, where the emphasis will be on the promotion and attainment of normality. Although brief anatomical and physiological descriptions are included, you are recommended to refer to specialist texts for greater depth.

Vision

If one of your senses was to be impaired, which do you feel would be the worst for you? The most important sensory input is often considered to be that of sight, although Hutchinson (1991) suggests that 'undue emphasis is often placed on the use of vision'. In fact, most of us will experience changes in our vision from around our mid-20s, with many of us needing to wear glasses for close work, such as reading and sewing, by the time we are in our 50s.

Damage to the eye is not caused by over-use, reading or writing for long periods with or without good light, watching television or carrying out fine visual discrimination tasks such as embroidery. Nor is it true that sexual practices damage the eyes!

Why then does visual acuity change? There is a gradual deterioration in the powers of accommodation of the eye, which starts around the 20s. Suspensory ligaments, which hold the lens in place, become slack and the lens becomes less elastic and harder; gradually the lens flattens, reducing the ability to focus on near objects (presbyopia). Visual acuity is further reduced as the muscle of the iris becomes less responsive, which decreases the size of the pupil, causing slower adaptation in poor light. Parallel to this is a reduction in the ability to discern colour, so that objects set in contrast are more easily discernible.

Hospital interiors have historically portrayed a blur of pastel shades, from wall decoration to floor covering, bed linen to nurses' uniforms. Gradually this is changing – a change which is often influenced by nurses. Research by Long, Rieser and Hill (1990) highlights the importance of contrast for effective and safe mobility. Contrasting floor coverings to wall decoration enable a person with poor vision to appreciate space and parameters. Contrasting uniforms enables patients to identify staff of differing status and role. These simple and logical considerations go a long way towards enhancing independence and empowerment of individuals.

The majority of people enter retirement with good sight, or at least with only a degree of presbyopia, yet sight threatening conditions are common among the older adult population (Long *et al.*, 1991), cataracts, glaucoma and macular degeneration presenting most commonly.

Cataract

Cataracts are considered the most common disabling eye condition in older people (Redfern, 1991), and are rare before the age of 50 except in those suffering with diabetes.

The lens is made up of numerous layers of protein fibres, arranged like layers of an onion. New fibres are laid on top of old ones, with the lens remaining transparent. Cataracts result from additional coagulation and necrosis of the fibres of the lens (Gould, 1987), the transparency being replaced by opacity. The person usually reports clouding, blurred or misty vision (Royal National Institute for the Blind, 1992) or of a permanent speck or wedge in the visual field. The increase in opacification of the lens is variable from one individual to another. Once a cataract is diagnosed it is usually some time before treatment, which is surgical removal of the lens, is carried out. This is generally not until the sight has deteriorated to the extent that normal activities of daily living, and therefore the quality of life, are significantly disrupted.

CASE STUDY 1

Mary Hartley, a 68-year-old lady, was referred to the ophthalmologist at the regional eye unit following a visit to her GP. Mrs Hartley was complaining of a permanent speck in her visual field. A cataract was diagnosed. Because it was small and causing her no significant difficulties in her daily living, her name was put on the waiting list for removal of cataract in two years time, when, it was thought, the cataract would be 'ripe' or 'mature' enough for removal, the assumption being that by this time it would be significantly affecting her ability to carry out her everyday activities, and therefore reducing her quality of life.

Duly, in two years time, Mrs Hartley received a letter from the hospital with details of her planned admission. However, at this stage, Mrs Hartley did not feel that she wanted to have the operation as, although the cataract had progressed slightly, it was still not having any detrimental effect on her quality of life.

This case study demonstrates that the advancement of a cataract is not easily predetermined, and that further assessment and consideration of the individual's perception of the situation is essential.

Glaucoma

Glaucoma is the condition in which the intraocular pressure of the eye is raised because of an imbalance between the production and drainage of aqueous fluid. Normally the pressure ranges between 18 and 22mmHg. There are two types of glaucoma: chronic and acute.

Acute glaucoma

With acute glaucoma the onset is fast, the pressure builds up quickly, the patient may complain of nausea and perhaps vomiting, halos or rainbows around lights may be seen, and headache and severe pain are common. Vision may become blurred as the cornea becomes oedematous, and the patient may complain of feeling dizzy. The efficiency of the blood vessels, retina and nerves is also compromised by the high pressure the fluid places on the internal surface of the eye. This is an emergency situation. Treatment must be given as soon as possible to prevent, or at least reduce, the amount of loss of visual field.

Although acute glaucoma is less common than chronic, it can affect the older person. However, because of overall physiological changes, particularly of pain perception, the older person may have difficulty in discriminating changes and identifying that there is a problem.

CASE STUDY 2

Joe Smith was 72 years old and enjoying retirement with his wife, Joy. One morning he complained that he felt 'a bit off', his head was woolly and he didn't have an appetite. Later he noticed halos around lights, had a headache and was having difficulty reading the paper. Joy became increasingly worried and, much against her husband's wishes, insisted he saw a doctor:

Mr Smith was diagnosed as having acute glaucoma and at the time of examination had an intraocular pressure of 80 mmHg (remember that the normal range is 18–22 mmHg). Joe received prompt treatment and thus retained good vision with only a limited loss of peripheral visual field.

Chronic glaucoma

This has a much more insidious onset, but eventually damage will occur to the optic disc owing to high pressure, which may remain asymptomatic for months or years. Eventually the patient realises that something is wrong because they have a blind area in their visual field. The sooner treatment is commenced the greater the chance of retaining the remaining vision.

A large proportion of blindness and visual deprivation is caused by glaucoma (Watson, 1992), and although glaucoma can be managed effectively by surgical or medical treatment it cannot, in itself, be cured. It is important that the patient and significant others appreciate the situations and activities which may cause a rise in intraocular pressure, such as emotional upset and stress, and constipation resulting in straining on defecation.

For the patient and family to be aware of the things that may be problematic, a good health needs assessment must be carried out. They should also be made aware of the hereditary context of this condition, and the need for family members to take advantage of the free or subsidised eye tests available.

Macular degeneration

Redfern (1991) describes this slowly progressive degenerative disease as one that contributes most largely to poor sight in those aged over 75 years. The blood supply to the macula is compromised by debris deposited from ageing pigmented cells, and as a result the cells are raised from the membrane underlying them. The vessels themselves may bleed or leak, in which case the disease will progress more quickly.

Macular degeneration is a common cause of loss of central vision, and activities such as reading, watching television, sewing and sports may become more difficult. Detailed observation of facial expression is part of normal communication, and thus this sort of visual deprivation adds further frustrations to everyday living.

Infections

Infections of the eye are little mentioned in the literature in relation to the older person, although this can be very serious indeed, and can lead to a loss of visual ability. The nurse has an important part to play in preventing unwarranted conditions occurring.

CASE STUDY 3

Sarah Jenkins was an 83-year-old lady suffering with dementia. She had a devoted family and despite having a severely reduced quality of life enjoyed watching her grandchildren play, even though she often asked whose they were.

A health needs assessment carried out by the care givers highlighted areas of vulnerability – a vulnerability which could be greatly reduced with conscientious care. Mrs Jenkins was a very proud lady who liked to maintain a smart appearance. Because she suffered with dementia Mrs Jenkins was not able to achieve this for herself in all respects; for example, she requested assistance in caring for her fingernails. The care givers appreciated this difficulty and facilitated this aspect of her care.

This sounds so simple, and indeed it is, but without concern to detail a vulnerability exists. We have all, at one time or another, found our nails to be 'dirty' or rough and in need of filing (and, indeed, nails are susceptible to breaking or splitting and to the accumulation of particles). Mrs Jenkins appreciated the attention given to this area of her care. But apart from the importance Mrs Jenkins placed on her appearance, and the therapeutic value, this area of care prevented her from sustaining accidental injury, such as skin damage which may be caused when scratching an irritating little itch, or corneal abrasion whilst rubbing an eye.

Nails pose a means of introducing infection and, with reduced sensitivity, accidental damage may not become evident for some time. Infections of the eye, such as conjunctivitis, are no more common for the older person than for any other, but an infection introduced via a corneal abrasion could cause serious damage and even loss of sight in severe cases. This is particularly so for the older person who may not notice a corneal abrasion.

Hearing

Older adults suffer with hearing difficulties and loss more commonly than is often appreciated, either by the individual or by health care professionals. This is possibly because hearing loss is not dramatic in its change, as it takes place slowly (Gould, 1987).

With ageing certain physiological changes occur and, like vision, these changes may begin early in life: sensory neural hearing loss, for example, begins between the ages of 30 and 40 (Jackson, 1988).

Any part of the hearing pathway can suffer changes that may cause hearing deficits. Hearing starts when sound waves from the air hit the tympanic membrane, setting up vibrations which are conducted through the ossicles (small bones) of the middle ear to the oval window, another membrane. The vibrations then reach the fluid of the cochlea (in the inner ear). This is a snail shaped structure that is the hearing part of the ear.

The inner ear contains a maze-like structure of tubes known as the labyrinth. This includes three semicircular canals associated with balance. These semicircular canals are at right angles to each other and contain sensory hairs. Movement of the head causes movement of fluid within these canals, the hairs move and stimulate nerve endings which transmit information to the brain regarding the position of the head in space. This is essential to our static and dynamic equilibrium.

Infection, or thickening of the fluid, causes distortion in the movement of the fluid, resulting in dizziness and vertigo.

Changes towards hearing deprivation

The slow decline in hearing throughout adult life results in a type of deafness, common in old age, known as presbyacusis (McKenzie, Chawla and Gordon, 1986). Presbyacusis is a sensory neural impairment, which is usually bilateral and associated with pathological changes due to ageing (Brunner and Suddarth, 1989).

The second form of deafness affecting the older person is conductive deafness, whereby sound waves are prevented from reaching the inner ear. Hardening of the tympanic membrane reduces transmission of sound vibration. Jaw movement, which normally promotes mobility of wax in the ear, may be reduced in frequency and intensity with the older person, with the result that wax remains more static, becomes hardened, and compromises the transmission of sound waves.

Changes in the outer ear, such as changes in ear wax consistency and dry scaling skin, increase the tendency to harden plugs of wax and debris. This can be easily diagnosed and treated (Webber-Jones, 1992). However Jackson (1986) suggests that removal of wax does not automatically lead to an improvement in hearing levels.

Occasionally the ossicles of the middle ear become calcified and more fixed, reducing their ability and effectiveness in conveying sound waves. Infections of the middle ear should never be neglected as they are potentially very dangerous (Murphy, 1987). Likewise, upper respiratory tract infections can lead to middle ear problems, with infections tracking along the eustachian tube. These also require prompt treatment.

Medical or surgical intervention may assist in overcoming conductive forms of deafness. Alternatively, some form of amplification may assist, as it is the loudness of sound which is lost in this instance.

Hearing degeneration tends to start with the loss of high frequency (or tone) sounds, which make it difficult to distinguish between the different pitches of sound. Confusion may arise between the consonants S and F, for example, with speech presenting as a jumble of sounds from which the vowels sounds are most discernible.

Understanding a patient's hearing perception and level of deafness is very important for health care professionals. The hearing deprivation a patient experiences may be sufficient to cause them extreme, and potentially serious, consequences, such as administering their medication wrongly or agreeing to something they thought they had heard correctly but hadn't.

Whatever the cause of the hearing deficiency in the older person it is important for health care workers to have the concern and knowledge that enables them to appreciate the distorted hearing which may be experienced by individuals, and to recognise the reactions, behaviours and emotions that arise from this. They also need the skills to design appropriate nursing intervention and to give care effectively.

Given that high frequency loss predominates, low frequency sounds prevail as those best heard. Unfortunately, 'noise' generally consists of mainly low frequency sounds. Therefore, when hearing aids are worn to amplify high frequency sounds and facilitate the hearing of speech, noise sounds will also be amplified.

CASE STUDY 4

William Shuttle, a 77-year-old diabetic bachelor, lived with his friend, and both were profoundly deaf. Mr Shuttle was admitted to hospital for investigations relating to circulatory problems of his legs. Mr Shuttle had been in hospital for ten days when the surgeons decided that the only course of treatment was an above-knee amputation of his left leg.

Ensuring that she had an appropriate quiet environment and the time to spend with Mr Shuttle, the nurse assessed his perception and understanding of his diagnosis, treatment and future. Mr Shuttle had obvious difficulty in hearing everything that was said to him. Further assessment revealed an accumulation of wax, which, after softening with ear drops, was successfully removed. He then had an audiology assessment and was subsequently fitted with a hearing aid.

Mr Shuttle was so pleased with the simplicity and success of his treatment and hearing aid that he insisted that his partner went to see his GP to arrange a similar assessment!

What problems can you identify in the following case study?

CASE STUDY 5

Miss Ellis is sitting in the dayroom. Her hearing aid is turned off. The television is on, a nurse is talking to the patient next to her, and the two patients adjacent are having a conversation. A nurse asks Miss Ellis if she wants a drink. Miss Ellis says she can't hear the nurse, so the nurse turns up Miss Ellis's hearing aid and speaks more loudly, directly into the hearing aid. Miss Ellis gets cross, jumps and tries to push the nurse away, saying 'Don't shout at me!'

For many people, sounds become too acute when hearing aids are used (Jackson, 1986), and the noise and sounds amplified in this way can be unbearable (Murphy, 1987). Not only is it unpleasant but it can also be very painful.

In this last case study, not only does Miss Ellis have a variety of amplified background and surrounding noises to contend with, but the nurse moves her head so that Miss Ellis cannot see her face, therefore giving her reduced facility to observe facial expression (which would help her to determine what is being said to her).

Taste and smell

The decline in sensitivity of the senses of taste and smell varies, but frequently occurs to some degree, with ageing. The number and functioning capacity of olfactory cells and taste buds declines owing to atrophy, although it is unlikely that this is the sole cause of diminished response.

We have all experienced to a greater or lesser extent the changes that occur to our appreciation of food when we have a cold or flu. The older adult may experience increased diminution of smell (and therefore taste) with increased nasal hair and crusting of nasal secretions in the air passageway, which obstruct the functioning of olfactory cells. This also means that they may not notice certain odours that a younger person may find unacceptable. This may leave them vulnerable to dangers such as burning and gas.

Aitken (1995) postulates that 'by age 70 a typical man has less than half as many taste buds as he had in his 20s'. This sort of decline in taste sensitivity would understandably affect the interest afforded to food. However, Gould (1987) also suggests that food may not appear to taste so good anymore because of 'modern food technology, with its highly processed products'. A further detraction from food clarity also occurs when rendering it suitable for a 'soft' diet. You can try a little experiential learning for yourself by liquidising one of your own meals!

Other factors that aggravate the situation are heavy cigarette smoking, chemicals in the air, poorly fitted dentures, a sore mouth and poor oral hygiene.

The decrease in these senses means that food can taste very bland and uninteresting. As a result, an older person may be found to be using an increased amount of salt, pepper and other condiments to 'spice up' the food and make it more palatable. The greatest loss of sensitivity is for sweet (Aitken 1995), hence the development of a sweet tooth as one gets older. Yet, particularly in institutional care, the older person may be denied the opportunity to order the spicy and sweet food they prefer, or they may not have the ability to add extra flavourings.

CASE STUDY 6

Jack Brown, 82 years old, was maintaining his independence well at home. He attended the day care centre twice a week for physiotherapy, after which he would stay for lunch and the afternoon's activities before returning home.

Mr Brown was amiable and easy going, but on one occasion he had obviously had enough. Lunch was served, and Mr Brown started eating. After a few moments Mr Brown looked up and said firmly

'Mince, . . . mince, . . . boiled fish, . . . boiled potatoes . . .. Oh, why don't they give us something we can taste, preferably with a bit of colour to it'.

CASE STUDY 7

Mrs Babbage, at 69, had been in hospital for three years suffering with motor neuron disease, which had progressed to the extent that she was paralysed from the neck down and her swallow reflex had become greatly affected. She enjoyed her food as a rule, but loathed the blandness of the liquidised diet she was receiving from the hospital kitchens.

How do you think you could help to make meals more appetising and pleasurable for Mrs Babbage?

Skin senses

The skin senses are associated with warmth and cold, pain and touch, or pressure. The older person may complain of feeling uncomfortable even in an environment where the temperature is kept fairly constant. The changes that contribute are the poorer blood circulation and the reduction in subcutaneous fat experienced with ageing. A change in activity levels may also occur.

Victor (1991) found that older people recognised their own activity changes, moving from the more athletic leisure pursuits to more controlled (although potentially energetic) forms of activity such as gardening. Of course, outdoor activity is as valuable for older people as for younger ones but there is the potential for heat exhaustion (even though you may think it only a slim chance in the UK), as the body takes longer to adjust to changes in internal and external temperatures. Equally, the effect can be as devastating if internal and external temperatures drop; if not corrected, this can result in accidental hypothermia. The difficulty is that the older person doesn't necessarily notice rising or declining temperatures as acutely as a younger person, and consequently doesn't respond to the condition.

The sensory nerve cells that supply the skin decline in number with ageing (Aitken, 1995), leaving the older adult susceptible to unnoticed knocks and cuts. Even burning of the skin from sitting too close to the fire is not an uncommon finding on assessment of an older person.

Pain acts as a warning sign. Unfortunately, with ageing, the perception of pain diminishes and not only may the elderly person not know how they obtained bruises or cuts (which occur more easily in the elderly due to increased skin fragility), but illness, internal injury and broken bones may present a patient with only discomfort, general distress or confusion (Gould, 1987).

Everyone's pain threshold and perception of pain is different, often influenced by culture, upbringing and personality, and this, Aitken (1995) suggests, can also affect the rate at which pain perception diminishes in old age. Assessment of pain is difficult at the best of times, and usually McCaffery's (1983) advice to nurses stands true, that pain is what the patient says it is, when and where they say they have it.

However, with older people it should not be assumed that there is no injury just because the patient is not focusing on, or complaining about, a particular pain: something could still be seriously wrong. The nurse's skills in communication and assessment are vitally important in helping to establish a diagnosis and the pain relief intervention that may be needed to achieve quality care.

It is well recognised that pain assessment and relief is an aspect of care not particularly well addressed by health care professionals. Rather than looking at a case study here, consider how *you* go about assessing whether someone has pain or not and what *your* feelings and attitudes are in these situations.

Discussion

It is fair to conclude that sensory changes are inevitable with ageing. These changes are slow and the onset can be early in life. Often, however, the progress of the changes does not become apparent until the deprivation starts to interfere with the activities of daily living. 'Researchers' typically focus upon personal care (e.g. washing, dressing and feeding) and household management activities, or instrumental activities, such as shopping or cleaning' (Victor, 1991). The concerns of nurses have also traditionally followed in this vein. This is a limited approach, particularly when the quality of a person's life is considered from their perspective.

The nurse's role is multifaceted. Part of the role is to work in conjunction with other members of the multidisciplinary team (Thompson, Melia and Boyd, 1994). It incorporates not just assisting in the carrying out of surgical and medical procedures and interventions and ensuring that prescribed treatment is given, but also promoting the optimum level of wellbeing for an individual, which may have a much greater nursing focus.

From considering these case studies it can be appreciated how the autonomy of a person can be seriously compromised through sensory deprivation. They also demonstrate how the professional's power base can further undermine or empower patient/client autonomy.

All health care professionals owe a duty of care: there is a moral (Brown, Kitson and McKnight, 1992) and legal requirement (*Bolam* v *Friern Hospital Management Committee*, 1957) for professionals to exercise their professed skills. By the nature of the position you hold as a nurse, patients/clients have an expectation that you will do the best for them, and that which is in their best interest.

It is not the intention here to describe corrective medical or surgical intervention, rather to consider how the nurse can empower patients/clients to reach their optimum level of autonomy, which is after all the basis of all health care (Seedhouse and Lovett, 1992; Beauchamp and Childress, 1989). If the barriers preventing a person from freely governing their own life can't be removed, it is often possible, through good management and education, to facilitate and achieve improvement.

Tyne (1994) states that 'people seem to mean different things by "empowerment" '. For nurses, empowering patients should mean helping the patient to recognise detrimental barriers and enabling or assisting them, to the extent possible, to use strategies to overcome those barriers, therefore empowering them to make life choices.

So much is taken for granted. That eyesight and hearing deteriorates with age is a fact accepted as commonplace and it is often considered that this should just be accepted. Further thought highlights risks, for example the increased likelihood of accidents and injury. Poor sight alone affects one's ability to understand and comprehend where we are and what is going on around us, which in turn 'affects our ability to communicate with others' (Windmill, 1992), as much of our understanding of what is said to us is conveyed through body language and facial expressions. When this is also compounded by hearing deprivation, vulnerability to accident, injury or the criminal in society is greatly exacerbated.

Knowledge of the changing senses is, for the most part, a neglected aspect of the person, being left, in the main, to the province of specialist nurses and physicians. This cannot be afforded, nor should we as nurses allow the deprivation of sensual experience to go unaddressed. Quality of life is essential and most disorders, if they cannot be cured, can at least be helped: they should never just be left and accepted as a part of ageing that has to be tolerated.

The risk of accident and injury comes quickly to mind, but what of the more subtle situations such as ensuring that the patient/client consents to the treatment and care proposed for them? Assessment, good planning and appropriate intervention are fundamental to the provision of quality care. For patient/clients and health care staff the outcome can be devastating if understanding and co-operation are not established. The older person may have some degree of sensory deprivation, but this does not render them incompetent.

Health care professionals have a duty to do the best for their patients, but it must be recognised that to do that without the involvement and consent of the patient is for the professional to act paternalistically, and it is questionable whether this can be justified in health care (Gillon, 1992). The nurses' code of conduct (UKCC, 1992) reinforces the nurse's duty towards patients. It states 'A registered nurse, . . . in the exercise of your professional accountability must: work in an open and cooperative manner with patients, clients and their families, foster their independence and recognise and respect their involvement in the planning and delivery of care'.

Because older people have limitations to the effectiveness of 'normal' communication channels, it does not follow that their capacity to understand and to continue to make their own life choices are also compromised.

It is the responsibility of nurses to use their skills and promote effective two-way communication, thus empowering older adults, and this may also go some way towards reducing some of the stereotypical attitudes held by some individuals.

MacFarlane (1994) expresses exasperation regarding the attitudes towards any older adult with disability, for it appears to her that once you have a disability it affects all your capacities to function as a rational independent person.

Lyon (1993) acknowledges that hearing is recognised as the 'social sense', where 'impairment may mean isolation and loneliness even in a crowd', and Allen (1991) points out that 'visual impairment is a threat to the social and personal existence of the individual'. Certainly a study by Barron *et al.* (1994) suggests that 'at a time of increased need, elderly people experience a loss of social support'. Spencer (1988) reflects that friends stayed away from him when he lost his sight. Although it is possible to reduce (if not alleviate) the sensory deficit, Thompson, Gibson and Jagger (1989) recognise that it is often the other social disadvantages that cause the greatest problems.

Lowell, Gerson and McCord (1987) recognise that the risks of imbalance in elderly people with impaired hearing or vision are substantial and serious. These sorts of incident can often be misconstrued as something they are not. Jackson (1988) recognises the potential for the misdiagnosis of dementia (a difficult diagnosis to correct), when the hearing impaired person, in becoming isolated, becomes distressed, perhaps depressed, and displays some apparent mental confusion.

Stimulation of the senses is important, but overstimulation can also have a detrimental effect. For example, speaking too loudly or increasing lighting to the extent that it becomes a glare to someone with cataracts can cause distress, frustration and increase vulnerability. To get the balance right can be difficult particularly, for instance, when auditory reception is variable. Involving the patient/client in establishing what works best for them, when and how, is essential, because unless we do we will not know how a situation or circumstance is viewed from their perspective.

The first step towards helping patients/clients help themselves seems logical and even obvious, but a review of the literature would suggest otherwise. Observation and detection is the first step, be this in a community or in an institutional setting. An individual may not notice their progressing impairment, but arguments between family members, patients or residents over the television volume control, for example, may provide some indicators for the onlooker.

An acute problem such as that experienced by Mr Smith in Case study 2 can also be missed, or at least treatment delayed, because the pain and sensory perception by the older adult is reduced, and signs and symptoms are muffled. What may present as a minor complaint should never be dismissed as something that will go away, or that is just part of getting old and therefore something that must be to put up with.

Behaviours suggesting a loss of interest (for example half-hearted attitudes towards dining and socialising) should trigger the need for further assessment. The solution to Mrs Babbage's dietary problem in Case study 7, by the way, was to order her an ordinary meal, let her see it presented on the plate, then liquidise it on the ward, adding a stock cube to it in the process to enhance flavour.

Diagnosis is frequently considered the province of the physician. Nurses seem reluctant to use the term 'nursing diagnosis', but diagnose we do. Webber-Jones (1992) describes the case of a lady who was 'moderately unco-operative', isolated and reluctant to interact. This lady was given a renewed quality of life once the nurse had made a nursing diagnosis following assessment. The problem was simply a build up of wax (or cerumen) in the external auditory canal, similar to that of Mr Shuttle in Case study 4. The nurse is in a prime position to identify such a problem and activate treatment.

Diagnosis is about observing and then asking questions on what has been detected. For example, Spencer (1988) (who had a visual impairment) found that when in hospital he had more accidents, such as knocking things over, because the nurses kept moving his things around trying to tidy up for him. If only the nurses had asked him what he felt the best arrangement was, a lot of frustration and loss of dignity could have been avoided.

To enhance communication and reduce the frustration and isolation generated by visual and auditory impairment there are several points that should be taken into consideration:

- Sit or stand so that the person can see you clearly. Both visual and auditory impairment can reduce or interfere with the ability to concentrate. Being a comfortable distance away, but in front of the person, aids their concentration, facilitates lip reading and their appreciation of the non-verbal communication and body language.

- Maintain a good position for the patient's benefit. Don't try to write and talk at the same time, for instance. This has two disadvantages. Firstly, dropping your head to write means that the other person cannot see your eyes, lips or facial expressions, only the top of your head. Secondly, it may be taken to suggest that you are not really interested, or have moved on to something else.
- Focus on the communication in hand, and remove or avoid barriers such as background noises and activity. Competing with these noises not only devalues an interaction but may compound an already anxiety provoking and traumatic time. Always consider that when there is no response to your calling a person's name it could be because they can't hear you or see you.
- Shouting can make things worse; so, too, can turning up hearing aids, as this amplifies all sounds (consider the case of Miss Ellis in Case study 5).
- Ensure that hearing aids and glasses are owned if they will improve a person's perception, and that they are in good working order. This may simply involve making sure that glasses are clean. There are, of course, those spectacle wearers who independently pursue their lives through the spotty mist and haze of dirty glasses, but it is unforgivable in a care situation.

Nurses have a responsibility to know how confidently and competently to deal with glasses and hearing aids, not only to provide care for those who cannot do it for themselves, but also to educate and facilitate the skills in those who can.

Liaison with specialist staff in the auditory department would afford you the opportunity of learning about the different types of hearing aid, how they work and how to maintain them. You would also have a chance to find out about other devices available. The Royal National Institute for the Deaf and the Royal National Institute for the Blind will also provide information upon request (their addresses are given at the end of the chapter).

The emphasis of concern in issues of sensory deprivation is appreciably given to visual and auditory loss. The frustration experienced by an older adult with reduced taste and smell can be seen in the case of Mr Brown in Case study 6. It is often assumed that young children and older adults all like, or at least are happy to accept, bland food. The reality is significantly different.

Our role is only partly associated with being the providers of care. By nature of our position, whatever the reason for that person being in our care, we have a responsibility to meet their own needs as far as possible. We have a responsibility to promote health.

People are now living longer, and older adults have just as much right to health care as anyone younger. Mrs Hartley in Case study 1, for example, knew her situation and her circumstances, and she had developed coping strategies, as so many people do (Allen, 1989), and did not feel that the quality of her life was compromised so significantly as to warrant surgery. There are times when the nurse may need to act as the patient's advocate, particularly when no-one appears to be listening to the patient (Ogden, 1992), and to encourage recognition by others of their autonomy, individuality and self determination.

With increasing resource limitations 'those who are not deemed sufficiently "rational" to have a view such as . . . older people' (Naidoo and Willis, 1994) may find their needs not easily met. It has already been identified that sensory deprivation can lead to misconceptions about an individual, and with a value system within society that stigmatises disability it can be very difficult for a person to be accepted as competent and potentially independent (MacFarlane, 1994). Allen (1991) considers that this group is particularly vulnerable.

Touch

Before closing it is worth considering one more aspect of sensory deprivation, which emanates not from an internal source, as the others have, but from an external source. When Spencer (1988) was reflecting on how the loss of vision had affected his life he commented on the physical withdrawal by others which he experienced, the loss of physical contact: touch.

I recall being told once that we need three hugs a day to keep us mentally and spiritually well. Whether this is true or not will be left for you to decide, but it is reasonable to conclude that touch is therapeutic; whether it is a hug or a pat on the back, it makes you feel good. Touch is to most people a common and vital part of our everyday lives, powerfully influencing our wellbeing and motivation. It would seem then a desperate waste of opportunity and (free!) resources not to make effective use of this caring gesture as an empowerment agent for our patients. The benefits are potentially countless and you are left to ponder and consider these for yourself.

Nurses are identified as a professional group who are in a position to help to change attitudes and perceptions (Barron *et al.*, 1994). We have a duty of care, and that means that we must help the older adult to receive those things which would improve their quality of life, and empower them to be as independent as possible. Certainly we should never simply accept that sensory impairment is a part of ageing and therefore that nothing can be done to improve the situation, when frequently it can.

References

Aitken LR (1995) *Ageing: An Introduction to Gerontology.* Sage, London.

Allen M (1989) The meaning of visual impairment to visually impaired adults. *Journal of Advanced Nursing* 14, 640–6.

Allen M (1991) Stigma and blindness. *Journal of Ophthalmology and Technology* 10, 147–52.

Barron C, Foxall M, Von Dollen K, Jones P and Shull K (1994) Marital status, social support and loneliness in visually impaired elderly people. *Journal of Advanced Nursing* 19, 272–80.

Beauchamp T and Childress J (1989) *Principles of Biomedical Ethics.* Oxford University Press, New York

Bolam v Friern Hospital Management Committee (1957) 2 ALL ER 118.

Brown J, Kitson A and McKnight T (1992) *Challenges in Caring.* Chapman & Hall, London.

Brunner LS and Suddarth DS (1989) *The Lippincott Manual of Medical-Surgical Nursing.* Harper and Row, London.

Gillon R (1992) *Philosophical Medical Ethics.* Wiley, Chichester.

Gould D (1987) The biology of ageing: the special senses. *Geriatric Nursing and Home Care* 7, 15–19.

Hutchinson J (1991) Living with visual handicap. In Hawker M and Davis M (eds) *Visual Handicap – A Distance Learning Pack for Physiotherapists, Occupational Therapists and Other Health Care Professionals.* Disabled Living Foundation, London.

Jackson C (1988) Now hear this. *Geriatric Nursing and Home Care* 8, 19.

Jackson J (1986) Don't shout nurse. *Geriatric Nursing* 6, 12–13.

Long CA, Holden R, Mulkerrin E and Sykes D (1991) Opportunistic screening of visual acuity in elderly patients attending out-patient clinic. *Age and Ageing* 20, 392–5.

Long RG, Rieser RR and Hill EW (1990) Mobility in individuals with moderate visual impairment. *Journal of Visual Impairment and Blindness* 84, 111–18.

Lowell W, Gerson D and McCord G (1987) Risk of imbalance in elderly people with impaired hearing or vision. *Age and Ageing* 18, 31–4.

Lyon S (1993) Alone in a crowd. *Geriatric Medicine* 23, 5 (commentary).

MacFarlane A (1994) On behalf of an older disabled woman. *Disability and Society* 9, 255–6.

McCaffery M (1983) *Nursing the Patient in Pain.* Harper and Row, London.

McKenzie AJ, Chawla HB and Gordon D (1986) *The Special Senses.* Churchill Livingstone, Edinburgh.

Murphy K (1987) Problems of impaired hearing. *Geriatric Nursing and Home Care.* 7, 9–11.

Naidoo J and Willis J (1994) *Health Promotion.* Baillière Tindall London.

Ogden V (1992) Advocates for the elderly. *Journal of Community Nursing* 6, 8–9.

Redfern SJ (ed.) (1991) *Nursing Elderly People*, 2nd edn. Churchill Livingstone, Edinburgh.

Royal National Institute for the Blind (1992) *Ten Things You Should Know About Visual Handicap.* RNIB, London.

Seedhouse D and Lovett L (1992) *Practical Medical Ethics.* Wiley, Chichester.

Spencer R (1988) Transitions: reflections on being blind in a sighted world. *Journal of Ophthalmic Nursing and Technology* 7, 220–2.

Thompson H (1989) An old problem. *Geriatric Nursing and Home Care* 9, 20.

Thompson I, Melia K and Boyd K (1994) *Nursing Ethics*. Churchill Livingstone, Edinburgh.

Thompson J, Gibson J and Jagger C (1989) An association between visual impairment and mortality in elderly people. *Age and Ageing* 18, 83–8.

United Kingdom Central Council (1992) *Code of Professional Conduct for the Nurse, Midwife and Health Visitor*. UKCC London.

Victor CR (1991) *Health and Health Care in Later Life*. Open University, Milton Keynes.

Watson J (1992) *Medical–Surgical Nursing and Related Physiology*. WB Saunders, London.

Webber-Jones J (1992) Doomed to deafness. *American Journal of Nursing* November.

Windmill V (1992) *Caring for the Elderly*. Pitman, London.

Useful addresses

The Royal National Institute for the Blind, 224 Great Portland Street, London W1N 6AA

The Royal National Institute for the Deaf, PO Box 266, London WC1E 6AN

4

Keeping active

Anne Hayes and Abebaw Yohannes

This chapter highlights some of the special needs of older people as well as some of the risk factors we must all be aware of. But, more importantly, it emphasises the need to take a dynamic and active approach in the treatment and management of older patients whether they be in a hospital or in a community setting.

One cannot be cured of ageing. However, although reduced mobility and function may be inevitable, we should adopt an optimistic and positive approach in order to minimise risks and allow for maximum potential. The longer we live the more prone we are to suffer from the effects of ageing and degeneration, and the everyday tasks of daily living become more difficult as our bodies become less efficient. But there is no fixed rate at which people age, and different parts of the body wear out at different rates, so how old a person is in terms of the number of years is immaterial. Senescence is a natural phenomenon. It is not a disease and will happen to all of us. 'Senescence is as much of a fact of life as its climax is death' (Gill, 1987).

Many older people greatly value their independence, even those afflicted with chronic diseases. It is the responsibility of all health professionals, social services, and families to support the older person's need to maintain independent living in the community.

Older people and mobility

Ageing is a natural process that happens in an individual's lifetime. It is important to have a comprehensive perception of ageing and to understand the impact of this natural process. The actual mechanism of ageing may have different biological, psychological and social implications. There is a need to consider how the mobility of older people is affected either because of normal ageing or as a consequence of diseases, which may lead to disability.

Most people reach retirement age in reasonable health (Guccione, 1993). The majority of older people live independent and active lives, unless affected by chronic disease. Many continue to work if they enjoy working, although they may have a few manageable medical problems. Many people regard the time of retirement as the start of a new life because children have left home and the routine of regular work is gone, which can lead to the freedom to develop an interest in leisure activities and to be involved in the community. However, these activities can be pursued successfully only if an individual is actively mobile. Activities that enhance physical and psychological wellbeing will encourage older people to lead life in more or less the same way as younger people. Generally, older people report their health to be good, and most describe a high level of satisfaction with their lives. Most of them are mobile, lead an active life and participate in social activities (Ruuskanen and Ruoppila, 1995).

Good health contributes to a satisfying and long life. It depends, in most cases, on having regular exercise throughout one's life span. Other factors that contribute to keeping the body healthy are, for example, a balanced diet, a clean environment, good housing and social activities. These factors help older people to have a sense of wellbeing in their lives. Older people should not be discouraged from participating in regular exercise because of their age: it helps to keep their joints mobile and to maintain physical fitness. Primarily, it is the responsibility of an individual to avert physiological decline with ageing.

Lewis and Bottomley (1990) suggest that there is a need to distinguish between bodily changes and functions due to ageing and changes attributable to disease. It is also important to recognise the effect of a sedentary lifestyle, which may contribute to a decline in muscle strength and functional reserve, common among older people. In general, this may lead to a decrease in the level of fitness and predispose to inactivity.

Older people who are active and participate in physical exercise have less physical disability and fewer consultations with their physicians each year than those who are inactive and do not participate in physical activities (Emery and Gatz, 1990). Many epidemiological surveys have shown that older people who have been active and participate in regular exercise have increased physical fitness. This may be a great benefit by decreasing the risk of cardiovascular disease (Paffenbarger, Wing and Hyder, 1978).

Mobility is essential for an older person wishing to live an active and independent life (Redfern, 1991). Physical exercise and activities that involve older people in the community are paramount. Health practitioners have a great responsibility to educate the public, whatever their age, to participate in physical exercise. Bortz (1982) claimed that regular exercise reduces the morbidity and mortality of ageing.

It would be naive to expect all older people to be physically active, agile and flexible throughout their lives. There is a natural process that we have to accept: ageing may predispose to a decrease of physical function in the body. The body regulatory mechanisms change with increasing age, and decline in physical health may be a limiting factor for older people when participating in physical activities. However, inactivity is the main factor for deconditioning of the body, with a gradual decline in physical strength and, at worst, a deterioration of health. Loss of physical strength and mobility may have an adverse effect on social relationships: some older people prefer to stay at home rather than to go out to visit friends or relatives, and hostile environments often discourage older people performing common activities such as going out for a leisurely walk (Guccione, 1993). When an individual has passed retirement age, they often adopt a 'take it easy' approach. This can have an impact on advanced ageing because of a decrease in physical activities, and may reduce the person's motivation and interest so that they stop becoming involved in physically demanding activities. Often an older person will explore alternative ways of doing things, which conserve energy and minimise activities. Many prefer spending their time watching television, which involves a lot of sitting, and other related sedentary activities.

Chronic diseases such as arthritis, and heart, chest and neurological conditions, which are common in old age, contribute to the decline and loss of physical mobility of older people. This may have a great impact on the activities of daily living (ADL). The success of chronic illness management in old age mostly depends on the integration of the primary health care team in the community. It is essential that rehabilitation started in hospital should continue at home. Hence, each team must clearly understand its role in order to co-ordinate effectively the support offered to the patient. The team should strive to make the older patient to become an active participant in the rehabilitation process rather than a passive observer. Carers and professionals should be readily available to give appropriate support whenever the need arises.

Assessment

Assessment is a systematic way of gathering data from a patient, and it requires the skill of an expert in a particular field (Rogers, 1980). Any assessment process may have two facets:

- Subjective assessment helps to extract relevant information about the patient's illness and behaviour, and the development of the disease process complaints, and to collect personal data.
- Objective assessment is a way of measuring the patients' problems and their functional limitations in ADL.

When assessing older patients with multiple pathology which is closely associated with social factors, there is a great temptation to be too broad or to be shallow. A problem solving approach to assessment is necessary to encourage logical thinking in order to direct the assessor to the patient's problems rather than to the diagnosis. It will also allow easy access to retrieve information when reviewing the patient's problems, and will assist in modifying the treatment programme. A problem solving approach may be an important tool when assessing an older patient. It is not enough to identify the patient's problems: the root cause of the problem should be investigated. For example, if the patient is unable to stand up, is this because of:

- Pain in the knees?
- Dizziness?
- The legs feeling weak?
- The bed or chair being too low?

Functional assessment

It is very important to assess each patient as an individual because each patient may have different needs. In addition, the needs of the carers must be taken into account. As already pointed out, there are various formats for assessment, but the emphasis should be on identifying the patient's ability to perform the basic activities required at home during a 24 hour period. This is the basis of functional assessment: for example, an older patient with dressing difficulties will need the same level of care and assistance regardless of whether the problem arises from a stroke, arthritis or mental health problems.

The following points are important in assessing an older patient for functional activities:

1. *Bed mobility:*
   - Turning to the right and to the left
   - Moving up and down the bed
   - Moving from lying to sitting
   - Moving from sitting to lying

2. *Balance:*
   - Sitting unsupported/supported
   - Standing unsupported/supported
3. *Functional activities:*
   - Getting in and out of bed
   - Transferring from bed to a chair or wheelchair
   - Getting on and off the toilet
   - Changing from sitting to standing and standing to sitting
   - Walking
   - Getting up from a floor
   - Climbing up and down stairs
4. *Activities of daily living:*
   - Washing
   - Dressing
   - Bathing
   - Eating
   - Combing hair
   - Cleaning teeth/dentures
   - Cleaning glasses

Establish the level of independence. For instance:

- Cannot do the task (or will not do it)
- Requires expert help, for example from the physiotherapist
- Needs some help, either verbal or supervisory
- Requires no help, but may need a walking aid
- Independent

The information gleaned from the assessment should be easily retrievable and for this purpose a chart or a functional grid (e.g. Table 4.1) will help not just to identify areas of need but also to monitor progress.

The assessment of an older patient should focus on functional abilities, rather than being specific about a particular joint or grading of muscle power. Factors that limit the patient's independent activities should be identified. For example, a stroke patient who sits in a low chair may have difficulties in standing up. In this case the main problem would be the low chair rather than the condition of the patient.

General guidelines

The following are general guidelines for the assessment of older patients:

- The patient requires the full attention of the assessor as *the patient* is the most important person during the assessment.
- The interview should be conducted where possible in an area of privacy.

Table 4.1 Functional chart to record activities of daily living

Activity/task	0	1	2	3	4	Comments
Bed mobility						
Turning to right and left						
Moving up and down the bed						
Function						
Lying to sitting						
Sitting to standing						
Walking						
Stairs						
Transfers						
Chair to commode/toilet						
Bed to chair						
ADL						
Washing						
Dressing						
Feeding						
Toileting						

Key: 0, totally dependent; 1, independent with maximal assistance; 2, independent with minimal assistance; 3, independent with supervision; 4, fully independent.

- Assessment should follow a multidisciplinary approach, and good communication is essential.
- Areas of overlap may occur among various professions, but the focus should be on the patient's problems. Professional jealousies hamper the team work spirit, and ultimately patient care.
- The patient should always be in a position to see and hear the assessor.
- All necessary aids for communication (dentures, hearing aids and glasses) should be available at the time of assessment.
- Appropriate walking aids (stick, walking frame and crutches) should be available. Special attention should be given to the ferrules: worn-out ferrules are as dangerous as a bald tyre.
- The patient's perceived problems should be taken into account.

Falls

Falls are defined as 'events that cause subjects to fall to the ground against their will' (Gibson, 1990). An older person who has experienced a fall may live in fear of falling again. This can lead to loss of confidence, reduced movements and a decline in activities of daily living. Falls are serious problems in the older population and they are major risk factors of morbidity and mortality (Dunn *et al.*, 1992).

Major injuries sustained in a fall may lead to hospital admission in all age groups. However, minor injuries such as bruising and swelling endured by older people may force them to stay in bed. It is important to keep time spent in bed to a minimum. Bed rest may have serious consequences: decline in strength, poor circulation and pressure sores. Patients should be advised to move their limbs frequently while they are in bed.

Risk factors

Risk factors are predictors of accidents most likely to happen in given circumstances. Blake *et al.* (1988) categorized falls into two main divisions: accident falls and pathological falls.

Accident falls

These are associated with environmental hazards. Gill (1987) notes that 95 per cent of patient admissions in the wards caring for older people are due to falls sustained at home.

Predisposing factors to falls at home include:

- Loose carpets
- Cluttered furniture
- Trailing wires

- Poor lighting
- Unsuitable footwear
- Unsuitable walking aids
- Slippery ground.

Pathological falls

These are the result of factors related to underlying debilitating illness and disabilities, for example Parkinson's disease, stroke, musculoskeletal disorders, and vision and hearing problems. They affect the abilities of older patients to control their balance and to maintain upright posture during walking.

Chronic illness → Physical decondition → Reduced balance reaction → Recurrent falls

Chronic illness may lead to decreased physical activities, which affects the individual's balance reactions, such as agility and flexibility. Hence, this may lead to recurrent falls.

However, there are other factors that cause falls, such as postural imbalance and 'drop attack', which may occur with sudden onset without apparent warning. The frequency of attacks increases with advancing age. This contributes to 12 per cent – 25 per cent of falls in the older population (Overstall *et al.*, 1977). Overuse or mis-use of drugs, for example diuretics, tranquillisers and some analgetics, may have side effects such as lethargy and drowsiness. This may contribute to recurrent falls.

Immobility

Immobility is functional incapacity for a period of time.

Older people who experience falls tend to suffer from post-fall syndrome, which causes loss of self confidence, reduction in daily activities, social withdrawal and depression (O'Loughlin *et al.*, 1993). A patient in pain will be unwilling to move because of depression and lack of motivation. If long-term dependency is to be minimised current levels of mobility should be maintained to prevent further deterioration.

Normally nurses spend more time with the patient than physiotherapists, and they are in a better position to observe realistically the patient's functional limitations. During the interdisciplinary meetings or on the ward rounds, nurses may be able to highlight the patient's physical disabilities and exercise tolerance. This would provide invaluable feedback to assist the physiotherapists to focus on the patient's main problems.

Non-injurious falls can be unpleasant and frightening for older people, who then fear further falls. Their effect can be profound, reducing daily activity and accentuating dependency. This may lead to 'gone off feet' syndrome. The cause of this is complicated and mixed in nature: it can range from a simple painful bunion to a complicated multipathology of age related diseases.

Functional incontinence is another factor that may make older people immobile. This can be the result of being confined to bed or to a chair owing to chronic illness. Because patients frequently feel shy and reluctant to ask for help, usually they wet their chair or bed, which may lead to functional incontinence. It is a common problem in the older population, especially for those whose mobility levels are reduced. This may reduce the person's dignity and independence pertaining to personal hygiene. Patients with Parkinson's disease may develop problems with continence due to reduced dexterity of their hands, and inability to manipulate underclothes on time. To be incontinent is not only very distressing, but also a humiliating experience leading to declining social relationships.

In older people functional incontinence can be managed by encouraging patients to go to the toilet at set times and gradually increasing the time intervals. Rather than employing conservative bladder training or a pelvic floor exercise programme, it is important to make sure that the environment is conducive with easy access to the toilet. It would be advisable to ask older patients whether they want to visit the toilet before meals or group exercise programmes. This should stimulate the bladder to expand, and encourages older patients to remain continent and to understand the importance of controlling their micturition.

Rehabilitation

Rehabilitation aims at enabling 'patients to achieve their maximum potential in terms of physical, mental and social recovery' (Barer, 1993). It should be a continuation of the assessment process, after identifying the patient's problems, to restore lost function, or 'alternatively to maintain or maximize remaining function' (Williams, 1984).

Many older patients who are referred to wards caring for older people have varied and complex needs. Because some older patients may suffer from one or more age related chronic conditions, which are clinically intertwined, it is important to perform a comprehensive assessment to plan realistic goals that will be achievable by the patient (Mulley, 1994). The rehabilitation process should never be delayed until after the period of acute care is over (Barer, 1993). It should commence as soon as possible when the patient's condition is stable, to prevent further deterioration. In the rehabilitation of older patients, old age itself should not be regarded as a disability, but as a factor that needs careful planning when realistic goals are being established.

The multidisciplinary team has to work in close co-operation to facilitate the rehabilitation programme. It helps the team members to share ideas, knowledge and experience that will be beneficial to the patient. If possible, a well co-ordinated approach that prioritises the patient's problems and shared care plans are essential. The attitude of members of the team towards older people should be positive so as to motivate patients and carers for the programme to be successful. It is essential that there is no conflict within the team; therefore, time must be allocated for proper training of all the team members in order to avoid misunderstandings, lack of co-ordination and problems with programme implementation (Rockwood, 1994).

Effective communication among the team members, with the passing on of relevant information to the patient, is essential if successful rehabilitation is to take place. The team should also be encouraged to pass appropriate instructions and information to the carers.

Setting realistic goals will motivate patients to co-operate in the rehabilitation process. If they see only things that they cannot achieve, they will become anxious, frustrated and depressed, and in most cases the easy option is to give up. Once this happens, patients are quickly labelled as unco-operative, unwilling to help themselves, or lazy. When care planning is devised, it is paramount to involve patient and carers in the decision-making process. The active participation of patients and carers in the early part of rehabilitation will stimulate motivation and compliance (Mulley, 1994). This will increase the patient's confidence in continuing with exercises at home and in the general success of the rehabilitation programme.

The patient's motivation may also be reduced if members of the team have different information, goals, or opposing ideas and opinions on the approach and treatment programme. Unfortunately, sometimes rules and regulations in the ward reduce the older patient's motivation and participation in the rehabilitation process. If patients are to be motivated, they need to receive appropriate explanation of their condition and the effect of treatments. Teaching the patient to perform ankle exercises ten times a day without proper explanation does not make the patient comply with the exercise programme. They are more likely to comply if it is explained to them that during normal activities muscles work as a pump to maintain circulation, and that when their mobility is reduced this pumping action is compromised, the circulation becomes sluggish and fluid collects in the extremities. However, simple exercises, which can be performed while sitting in a chair or in bed, stimulate the muscle pumping action. This will minimise the risk of ankle oedema.

Rehabilitation is a re-learning process, and we learn by doing; so patients must be given opportunities to practise and to incorporate newly acquired skills in their everyday activities. The patient who is always wheeled to the toilet or walked between two people to save time may lack the confidence and the strength to walk alone. Active participation of older patients in the daily activities will boost morale, confidence and self esteem.

However, at the start of the programme, they may need a lot of support, guidance and encouragement. When they feel confident, this help can be gradually reduced until they maintain full independence. Early withdrawal of support may have devastating consequences: loss of interest to participate in the exercise programme, proneness to accidents and lack of confidence in performing functional activities. Each patient should be treated with respect and dignity and should be seen as an individual with a variety of needs.

Hesse and Campian (1983) describe one of the most frustrating experiences in geriatric medicine as that of caring for the patient who has the physical capacity but lacks the motivation to participate in a rehabilitation programme. To blame the patient is an easy option, but it does not solve the problem. It is important to investigate the cause of this lack of interest. Physiotherapy to improve mobility should not only aim at improving functional independence and the self care of patients but also provide training, advice, guidelines and practical help to all those actively involved in the patient's management.

In hospital, the nurse is in a unique position to have close contact with older patients and to observe their needs: that is, washing, dressing, transferring from bed to chair, and walking about around the bed. Nursing staff will be with the patient all the time, and physiotherapists like to observe functional limitations and facilitate activities that are required to make the patient independent. When dealing with older patients, nurses should adopt an active participatory approach. This will help older patients to feel that they are in control of their lives. Self esteem is enhanced and confidence improved to participate in the exercise programme.

For patients with long term or debilitating (chronic) diseases, the roles of the carers are paramount in achieving a successful rehabilitation programme. It is important to teach carers how to motivate the patient, when to give support and how to encourage the patient to continue with the exercise programme at home.

Rehabilitation is about what happens 24 hours a day in the patient's life. It starts on day one of admission, so a large proportion of the workload falls on nursing staff; they are close to the patient and provide a 24 hour service (Watson, 1993). Hence, good staffing levels at all times are essential to combat staff exhaustion and frustration when caring for older people in the hospital. Costello (1994) describes the nurse's role in the multidisciplinary team working with older patients as that of being 'a facilitator of care, patient advocate, counsellor and the primary care giver'. The nurse who works in the wards caring for older patients should explore resources that are available and liaise with the other disciplines involved in the care of the patient.

The nurse's role in the older patient's rehabilitation is multidimensional, nursing the patient while in hospital and working with other team members to ensure that the rehabilitation process continues when the patient is discharged home. Many older patients suffer from multiple pathology that requires the 'multidimensional patient assessment, treatment, rehabilitation and discharge planning that is a reflection of the combined efforts of experts in the field of elderly care' (Costello, 1994).

Discharge

Discharge planning is defined as 'the amount of notice given before discharge and the discussion of the patient's return home by hospital staff' (Victor and Vetter, 1988). It is an integral part of the rehabilitation process in the management of older patients, and special consideration is essential.

Older people who have been admitted to hospital without notice are more likely to find the atmosphere and environment very confusing, and equally their discharge may be traumatising. Once optimum function has been achieved, older patients and carers should be involved in the decision process of discharge. To maintain the achieved function, active participation of the patient in physical activities and regular exercises is essential. This requires the support of carers, and liaison between the hospital, and community team workers and social services (Jones and Lester, 1994).

Discharge planning should start once the patient's condition is stable in order to stimulate the patient and carers to play an active role in the process of reintegration back into the community (Victor and Vetter, 1988). Time spent in planning discharge is time well spent if readmission is to be prevented. Victor and Vetter (1988) and Tierney and Worth (1995) suggest the following guidelines for discharge planning:

1. Inform the patient of their discharge, with sufficient notice, in the presence of carers.
2. Involve the patient and carers in any decisions that may require a change of accommodation.
3. Provide adequate information to the GP about the state of the patient.
4. Liaise with social services.
5. Ensure that the primary care team will continue with the rehabilitation process at home.
6. Arrange post-discharge support, especially for older patients who live alone.

Walking aids

Walking aids are appliances that help in 'transferring weight from the upper limbs to the ground to assist balance' (Hollis *et al.*, 1989). They also increase the area of support, to enhance locomotion in patients who are suffering from musculoskeletal and neuromuscular disorders.

When walking aids are required by the patient, the following points should be considered before supplying the aids (Wagstaff and Coakley, 1988; Mulley, 1988):

1. Assessment should confirm that the aid is required by the patient.
2. Assessment should ensure that the aid is needed to assist the patient's independence during walking.
3. The aid should be light to handle, comfortable, durable and socially acceptable.
4. The aid should be appropriate and of the correct size for the patient.
5. The aid should be provided with the necessary 'gadgets' to satisfy the patient's needs.
6. Proper instruction and demonstrations in the use of the aid must be provided.
7. The aid must be always safe for the patient to use.

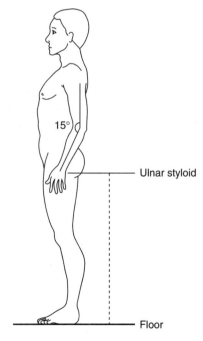

Figure 4.1 Measuring for walking aids.

The provision of an unsafe or unsuitable aid can be hazardous. It may reduce the patient's confidence, impair progress and be dangerous. As older patients tend to lose their balance easily, they should be advised not to borrow other patients' aids even for a short period of time. It is sometimes difficult to meet the ever-increasing physical and material demands of older patients. However, essential and appropriate equipment such as walking aids and appliances should be provided whenever the need arises. There are many and different types of walking aid available, so only a few of them will be discussed in greater detail here.

Walking frame

Walking frames are light in weight and are available in a wide range of different sizes, widths and adjustable heights. The most commonly used walking frames are known as Zimmer frames after one of the manufacturers. They stimulate safer mobility in frail older patients. Walking frames relieve 'pain by taking some of the body's weight through the arms; they also provide confidence and stability' (Mulley, 1990).

The usually accepted and appropriate way of measuring walking frames is from the ulnar styloid to the ground with the elbow in 15° flexion (Mulley, 1988). To prevent an abnormal gait pattern developing and to minimise falls, the patient must be taught how to use the frame. Mulley (1990: 925) describes that 'to use it correctly the patient lifts the frame, puts it down in front without overstretching, takes two even steps into the frame, and stops'.

Walking sticks

There are several types of walking stick, including metal, wooden and special handled sticks. Many patients find metal sticks light in weight, durable and easily adjustable according to the patient's height. However, they tend to be more expensive than wooden sticks, and many patients prefer the wooden variety which they consider less obtrusive. For rheumatoid patients there are separately shaped handles, which allow for the weight to be taken in the pad of the thumb and palm, thus relieving stress through the wrist joint.

Measurement for a walking stick is similar to that for a walking frame. The patient should wear normal walking shoes. The stick should be held in the hand opposite to the bad leg. A walking stick of incorrect height is a major cause of falls and accidents.

Wheelchairs

If an older person's ability to get about is limited, a wheelchair is a useful piece of equipment to have, provided it is used sensibly. It is sometimes much easier to use a wheelchair to go shopping, to go on holiday or to go on a leisurely outing in the park. This would create a useful social interaction for an individual in the community. A wheelchair should not be used just because it is easy to do so. Before issuing a wheelchair serious thought and considerations must be given. If a wheelchair is deemed necessary, there are some general rules to be observed when using one:

1. Always make sure that the brakes are on before sitting in or standing from a wheelchair.
2. Never stand on the foot plates because this may lead to falls. To avoid accidents, the foot plates must be removed.
3. When pushing a patient, always ensure that their feet are on the footplates.
4. Before getting out of a wheelchair, make sure that the feet are on the ground with the footplates out of the way.
5. Remove the arms of the wheelchair to make transfer easier.
6. Make sure that the wheelchair is close to the bed or chair, and preferably at the same level.
7. Give adequate instructions when assisting a person in and out a wheelchair. Do not make sudden movements: this can induce fear and make it more difficult for the patient to be helped.

General guidelines for pushing someone in a wheelchair include the following:

1. When pushing someone in a wheelchair, do remember to talk to them.
2. Do not go too fast or suddenly change direction without word. This can be a frightening and unacceptable experience for the patient.
3. When negotiating doorways, make sure that the patient's hands and feet are well tucked in to prevent awkward bumps and grazes. Watch out for hidden steps.
4. Warn the patient when negotiating slopes, turns and steps.
5. Make sure that the chair is properly maintained.

Sensible use of a wheelchair can be a great asset, but a wheelchair unwisely used this decreases mobility and reduces the patient's independence.

Footwear

An older person's lifestyle may change, mobility may be reduced, and independence in ADL compromised by bad footwear. Simply issuing walking aids will be of no help unless appropriate footwear is available.

Suitable shoes are considered a fundamental prerequisite for safe mobility. On admission, footwear is often found to be missing. Very few older patients are safe, or feel confident, when walking in bare feet or in slippers. Any delay in providing suitable footwear may cause a temporary loss of mobility and make the patient permanently dependent, thus minimising the effects of the rehabilitation programme. It is important to provide appropriate footwear to improve the patient's confidence, to keep the feet warm and to protect the patient from environmental hazards.

Conclusion

Society during the past two decades has encouraged many older people to participate in exercise programmes either privately at home or in the community. Regular exercise can improve general condition, maintain the range of movement of joints, and stimulate heart and lung function. This helps to keep an individual physically and mentally active.

When care planning is devised for older people, the primary aim should be for care to be home based and tailored to the individual's needs. The emphasis should be on a self-care management programme. When handling and helping older people, an active participatory approach should be adopted. This helps the older person to feel that they are in control of their lives. Self esteem is enhanced and confidence to participate in the exercise programme improved. Increasingly, hotels, shops, theatres and public transport are providing disabled access. This is encouraging because, despite illness and disability, many older people are determined to retain their independence and continue to live in the community. For those who need help, professional services must be flexible to assist them in their daily activities. Often carers as well as the individual need encouragement to ask for access – despite the fact that so many agencies are willing to help.

There is now less emphasis on illness and hospitalisation, and more recognition of the wellbeing of older people and health promotion in the community. Doctors, nurses and therapists are more likely to be facilitators of a training programme of untrained non-professional carers in identifying patients' problems. This will include referrals to appropriate agencies.

In the past, the disabilities of older people have been treated with passive and negative attitudes. It must be recognised that a well organised team approach is essential for assessment, accurate diagnosis and intervention in the management of older people in order to have impact on the prospect of continuing good health for the ageing population. Collaboration and co-ordination of all professional services is a key factor in achieving independence, wellbeing and a better future for older people.

References

Barer D (1993) Assessment in rehabilitation. *Reviews in Clinical Gerontology* 3, 169–86.

Blake AJ, Morgan K, Bendall MJ, Dallosso H, Ebrahim SBJ, Arice THD, Fentem PH and Bassey EJ (1988) Falls by elderly people at home: prevalence and associated factors. *Age and Ageing*; 17, 365–72.

Bortz WM (1982) Disuse and ageing. *Journal of the American Medical Association* 248, 1203.

Costello J (1994) The role of the nurse in the multidisciplinary team. *Reviews in Clinical Gerontology* 4, 169–76.

Dunn JE, Rudeberg MA, Furner SE and Cassel CK (1992) Mortality, disability, and falls in older persons: the role of underlying disease and disability. *American Journal of Public Health* 82, 395–400.

Emery C and Gatz M (1990) Psychological and cognitive effects of an exercise program for community residing older adults. *Gerontologist* 30, 184–8.

Gibson M (1990) *Falls in later life. Improving Health of Older People*, pp 296–315. WHO, Geneva.

Gill G (1987) Health needs of the elderly. *The Essentials of Nursing*, 2nd edn. Macmillan Education, London.

Guccione AA (ed.) (1993) *Geriatric Physical Therapy.* CV Mosby, St Louis.

Hesse K and Campian E (1983) The geriatric patient for rehabilitation. *Journal of the American Geriatric Society* 31, 586–9.

Hollis M, Kitchen SS, Sandford B and Waddington PJ (1989) *Practical Exercise Therapy*, 3rd edn. Blackwell, London.

Jones D and Lester C (1994) Hospital care and discharge: patient's and carers' opinions. *Age and Ageing* 23, 91–6.

Lewis CB and Bottomley JM (1990) *Musculoskeletal Changes with Age: Clinical Implications*, 2nd edn. FA Davies, Philadelphia.

Mulley GP (1988) Everyday aids and appliances – provision of aids. *British Medical Journal* 296, 475–6.

Mulley GP (1990) Everyday aids and appliances: walking frames. *British Medical Journal* 300, 925–7.

Mulley GP (1994) Principles of rehabilitation. *Reviews in Clinical Gerontology* 4, 61–9.

O'Loughlin JL, Robitaille Y, Boivin JE and Suissa S (1993) Incidence of and risk factors for all injuries and falls among the community-dwelling elderly. *American Journal of Epidemiology* 137, 342–54.

Overstall PW, Exton-Smith AN, Imms FJ and Johnson AL (1977) Falls in the elderly related to postural imbalance. *British Medical Journal* 11, 261–4.

Paffenbarger RS, Wing AL and Hyder T (1978) Physical activity as an index of heart attack risk in College of Alumni. *American Journal of Epidemiology* 108, 161–75.

Redfern SJ (ed.) (1991) *Nursing Elderly People*, 2nd edn. Churchill Livingstone, Edinburgh.

Rockwood K (1994) Setting goals in geriatric rehabilitation and measuring their attainment. *Reviews in Clinical Gerontology* 41, 141–9.

Rogers JC (1980) Advocacy – the key to assessing older clients. *Journal of Geriatric Nursing* 6, 33–6.

Ruuskanen JM and Ruoppila I (1995) Physical activity and psychological well-being among people aged 65–84 years. *Age and Ageing* 24, 292–6.

Tierney AJ and Worth A (1995) Review: readmission of elderly patients to hospital. *Age and Ageing* 24, 163–6.

Victor CR and Vetter NJ (1988) Preparing the elderly for discharge from hospital: a neglected aspect of patients care? *Age and Ageing* 17, 155–63.

Wagstaff P and Coakley D (1988) *Physiotherapy and the Elderly Patient: Therapy in practice.* Croom Helm, London.

Watson R (1993) *Caring for Elderly People.* WB Saunders, London.

Williams TF (ed.) (1984) *Rehabilitation in the Ageing.* Raven Press, New York.

5

Cognition of self-awareness

Ian Jacques

Those of us who have yet to reach retirement age frequently perceive old age as a time of ill health and disability; indeed, much of the literature relating to the planning of care services for older people has been presented in apocalyptic terms, the reader being encouraged to believe that society is about to be overwhelmed by hordes of dependent older people whose needs will drain the public purse. However, when asked, older people themselves report general satisfaction with their state of health: see, for example, The British Gas Report on Attitudes to Ageing (Midwinter, 1991).

Why should there be such a gap between the perceptions of policy makers and of care professionals and older people themselves? Part of the answer to this question lies in the manner in which health is defined and our own ability to interact effectively with the world within which we live.

Perception and behaviour

Each of us has our own view regarding our state of health. Medical students and student nurses invariably believe that they are suffering the early stages of whatever condition they have most recently studied. Where there are gross pathological conditions, of course, there is little room for perception and debate. A tumour is a tumour no matter what we decide to call it. How we react to its presence may affect our subsequent quality of life, but it is unlikely that the power of positive thought can physically destroy a cancerous growth. Many conditions are, however, less obvious and accessible to objective observation. The diagnostic test for many conditions is dependent on the perception of either the sufferer or the observer. In the absence of any pathology, how should we react to someone's claim to be in pain? Pain levels are clearly dependent on the sufferer's perception.

Each of us interacts with the world via the special senses of vision, hearing, taste, touch and smell. Studies of physiology teach us that the messages received by the eyes, ears, mouth, skin and nose are relayed via nerve pathways and synapses to be interpreted by the brain. The eyes, for example, contain cones and rods which are stimulated by light. In scanning this page the cones and rods within the eyes of the reader are each individually stimulated by the light reflected from the page. The degree of stimulation is then analysed by the brain and a recognisable picture is established: initially, in this case, a picture of print on a page. The example of television further illustrates this point. A still picture on a television screen consists of some 625 separate horizontal lines of data, each line being made up of many hundreds of separate points. The viewer, however, does not register the thousands of dots but, instead, 'sees' a complete picture (see, for example, Hilgard, Atkinson and Atkinson, 1979). In a similar manner, the ear sends messages to the brain, but this is not heard in terms of separate tones. Music is not heard as a series of individual notes but, rather, as melody and symphony. The way in which we interpret this sensory input can become extremely complex. The mechanics of the sense of smell are reasonably straightforward: air breathed in through the nose passes over the relevant receptors and we learn to assign a name to the resulting sensation. As the years pass, however, we also learn to associate whole memories and emotions with the odours we encounter. The smell of our favourite food drifting from a restaurant will make us ravenously hungry. The smell encountered when entering a room may bring flooding back memories of long Sunday afternoons spent with a favourite grandparent, and a tear will appear as we silently grieve for our lost childhood. We may also wish to consider how the temperature and pressure of a hand on our shoulder can evoke feelings of belonging, value and comfort or alternatively can be perceived as being threatening and invasive.

It is clear that the brain seeks to interpret stimuli so as to create a whole sensation. It is further argued that, where gaps appear in the messages received from the relevant senses, the brain will seek to fill those gaps so that we see a whole picture, even though a part of that picture does not actually exist. The interpretation of stimuli is then apparently dependent on expectations derived from previous experience. Hilgard, Atkinson and Atkinson (1979) illustrate this point by drawing on the experience of young children, who have difficulty in interpreting the size of objects at a distance: very young children viewing cars from the top of a tall building may perceive the cars below as toys – to the extent that they may reach for them.

Hilgard, Atkinson and Atkinson also illustrate that perception is dependent on the context within which sensory stimulation occurs. A white light shone on black velvet does not make the velvet appear anything other than black when the velvet is viewed against a white background. View the same velvet through a cardboard tube which excludes all background, however, and the result will be that the velvet appears white.

Thus far, perception has been viewed as an unconscious process. The brain receives nervous impulses from the five senses and seeks to produce a sensory picture which, on the basis of previous experience, makes sense. Optical illusions play on this process by seeking to convince the viewer that there is, in fact, no one particular interpretation of events. The brain thus presents first one interpretation then another. The way in which messages are interpreted is also influenced by our level of motivation. When at a party or perhaps in a busy work environment we may have to concentrate to hold a conversation: we filter out the background noise of other conversations. When our name is mentioned across the room, however, we will, metaphorically, drop everything to find out what is being said. Subsequent perception depends on a higher level of consciousness, and in the example given interpretation may depend on personality and recent history as well as the social context.

Perception, cognition and behaviour

During an award ceremony, the winner of the major award will find nothing unusual in the fact that people across the room are talking about his or her achievements. The more vain winners may even pay only slight attention to the immediate conversation, so keen are they to hear flattering remarks in the background. In other circumstances, however, the overheard remark can be taken as evidence of an undisclosed threat. The interpretation moves from one of satisfaction to one of anger. The behaviour of the protagonists depends, then, on the interpretation placed on events. The person who feels that the overheard remark implies a threat will react with suspicion or anger, whereas the award winner may seek to provoke further flattering comment.

Woods and Britton (1985) have noted that our behaviour is determined by our level of competence, our relationships and interactions with other people, and the culture and environment within which we live and work. It is argued that in addition to the subconscious meaning attributed to sensory input, the brain also ascribes meaning on the basis of past behavioural experience. Theories of socialisation are based on just this point. Giddens (1993) discusses in great detail the processes by which we learn to interpret perceptions and thus to behave in ways that will be socially acceptable.

The process of socialisation begins to illustrate the pressure to conform. To be able to conform, however, we must first be able to predict the acceptability of any given response, and to do this we must first be able to understand the immediate environment. Schachter and Singer (1962) refer to this process as 'evaluative need'. In essence, our behaviour is determined by our understanding of the immediate circumstances, based on previous experience and environmental cues. Aggleton and Chalmers (1986) note that 'people behave as they do, not because of the workings of systems within them, but because of meanings attached to the actions they perform.'

We assign meaning to events and act accordingly. Mead (1934) takes this further and suggests that we derive this meaning from symbols drawn from our environment. The interpretation of such symbols can, however, be based on meanings that are unique to the observer. Case studies provide an insight into this process.

CASE STUDY 1

Now in his seventies, Joe Ogden is resident in a nursing home in South London. Joe was born in the East End of London, where he has lived throughout most of his life. Usually employed in the local docks, Joe has spent some years as a semi-professional boxer, and throughout the early 1960s lived in an environment in which violence and crime were never far away. When Joe developed Alzheimer's disease his family rallied around and looked after him as best they could. When his wife became ill, however, it was clear that Joe required a level of care that could not be provided at home. In seeking to reach an understanding of his current circumstances, Joe wanders the corridors of the nursing home on a regular basis. Such wanderings invariably cease when he reaches a locked door. Joe clearly interprets the door in a manner that supports the view that he has been imprisoned. The fact that he cannot remember why he should be imprisoned adds to a growing sense of fear, for failure to recall such an event must mean that he has carried out a crime too awful to remember. The fact that the doors are locked must mean that all of the other residents have also committed some crime. The staff, then, must be warders of some sort. Having reached this conclusion, which he does on a regular basis, Joe becomes suspicious of staff and treats fellow residents as though they have carried out terrible crimes.

CASE STUDY 2

Suffering from an intractable depression, Victoria James is being cared for in an assessment ward of an inner city hospital. The hospital had, in the past, been one of the original Poor Law workhouses and Victoria remembers it as such. Victoria was born towards the end of the last century and enjoyed a relatively successful life before her admission. Although she would argue that she has always been staunchly working class, Victoria managed to buy her own newsagents many years earlier. She had taken pride in her ability to pay her way and had made sure that her children wanted for nothing. Admission to the 'workhouse' has come as an enormous blow. The workhouse was for those who could not pay their way, who did not have family and friends to help when things became difficult. Despite the fact that the hospital was, internally, a modern homely establishment, Victoria correctly associated the name and the structure of the building with the old workhouse. This meant that her family had abandoned her (although they visited regularly) and that a lifetime of hard work had all been in vain. Victoria's perception of events left her depressed and totally unmotivated.

Interpretation of behaviour

Having illustrated how our behaviour is dependent on the meaning that we attach to sensory input, it must also be noted that the meaning of behaviour is, itself, dependent on the context within which it takes place. It further follows that the meaning of behaviour is defined by those observing our actions.

Mary Marshall (1993) succinctly illustrates the point when reminding her readers that the view of the community nurse concerning a new patient will be influenced by the venue of their first meeting. The patient viewed in his or her stately home is regarded somewhat differently from the patient viewed in a hostel for the homeless. The context of the first meeting greatly influences subsequent assumptions, and the same assumptions can then greatly influence the patient's subsequent behaviour. A 1994 advertising campaign made on behalf of SCOPE vividly illustrates the dangers. A full page advertisement in the national press had as a headline 'My son has cerebral palsy, he has a mental age of twelve . . .'. The final part of the sentence demonstrated the dangers of the assumption: '. . . he is ten years old'.

Rosenhan (1973) carried out a number of experiments that expand on this. In his research a number of people gained access to psychiatric hospitals in the USA. Admission was organised on the basis of one conversation, during which the prospective patient claimed to have had an auditory hallucination. Once admitted, the patient behaved in precisely the same manner as they had while living successfully at home. None of the participants had a previous diagnosis of psychiatric illness. The research showed that clinicians failed to identify normal behaviour: discharge was denied to the participants despite the absence of any behaviour indicative of a psychiatric condition. As a follow-up, clinicians were warned to expect a situation in which a 'normal' person would attempt to gain admission by feigning mental illness. In this case, the clinicians tended to misdiagnose in large numbers, identifying as normal those who were referred with genuine problems. Rosenhan (1973) thus demonstrated that the meaning ascribed to behaviour is, in part, dependent on the observer's expectations.

Rosenhan also noted in the same study that patients' actions were reported in medical and nursing notes in such a way that they were seen to support the original diagnosis. The participants' maintenance of continuous notes detailing their experiences throughout the experiment was reported as evidence of potentially psychotic behaviour. The fact that staff did not see a reason to enquire as to the nature of the note keeping should perhaps raise questions as to the normality of their own behaviour, rather than that of the participants.

It can be seen from this example that behaviour which has been successful throughout one's life takes on a different meaning in certain circumstances. If care professionals feel, for example, that there is reason to doubt a patient's abilities, it is possible that they will give new meanings to old behaviours. Alternatively, behaviour which is successful in one environment can be extremely unhelpful if that environment should change. How is it, for example, that an 80-year-old man living at home alone is regarded as amazingly independent and yet when he attempts to live in privacy in a nursing home his behaviour is regarded as maladaptive? Having spent the past ten years of his life living alone in a council flat, this gentleman has learned to adapt to a solitary existence. Admission to a nursing home should present this man with few problems, and yet the very thing that he is not allowed to pursue is a solitary existence. He is at best encouraged to join the other residents in the lounge; at worst, mobility problems that necessitated the admission may prevent a return to his room once he is placed in the lounge area.

Normal behaviours in abnormal environments are viewed as aberrant by those living in such environments. To survive in the new environment, the individual must understand the norms of the new regime and adapt accordingly. The classic text in this regard is Goffman's *Asylums* (1968), in which the author explores the extent to which our ability to act in an independent and individual way is whittled away to the point where we adapt our own needs to the needs of the organisation. The process of adaptation is poignantly illustrated by Primo Levi in his accounts of his time in Auschwitz (see, for example, *If This Is a Man* and *Moments of Reprieve*). A similar point is made by Giddens (1993), who notes that those who survived the atrocities of the Holocaust displayed, during their incarceration, behaviours that would be insane in any other circumstances.

Roy's (1980) stress adaptation model of nursing is based on the concept that each of us will seek to understand the circumstances in which we find ourselves and then adapt accordingly, although we may be entirely unaware of this process. The difficulty is, however, that at certain periods of our life, due to our stage of development, illness or disability, we may be unable to adapt in a manner that will maintain our healthy existence. The role of the nurse, according to Roy, is to assist the individual, in times of stress, to reach a healthy adaptation to his or her circumstances, through education or the manipulation of contextual stimuli. It is with this in mind that we now turn our attention to the effects of sensory impairment and physical disability in relation to perception and health status.

Sensory impairment and loss of mobility

The difficulties in reaching a correct interpretation of the events around us have been illustrated above. We may wish to ponder, however, on events in our own experience that have demonstrated this point. How often has a slightly mis-heard request resulted in the wrong items being bought from the supermarket? How often has a rushed telephone conversation resulted in work being overlooked or replicated? Why is it that those arriving for a meeting can *never* agree whether the meeting was scheduled for 2 p.m. or 3 p.m.? The results of such misinterpretations are frequently comical and usually inconsequential – only occasionally do they cause us problems. How much easier, though, to make such mistakes when one has difficulty hearing the telephone message. Does the age of the person making the mistake have a bearing on how that mistake is perceived by others? How many mistakes does it take before someone attributes a meaning to the mistakes themselves? At what age does the slightly scatty woman become the senile lady? The answer to those questions is that it rather depends on the individual and the circumstances. Once the connection has been made, however, the label tends to stick and subsequent behaviour is interpreted so as to reinforce that label.

This is not simply a problem of stereotyping, however. Disability, genuine problems with the maintenance of continence, lack of financial resources, even the lack of decent public transport, can all lead to gradual social isolation. This is not a matter of age or pathology but rather a matter of circumstance. To illustrate this point let us examine a case study.

CASE STUDY 3

Mrs Ella Shaw is in her mid-60s. She has recently been widowed and lives in a block of flats on an inner city estate to which she and her husband moved after her children left home as part of a council redevelopment scheme. She has two daughters: one lives about an hour's drive down a busy motorway; the other lives locally but has two pre-school age children. Ella is physically in good health and has coped well with her bereavement. She has little money and survives on her state pension. Initially, Ella coped well in her new circumstances. Over a period of time, however, she found it difficult to get to the shops and she realised that she goes for longer periods without seeing friends. Ella is still fit and active but the local shops have closed. Her friends have moved closer to their families or are finding their own difficulties in getting about. Ella spends more and more time in her flat. Her contact with the outside world is made through the television, although one of her daughters visits once or twice each week. Ella is happy with this scenario. She has enough food in her cupboards and although it is nice to see her children they have their own life to live. Anyway, she speaks to them on the telephone quite often. Ella is happy in her own cosy little flat: she does not need to worry about what is going on outside.

It can be seen that in the absence of pathology or disability Ella is adapting to social circumstance in a manner that maintains her personal integrity and self concept. What may be less obvious is the insidious onset of a process of gradual sensory deprivation. Holden and Woods (1984) note that sensory deprivation is not simply the absence of sensory stimulation, but also a function of sensory monotony. They further identify the consequences of sensory deprivation as including '... difficulties in thought and concentration, perceptual distortions, thought disorder, hallucinations, deterioration in reasoning, logic and word finding ...'.

But consider Ella's case further.

Age and sensory ability

Ella will face the same assault on sensory ability that each of us has, or will in the future – a process that begins in one's teens or early 20s. Physiological changes to the inner ear include a loss of neuron activity, cell degeneration in the cochlea, and sclerosis of the tympanic membrane. The normal hearing range at ten years of age, for example, extends to 20 kHz. By the time we are 50 this has already dropped to 14 kHz, and in our mid-60s this drops to about 5 kHz (Kenney, 1989).

The good news for Ella is that she can no longer hear the screaming guitar solo from the neighbours' hi-fi. The bad news is that she continues to hear the monotonous base thud. Physiological changes in the eye mean that Ella is now slightly colour blind in the green–blue spectrum. Her eyes are less responsive to changes in light levels. The lenses of her eyes have thickened somewhat, which makes focusing a little more difficult – but no matter, she can find her way around the flat perfectly well. The number of taste buds in one's mouth reduces by some 70 per cent between childhood and 80 years of age, but this does not bother Ella because she is not really interested in food very much. It has very little taste these days no matter how much salt she puts on her dinner or how much sugar in her tea. She eats the same things most days anyway, now that food is getting to be too expensive and the shops too far away.

Ella is still free from any illness or disability, but she is unaware of the nutritional problems caused by her monotonous diet of tinned foods, and she does not notice the physical and mental decline that has resulted from her poor diet. Ella is also unaware of the looks that she gets from her neighbours when she responds oddly to their comments. She did notice that her daughter sounded a little exasperated on the telephone recently; in fact, this is getting to be a regular occurrence. Perhaps, Ella thinks, the kids are getting to be a handful – but she does wish that her daughter would stop nagging about a hearing aid. Surely Ella has explained a million times that the hearing aid does nothing to stop the high pitched buzzing that she hears all the time.

The accumulation of normal sensory impairment can quickly lead to the accumulation of minor misinterpretations, the consequences of which vary in terms of seriousness according to the context in which they occur. Living alone in her own home, Ella can afford to mis-hear the television and she can usually predict her telephone conversations, being caught out only when her daughters move away from their well rehearsed script. Shopping in the late autumn dusk, the relatively minor sensory difficulties which are encountered by everyone take on a more sinister significance. The inability of her eyes to react quickly to light changes perhaps contributes to the fall that leaves Ella with a broken leg. Ella must now cope with the pain of her fracture and, perhaps of more concern, she must adapt to the strange environment of the busy hospital ward.

Adapting to environmental change

Ella is not used to the pace of the ward, nor is she used to the speed with which information is received and required. Ella has always been nervous of hospitals. Although admissions have brought joys in the distant past, bringing her two beautiful daughters, they have also brought great pain, and memories of her husband's final days are brought into focus once more. The pain in her leg makes it difficult for Ella to concentrate, and at night her head is filled by a buzz of whispered conversation punctuated by the snores and gentle moans of fellow patients. Morning often brings an empty bed with no-one able to tell her whether the woman in bed 4 has been discharged or whether she has died during the night. No wonder that Ella's questions of the staff become more insistent. No wonder that the lack of a satisfactory answer is taken as evidence that staff do not wish to tell her the truth for fear that this will upset her. The staff, who do not have time to answer questions about the woman in bed 4, fail to see why a routine discharge provokes such anxiety in Ella. Ella's behaviour, in fact, appears rather odd. Why is she becoming so difficult? The nurses and doctors agree that Ella's responses to some of their questions appear rather vague. She sometimes acts as though she does not hear their questions although she must have good hearing because she could hear her name being mentioned when the Registrar was talking to Sister about her case, even though they were at the other side of the ward. Still, she is due for discharge the next day so it is probably best not to delve too deeply into the fact that she is a bit paranoid: further assessment will only block a bed for a few more weeks. Better simply to add a line to her notes and discharge her to the care of her daughter.

Ella's case is entirely fictional, but you may wish to reflect on your own experience before deciding how close the case is to the truth. Misinterpretation of events is common in the most able of young bodies. The pace of life and the extraordinary complexity of communication makes this inevitable. Imagine, then, the difficulties encountered where pathological changes occur within the sensory organs or where illness or disability intervene.

The process of presbyacusis, described in Chapter 3 gradually impairs an individual's hearing. This process can be exacerbated by the onset of tinnitus, the high pitched buzzing in Ella's ears. Physical damage to the inner ear can be caused by exposure to noise over a prolonged period or can result from infection.

Visual impairments are common across the population, the problems of short sightedness occasionally being magnified by the onset of cataracts as we become older. More serious conditions may include glaucoma and diabetic retinopathy. The point here is *not* to catalogue the illnesses and infections that affect the senses. Common conditions such as cataract can be treated with relative ease, but older people especially may have physical difficulties in accessing the appropriate services. This may result from something as simple as the location of the doctor's surgery, even though this is only a mile or so from home. Lack of money, the absence of public transport, the location of bus stops or even the number of stairs to be traversed may discourage us from attending the consulting rooms. Psychologically we may feel that poor eyesight and deafness are the natural correlates of old age. Perhaps health care professionals no longer say 'what do you expect at your age?' – but it is not unknown for older people to feel that this is how they are perceived. Society generally sends messages to older people that indicate their relative lack of value in the eyes of the world at large. Older people are not allowed to work, for example, being effectively forced to retire at an arbitrary age regardless of ability. As a result they are forced to depend on the gift of government in the form of a pension. Phillipson and Walker (1986) illustrate the process whereby society has created a dependent generation, and this message is received clearly by older people. One result of this may be a feeling that to seek treatment for conditions that are not life threatening is a waste of time and energy. Far better to suffer in silence and maintain one's dignity. Treatable conditions are thus ignored, and the information required to orientate oneself becomes ever more limited. We adapt to this situation, of course, filling in the gaps left by failing senses.

Pathology and perception

Organic damage to the central nervous system takes this process a stage further. Striking examples of this are seen in stroke victims. Jacques (1992) notes that stroke victims and others who are affected by speech disorders can demonstrate that they are able to form complex and cohesive thought patterns despite their underlying pathology. The difficulties encountered by those affected are found in the interpretation and communication of information. Those who suffer from a receptive dysphasia appear to have difficulty in correctly decoding the messages received from the ear, and they also appear unable to identify objects correctly, finding new names for objects when pressed. We do not necessarily recognise that we have incorrectly named something, but we may recognise the lack of understanding apparent in the person to whom we are talking. Others may easily view such behaviour as evidence of a much more malignant condition, mistaking a speech deficit for a dementia. Once again, you may wish to pause and consider the difference that age makes to this interpretation and the subsequent efforts made to treat the condition. One can easily see a successful young business man receiving an extremely vigorous treatment regimen following a road traffic accident which has left him with a communication deficit. The same confidence is not inspired in the treatment of the 70-year-old widow who is recovering from a mild stroke.

Expressive dysphasia often leaves our understanding of events completely intact, but with difficulty in finding the words to communicate our thoughts. This may leave us completely speechless or may result in only the odd word being lost. The reader may have little difficulty in being able to relate to the frustration encountered by the person suffering from dysphasia. Less obvious, however, is the extent to which such a condition drives us back into our own private world. Few people have the strength or motivation to continue attempts at communication when met with a response which does anything but invite further conversation. The most caring of people will occasionally, and inadvertently, respond in a manner that could have been calculated to raise our blood pressure. Less caring, or less skilled, people will simply cut short a difficult conversation claiming pressure of work. Some will cover their own embarrassment by making light of our efforts or their own inability to understand, further adding to our frustrations. At its worst, a reaction indicates that the speech impairment is indicative of a more general intellectual deficit.

The various forms of agnosia can severely affect our ability to interpret the messages received via our senses. Visual agnosia relates to a difficulty in recognition. Holden and Woods (1984) give an example of a sufferer describing in detail a lipstick as a cylinder which extends on rotating, containing a red paint-like substance. The observer recognises the constituent parts but is unable to see the object as a whole. Other forms of this condition include spatial and auditory agnosia as well as autotopagnosia. The latter condition can be seen in stroke victims who appear totally unaware of parts of their own body. Anosognosia leaves the victim unaware of one entire side of their body, to an extent where food will be eaten from only one side of a plate or perhaps only one side of their face is shaved.

Successful interaction with the world, and perhaps also the process of thought itself, requires constant rehearsal and practice. The development of ideas often requires argument, and each of us is constantly engaged in a process of reality testing through communication with others. We orientate ourselves to the world according to the messages received from our environment, and survival in the world requires that our behaviour fits broadly within the limits expected and is accepted by the society within which we live. Any condition that limits contact with the world will have serious consequences on our ability to interact successfully. Physical barriers to sensory input limit both our understanding of events and the way in which our responses are received.

Orientation, behaviour and Alzheimer's disease

Consider the process by which we orientate ourselves to the world. Consider, for example, who you are. The immediate response to this question will produce a name. Further thought may produce a response that identifies you in terms of the major roles which are played out in the course of your life. Ponder for a moment on the roles that you fulfil and the behaviours expected within those roles, then consider how your lifestyle might change were your National Lottery ticket to produce a jackpot prize. In simple terms our identity is, to some extent, defined and reinforced by those with whom we interact. A common exercise used to demonstrate this point is to think back to your last holiday. How clearly could you identify the day of the week? To what extent could you follow events discussed in current affairs programmes following a fortnight's holiday abroad? If abandoned, alone, on a desert island, for how long could you maintain a clear image of yourself? The answers to these questions depend on two things: your level of motivation and the availability of environmental cues. If an eagerly anticipated event is to happen on a given day, you may literally count down the days. If there is no-one to call you by name, however, it may become difficult to identify yourself by name alone.

For those who suffer from Alzheimer's disease the dangers in this situation are clear. We have already seen that sensory impairments can limit our ability to interpret incoming data correctly. The result can be that we become genuinely confused by conflicting interpretations while our best guess at a situation is itself given a false emphasis by those observing. It will be remembered that Ella's initial confusion was reported in a form that suggested the onset of a mental illness. Her notes spoke of an unusual level of anxiety, an unhealthy preoccupation with the imagined death of fellow patients and an apparent confusion suggesting the early stages of dementia. At that time Ella was, in fact, mentally alert with no underlying psychiatric illness. Some time later, however, she was visited at home by her GP, who felt the need to test for Alzheimer's disease. Ella did badly on the test, not having the faintest idea as to the identity of the President of the United States and assuming that 'that Thatcher woman' was still the Prime Minister because her face kept appearing on the television. As far as the day of the week was concerned she knew it was not the weekend but beyond that she was not really too concerned. Kitwood and Bredin (1992) note that tests for dementia are concerned with information which is irrelevant to the person being tested. They further note that the care of those suffering from dementia has, in the past, also been measured in terms of changes in the physical functioning of the dementia sufferer. By using inappropriate criteria for success, treatment regimens are doomed to failure at the outset and as a result the medical profession, in particular, has regarded the care of those with dementia as something of a lost cause. Care regimens have, in effect, attempted to force those suffering from dementia to comply with behavioural codes that the sufferer can barely begin to understand. In addition, carers have interpreted the behaviour of sufferers in terms that have a meaning only to the carers. Kitwood and Bredin (1992) argue that the care process consists of 'us' and 'them' where 'they' are somehow damaged while 'we' are intact, 'they' bring problems whilst 'we' are sane and problem free. Kitwood and Bredin's point is that everyone participating in the care dynamic brings their own problems to the situation. One can add that each brings their own interpretation of events, and each brings their own idea as to the correct behaviour to adopt according to that interpretation. All too often, however, the carer has difficulty in seeing beyond his or her own interpretations of events and beliefs as to how one ought to respond to those events. In reality, it is extremely difficult to imagine how any of us is seeing the world. It is even more difficult to predict how we will react and therefore how one can perhaps manipulate sensory stimuli so as to assist a healthy adaptation on the part of the person suffering from dementia. Jacques (1992) notes that one cannot possibly know the thoughts of a severely demented person. To recall Joe as an example, all one can hope to do is guess at the thoughts going through his mind. To make an educated guess, it is useful to know something of Joe's pre-morbid personality, that is how he behaved before to the onset of the illness. We must be able to estimate how much insight Joe has regarding his condition and what his expectations are concerning that condition. Finally, we must consider the personality changes brought about as a result of the dementia. Jacques (1992) suggests that previously extrovert personalities may cope well with dementia, particularly if admitted into long term care. They are likely readily to accept the help of others and, being previously gregarious, may enjoy the company of staff and residents. There is a danger, however, that this person receives more care than is actually required because they welcome such input. The more introverted personality may cope well with the isolation that results from the dementia but may not welcome the intensity of long term institutional care. We may also wish to consider the defence mechanisms that we employ. The person who accuses the home help of theft has not necessarily undergone a major personality change as a result of dementia. It may be that the thought of losing our purse or wallet is too much to bear. How can we be so stupid as to lose something so important? Some may respond with humour, 'I must be losing my marbles'; others may deny that they could be so stupid. In the latter, the only thing that makes sense is that someone must have stolen the purse. This is partly a defence mechanism and partly evidence that one makes a best guess as to the meaning of events, filling in any gaps that may have occurred in the messages received.

Jacques (1992) goes on to note that we adapt to situations in different ways. Some of us react by 'turning our face to the wall'. This response is characterised by a total withdrawal from the world, to the point where we refuse to eat and appear engaged in a process of prolonged suicide. Others will react to their situation with aggression; others will search for something familiar.

Kitwood (1993) argues that the way in which events are interpreted depends on temperament, experience and mood. The interpretation is also influenced by the situation itself, as well as the assumptions and basic intentions of those involved. Where Jacques (1992) proposes that the role of the carer is tactfully to develop insight in the sufferer, Kitwood and Bredin (1992) urge the carer to seek to assist in the process of understanding both the world and our reactions. The approach requires that the carer helps to explore and ventilate emotional responses. Note that this does not necessarily mean that the sufferer must articulate those emotions in words. Such an approach requires that carers accept and reinforce the individual personality of the sufferer. In part this means that the carer must begin to make efforts to see the world through the eyes of the person suffering from dementia. No general assumptions can be made that will help in this regard. The rule must be that each of us will see the world in our own unique way. This view will change as events themselves change. The carer must be aware of the cues taken from the environment and must attempt to understand the way in which environmental symbols are given meaning by the individual. One must also be aware that having begun the construction of a reality that explains current circumstances, we seek to interpret future events in a manner that supports the new reality. The carer must seek to manipulate sensory stimuli so as to limit the damage caused by sensory impairment. That manipulation must also attempt to provide clues, cues and symbols that help us to reach conclusions which encourage healthy adaptation to dementia. (The reader is strongly urged to adopt the approach detailed in the Dementia Care Mapping process. Details are available from Bradford University.) A short case study illustrates the point.

CASE STUDY 4

Jack Rubens would wake every morning at about 7.30 a.m. The staff of the nursing home in which Jack lived would know of his awakening because Jack would walk naked down the corridor muttering 'God, I may as well be dead. I don't even know who I am'. The response to this was to acknowledge what Jack had said without making any comment that could be seen to pass judgement on his remarks. No attempt made to impose a 'normal' behaviour. In other circumstances carers might have responded along the lines of

'You don't really mean that'. With Jack the appropriate response was slowly to work through the process of helping him to wash and dress. During this process the member of staff would prompt Jack to discuss a series of some five or six memories which had been gathered from Jack and his relatives at various times. The memories focused on the childhood holidays that Jack had spent hop picking in Kent, an anecdote about the relationship between his mother and father, something about his marriage and a little about his work. Jack's response to this conversation was invariably 'God bless you, mate, you've made me a new man'.

Again, let's consider Jack's case further.

The use of reminiscence

Jack's story introduces the concept of reminiscence which can, when used with care, provide a most effective intervention. The success of reminiscence rests on a number of key assumptions. First, reminiscence is about personal memories. You cannot possibly know what I was doing on the day that J.F. Kennedy was shot (or should that now be the day that Margaret Thatcher resigned?). Indeed, my companions on that day cannot recall the event as I lived it at the time. There can, then, be no *correct* reminiscence and hence no sense of failure when we discuss our personal reminiscences. Second, as we grow older, so our long term memories become stronger. Unlike a tape from which a message slowly fades, the recall of memories appears to etch events more deeply, making the picture more bold as time passes. When working with someone who is struggling to understand immediate events it is often less threatening to focus on memories that are easily accessed. In a sense, each of us carries a traveller's guide to help us negotiate social encounters. We may refer to the weather as a means of engaging in short conversations or, for more tricky situations, we may have a bank of 'soap' conversations, the latest events of *Eastenders* or *Coronation Street* being good for a wide range of circumstances. When working with people who are suffering from dementia, reminiscences can take the place of such conversational devices, allowing the sufferer to engage in a normal conversation. It cannot be overemphasised that it is the lack of such opportunities for engagement which both undermines the self confidence of the person suffering from dementia and reduces in the eyes of the carer the abilities of those suffering from the dementia. Indeed, many of the symptoms attributed to dementia can, in fact, be the result of an undiagnosed and untreated depression. Reminiscence offers an opportunity to both test out a diagnosis and alleviate a more malleable depression.

Each of us is nothing more than the sum of our memories and experiences. We orientate ourselves according to the information received from our environment and the demands placed on us in our daily lives. If we are taken out of our normal environment and the clues to our identity are removed, we struggle to maintain our sense of self and we lose contact with concepts of social norms. Reminiscence can help to reinforce who we are and how we have chosen to behave. In Jack's case this process clearly worked and the reminiscence became something of a ritual. Jack quite literally reconstructed his personality each morning.

Before leaving the subject, a word of warning must be sounded. Reminiscence can produce extremely powerful emotions, not all of which are pleasant. Jack, and indeed Joe and Victoria, were natives of the East End of London. For a time reminiscence sessions were of the 'what did you do in the war?' type. It quickly became obvious that few staff were sufficiently skilled to deal with the pain and heartache that was re-lived during those sessions.

Validation, acknowledgement and value

Jack's story is based on a genuine case, in which it took some months to arrive at this strategy. Kitwood and Bredin (1992) argue that carers, both at home and in institutions, must seek to develop a model of care that is not determined by how well the 'sufferer' conforms to the accepted norms, and that the model should not seek simply to contain, ensuring safety at the expense of emotional health. Rather than measure the success or failure of care in terms of ability to pass irrelevant tests (tests that are structured in a way in which those suffering from dementia are destined to fail), we should, instead, evaluate care in terms of the wellbeing of those in receipt of that care. In developing this model, Kitwood and Bredin have drawn on some aspects of validation therapy, as proposed by Naomi Feil (1992). Once again, a case study may help to clarify what this means.

CASE STUDY 5

Sylvia would wake many times during the night. At first she would wake and ask for her husband. 'Where's Bill? He should be in by now'. Bill had died some years previously, after sixty years of marriage. After several weeks, Sylvia became increasingly distressed during the night – calling for Bill, then crying inconsolably for the rest of the night. The night staff began by orientating Sylvia, gently telling her that Bill had passed on and that she was in hospital. Cups of tea did not help, and the staff were reduced to asking for

---

additional night sedation. Sylvia became drowsy during the day and cried whenever she was awake. Realising that Sylvia did, at times, recognise where she was and could recall her husband's funeral, the staff tried a different approach. They began by trying to focus on why Sylvia felt the need for her husband, and quickly concluded that she was feeling lonely and frightened. She missed Bill's warmth and physical presence alongside her in bed, and in the quiet of the night recognised the truth of her position. She knew that she was in hospital and that she was alone. She also felt that she would die alone. With care and patience much of this was tested out with Sylvia who, although not always able to articulate her feelings in words, could through emotion, gesture and behaviour confirm many of the conclusions. Once this was confirmed less skilled carers were taught simple management techniques, which 'validated' Sylvia's feelings and helped her to feel physical warmth and comfort. In practice this meant that the carer sat with Sylvia, placing an arm around her shoulder: a photograph album was used to help Sylvia to recollect happier times spent with Bill and, by following a series of pictures that depicted the growth of her children, Sylvia was able to appreciate that time had moved on.

Feil's discussion of validation is based on a belief that many of the behaviours exhibited later in life result from unresolved conflicts from one's early years. Where the Kitwood and Feil models overlap is in the suggestion that as carers we recognise the validity of the emotions exhibited by those in our care. Rather than try to run away from those feelings we must acknowledge that the feelings exist and hold our clients rather than block them. In such a model physical and psychological withdrawal is not greeted with relief that the sufferer can no longer appreciate his predicament, and the carer should not feel that life will now be easier as a result of the absence of difficult situations. Withdrawal should, instead, be regarded as the ultimate maladaptation in which sufferers have decided that the only way of making sense of their surroundings is to block all sensory stimulation.

Conclusion

To behave in the manner appropriate to any given set of circumstances, we must first understand the situation in which we find ourselves. Understanding is influenced by the data collected through our eyes, ears, skin, nose and mouth, which is then analysed and interpreted by the brain. The analysis of raw data is compared with our previous experience before a picture is presented which represents the brain's best guess as to the reality of the situation. How we then react depends on the meaning that we give to that situation and the estimated outcomes of possible responses.

Our interaction with the world is, then, a complex function of our physical ability to gather sensory data, the meaning that we attribute to the data and the social context within which the interaction takes place. A failure at any stage of this process can have a significant impact on our functional ability. This may be due to an internal dysfunction brought about by inadequate data reception, or it may result from the actions of others. The expectations and assumptions of those around us affect both the messages we receive and the meaning attributed by others to our own behaviour.

Those of us who have difficulty with the collection and interpretation of data thus face twin dangers in that we are likely to act in a manner which does not sit comfortably with events, while our behaviour will be judged by others who may then act in such a way as to hamper severely our chances of further successful interaction.

This cycle of events can be inhibited and the dangers reduced. Perhaps the first step in this process is for those involved to consider their own perceptions and the underlying assumptions that motivate their response. We may then perhaps judge how our own emotional state adds to the interaction, while also considering how others regard our own personality, skill and experience.

Poverty of sensory input can be caused by sensory impairment or by a reduced range of sensory stimuli. Those suffering from such a reduction in stimulation can be found in their own homes or in institutional care. They may be functionally able or they may be suffering from a severe form of Alzheimer's disease. In the former case continued sensory reduction may result in a drift towards confusion; in the latter it may exacerbate the underlying dementia. The role of carers in this field should be to work with the individual with the aim of correcting sensory deficits where possible. Alternatively, information and stimulation should be provided in a manner appropriate to that person. This may involve bringing the outside world into the realm of the physically immobile person living at home. A television set or radio, talking books or a telephone may be all that is required to maintain an active and informed interest in life. Alternatively, a more complex regimen may involve the dementia sufferer in sensory stimulation programmes, periodic use of a Snoezelan, regular contact with the local community and careful use of personal reminiscence.

All care workers should, however, give serious consideration to the expectations that they place on the behaviours of others. Traditional definitions of the medical and nursing professions place patients in the role of passive recipients of care. Their position in this regard is, however, a product of the model constructed by the caring professions. Medical study of the ageing process has concentrated on organic failings associated with older people, and the failure of medicine to offer constructive assistance to those with dementia has left sufferers and carers in a vacuum. The result is that older people in general are regarded as functionally inferior, whereas those who suffer from Alzheimer's disease are expected to degenerate into a vegetative state.

An alternative model for nurses may more usefully focus on theories of psychological development. The layman could be forgiven for assuming that development stops in early adulthood. Indeed, Alzheimer's disease can surely be described as the complete antithesis of development, given that sufferers are perceived to regress into a 'second childhood'. The truth, of course, is that we continue to develop to the point of death. Perhaps those working with older people should consider how to achieve a healthy development in old age. Perhaps those working with dementia sufferers should consider the development needs of those who suffer from Alzheimer's disease and related conditions.

References

Aggleton P and Chalmers H (1986) *Nursing Models and the Nursing Process*. Macmillan, Basingstoke.

Feil N (1992) *Validation: The Feil Method*. Edward Feil Productions, Cleveland, Ohio.

Giddens A (1993) *Sociology*. Polity Press, Cambridge.

Goffman E (1968) *Asylums*, 2nd edn. Doubleday, New York.

Hilgard ER, Atkinson RL and Atkinson RC (1979) *Introduction to Psychology*. Harcourt Brace Jovanovich, New York.

Holden UP and Woods RT (1984) *Reality Orientation: Psychological Approaches to the 'Confused' Elderly*. Churchill Livingstone, Edinburgh.

Jacques A (1992) *Understanding Dementia*. Churchill Livingstone, Edinburgh.

Kenney RA (1989) *Physiology of Ageing: A Synopsis*. Year Book Medical, Chicago.

Kitwood T (1993) Towards a theory of dementia care: the interpersonal process. *Ageing and Society* 13, 51–67.

Kitwood T and Bredin K (1992) Towards a theory of dementia care: personhood and well-being. *Ageing and Society* 12, 269–87.

Levi P (1969) *If This Is a Man*. Orion Press, London.

Levi P (1986) *Moments of Reprieve*. Michael Joseph, London.

Marshall M (1993) Designing for confused old people. In Arie T (ed.) *Recent Advances in Psychogeriatrics*. Churchill Livingstone, Edinburgh.

Mead GH (1934) *Mind, Self and Society*. University of Chicago Press, Chicago.

Midwinter E (1991) *The British Gas Report on Attitudes to Ageing 1991*. Centre for Policy on Ageing, London.

Phillipson C and Walker A (1986) *Ageing and Social Policy: A Critical Assessment*. Gower, Aldershot.

Rosenhan DL (1973) On being sane in insane places. *Science* 179, 250–8.

Roy C (1980) The Roy adaptation model. In Riehl JP and Roy C (eds) *in Conceptual Models for Nursing Practice*. Appleton–Century–Crofts, Norwalk, Connecticut.

Schachter S and Singer JE (1962) Cognitive, social and psychological determinants of emotional state. *Psychological Review* 69, 379–99.

Woods RT and Britton PG (1985) *Clinical Psychology with the Elderly*. Croom Helm, London.

6

Social interaction

Maria Scurfield

The need to communicate is an essential human drive for all individuals. As people grow older, social opportunities can decrease and they may develop problems that make communication difficult. It is essential for the nurse to develop skills in communication to enhance the quality of interaction and the life of the older person. This chapter will discuss the value of the older person and their life experience and how being valued by others is influenced by positive communication. The complex range of non-verbal and verbal communication and how the use of such skills can hinder or enhance the nurse–patient relationship will be explored. Common communication problems that older people experience will be described and suggestions of positive strategies to enable effective assessment and management will be offered. Finally, ways in which the nurse can work with the carers to maximise social opportunities for the older person will also be addressed.

The value of older people

Older people are very special: they are unique individuals with their own life experiences, values and needs. They have faced enormous changes throughout their life and have had to adapt and adjust their lifestyle to cope with poverty, deprivation, two world wars, global changes, political changes, economical changes and the development of technology. Indeed, many older people have been influential in the development of technology and political and social change. There has been massive change in culture and roles, which can be disturbing to people brought up with different values.

The majority of older people have experienced worthy positions within our society. They have been parents, partners, grandparents, employees, employers. Their life experiences has given them a richness of perspective and a set of values which can be distinct from those of other groups (Royal College of Nursing, 1993). Old age is part of the development process in life. It should be viewed positively as a time when health, happiness and self fulfilment are achievable.

Changes that occur in life require adjustment, and older people have had to adjust to many unwanted changes and losses in life, which they have often been unprepared for (such as loss of family or friends, loss of work role, decreased income and increased physical needs). Yet older people have enormous resilience in the face of difficulties and many older people cope well with loss.

Consideration of the environmental and social circumstances in which older individuals find themselves is necessary, as these factors have the ability to hinder or promote the growth of lifestyle. Many older people maintain their respected roles within society and within their families; however, for many older people such roles are lost and they may face social decline.

As the social circle of older people contracts, so does their ability to share experiences with others. Indeed, many older people may be living in circumstances in which they are isolated and deprived of stimulation. In such situations the older person is at risk of loneliness, loss of morale and self esteem, and lack of interest and motivation. Disorientation and confusion are also common effects of social and sensory deprivation.

Nurse–patient interaction

Older people are the largest client group within the health service and their health, psychological and social needs are extremely diverse. Nurses care for older people in a variety of health care settings. The ways in which nurses communicate with older people is vitally important because nurses are in a pivotal position in the determination of the quality of people's lives. Despite this, many studies have shown that communication between nurses and older people tend to be infrequent and brief, confined to physical care and treatment, and initiated by the nurse performing a physical task (Macleod-Clark, 1983). The low level of social interaction in clinical settings is reinforced by the traditional task approach to nursing. Recent studies also confirm the low level of staff patient interaction outside expected routines of care (Armstrong-Esther, Browne and McAfee, 1994). One has to question why nurses spend so little of their time in contact with their patients outside the routines of nursing care, treatment and meals. Nurses may focus on task centred care as it enables the nurse to avoid unhappiness at being unable to cope with the patient's feelings and needs. The life experiences of nurses and older people are extremely different, which may inhibit the nurse from understanding the older patient's needs. Wolfensberger and Thomas (1983) suggest that how a person is perceived and treated by others determines how that person behaves. The more a person is seen as passive and unable to make choices and decisions about their care, the less the person expects to have these responsibilities. In contrast to this, the higher the social value accorded to an individual, the greater the expectation for them to make choices.

In recent years there has been a move away from task allocation in nursing towards approaches that involve individualised care. Primary nursing and named nursing offers the opportunity to acknowledge that older people are individuals who benefit from a personal relationship with their nurse. This type of approach assumes that social interaction between the nurse and the older person is an important and frequent element of the nurse–patient relationship.

Communication

Communication between people involves a complex interaction of verbal and non-verbal behaviours. Increasing emphasis has been placed on the significance of communication skills to health care workers. There is much evidence to suggest that communication in health care is frequently inadequate. Failures in communication in health care have been related to patient dissatisfaction and distress. Owing to the nature of nursing, nurses are in a position to spend more time with the patient than any other health care worker. Macleod-Clark (1983), states that there are four main communication needs of older people in hospital:

- The need for social contact and interaction
- The need for explanation and confirmation
- The need for advice, education and support
- The need for comfort and reassurance.

Knowledge of communication skills is important in increasing the awareness of the communication process, thereby leading to improved nurse–patient relationships.

Non-verbal communication

In the last decade there has been a great upsurge of interest in the process of non-verbal communication between health professionals and patients. This is not surprising as Birdwhistell (1970) estimates that only 30 per cent of the social meaning of a conversation is carried by words alone. It has also been argued that non-verbal communication has five times the effect of words on a person's understanding of a message (Argyle, 1978). It is therefore imperative that nurses increase their knowledge and skills in developing their own non-verbal repertoire and ability to assess and respond to patients' non-verbal communication. Greater knowledge and skill will enhance therapeutic communication between the nurse and the older person.

Non-verbal communication describes all behaviours that convey messages without the use of verbal language and consists of vocal non-verbal communication and non-vocal communication. Vocal non-verbal communication contains all the voice qualities that accompany the transmission of words: pitch, tone and voice, rate of speaking, duration and pauses all convey meaning. Non-vocal non-verbal communication includes body movements, physical appearance, personal space, facial expressions, positive orientation and touch.

Non-verbal communication serves a number of functions:

- *Communicating emotions and attitudes.* In many circumstances feelings are communicated not by what is said but by facial expressions. Similarly, relationships between individuals are often assessed by looking at the non-verbal communication between them.
- *Synchronising conversation.* An individual wishing to start a conversation may hope to 'catch a person's eye' to indicate to the other person that they wish to say something. Similarly, conversations may be terminated using non-verbal channels. The flow of the conversation is regulated by glancing away from the speaker or nodding agreement to her, thus providing feedback.
- *Supplementing speech.* When a speaker puts more stress on certain words than others, or pauses between words, or varies the tone and speed of speech, they are supplementing the conversation non-verbally. In some circumstances the speaker may even contradict what he is saying verbally by his non-verbal expressions.

Facial expressions

Humans share six primary emotions (happiness, sadness, surprise, fear, anger and disgust) and these are easily recognised via the face. There is evidence that facial expressions tend to have a universality of meaning; for example, smiles are recognised as a sign of happiness and frowns are recognised as a sign of sadness all over the world (Ekman and Friessen,

1975). An important issue in the field of interpersonal skills is the extent to which facial expressions can make people feel differently. Exaggerating one's facial expressions increases feelings, whether positive or negative, and suppressing facial expressions decreases feeling.

Physical proximity

Conducting a conversation too close to an older person can cause them to become nervous and apprehensive. The normal degree of physical proximity varies between cultures. Nurses should be aware of cultural and individual differences in physical proximity because speaking too close to an older person can appear intrusive, but speaking too far away can appear cold and impersonal. Nurses perform many tasks that invade the older person's personal space. It is necessary for nurses to be able to assess the degree of proximity that is appropriate for each interaction. One important positive factor of the closeness of interventions by nurses is that it can help in developing close relationships with patients (Porrit, 1984).

Orientation

Orientation refers to the angle at which people sit or stand in relation to each other. People may sit or stand face to face, side by side or at an angle. Nurses can promote conversation with an older person by sitting or standing at the same level as the person.

Eye contact

Engaging in eye contact usually signifies that a person wishes to appear friendly or that they wish to engage in some form of interaction. Because eye contact is important, nurses must be aware of the cues that older people employ either to initiate a conversation or to avoid it. Davies (1994) states that nurses fall into two categories: those whose ability to decode non-verbal signals is poor, and those who can choose to ignore signals. Nurses can also give contradictory messages; for instance, if the nurse asks the patient how she is but fails to have eye contact, an insincere message results.

Failure to maintain direct eye contact may be interpreted as lack of attention, lack of interest or lack of trustworthiness (Altschul, 1972).

Posture, gesture and nods

The ways in which people stand, sit and lie convey a variety of social meanings. Emotional state may be signalled by specific postures; for example, depression in an older person may be signalled by a drooping, listless pose, whereas anxiety can be seen in a tense, stiff, upright older person. Nurses who lean forward in their chairs usually have a more positive attitude towards older people than those nurses who tend to lean backwards.

Gestures may be used to supplement and replace speech. It is very difficult to communicate with someone without using gestures of some sort. In many circumstances, individuals are not aware of the gestures they use, and therefore it is important for nurses to examine their non-verbal repertoire to gain insight into the sorts of message that are being transmitted unknowingly to the older person. It is also important for the nurse to be aware of the older person's gestures as these can indicate their emotional state. Patients may try to hide their feelings, but if a nurse observes older people wringing their hands or touching their face (which can indicate feelings of anxiety) and the nurse can respond appropriately to the person. Head nods promote the vision of reinforcement. Nods can be used by the nurse to encourage an older person to talk more about a certain topic, and often they signify to the patient that the nurse is actively attending to what they are saying.

Appearance

Appearance refers to self presentation and outward appearance. It can be used to convey strong messages about both our social status and our psychological state (Argyle, 1972). Both nurses and patients are influenced by the appearance of a person. However, too much attention can be paid to appearance at the expense of more reliable indictions of character. Porrit (1984) warns nurses not to fall into the trap of making assumptions about a person on the basis of appearance. The sense of smell is also an important aspect of communication. The presence of body odour often produces negative observations and it may lead the nurse to make assumptions about the older person's hygiene (Wright, 1988).

Voice quality

There are six main qualities of voice: volume, tone, pitch, clarity, pace and speech disturbances. Variations in volume can convey the following meanings: soft, sadness; affection, kindness; loud, dominance, confidence. The tone of the voice can be pleasant or unpleasant. Clarity of speech refers to clipping and drawl. Clipped speech may indicate anger and impatience, whereas drawl may indicate sadness or boredom. Pitch often varies with volume so that high pitch and low volume may indicate submissiveness or grief, whereas high pitch and high volume may indicate anger. Pace of speech varies from fast to slow: fast speech may mean anger, animation or surprise; slow speech may mean sadness or boredom. Speech disturbances may be classified into pauses and filters.

Too many pauses can be interpreted as boredom; too few can indicate anger or contempt.

Bodily contact

Bodily contact refers to physical contact, which may serve to get the attention of others or be used to convey emotion or understanding. Touch is an essential means of communication throughout childhood, fostering love and providing comfort, and enhancing psychological and physiological development (Oliver and Redfern, 1991).

Touch

It is important that nurses should consider how they can use touch as an effective means of communication. Touch can serve as a means of providing sensory stimulation, reduction of anxiety, reality orientation, relief of physical and psychological pain, and comfort in dying as well as sexual expression (Barnett, 1972). Further studies have indicated that affective touch promotes trust and empathy, and enhances self esteem and enhances communication generally among older patients (Burnside, 1973; Copstead, 1980). Touch also provides an opportunity to promote the older person's adaptation to their environment. It has been suggested that many older people suffer from touch deprivation; this increases when the person is separated from caring people. Men are more likely to suffer experience touch deprivation because of culture and lifestyle. Older women are allowed more freedom to touch, although they may lack the opportunity. Ebersole and Hess (1990) state that it is not uncommon for older men to be wrongly accused of sexual offences because they dared to give a child an affection pat on the buttocks.

Despite the enormous value of touch to older people, many studies confirm that nurses do not often use affective touch when caring for older people (Watson, 1975; Oliver and Redfern, 1991). Because of the nature of nurses' work, touch is often a deliberate physical contact required to perform specific tasks such as taking a pulse or cleansing a wound. It is important to distinguish between touch that is to perform a task and affective touch, which can be spontaneous and does not necessarily form part of a task (Oliver and Redfern, 1991). Nurses may also use touch in a condescending way, such as patting a patient's head. It is also important to consider that touch is an intimate process that not all older people would like: the comfort of touching depends on place, situation, life experiences and age. One way of assessing whether an older person will respond positively to touch is by observing their reaction to a handshake. If their reaction is positive it will feel relaxed; if not, it may feel tense. Touch is an extremely important means of communication with older people who have dementia. Studies have indicated that touch can enhance the confused patient's ability to relate and respond to the nurse (Beck and Heacock, 1988). Nurses need to examine their own feelings and attitudes towards positive means of non-verbal communication with these patients.

Massage

The use of touch can be extended to include massage. Massage allows the nurse to touch older people effectively in a very meaningful way. Massage for older people offers the opportunity to encourage reminisence, promote relaxation and enhance communication (West, 1993; Mason, 1988). The move to a more holistic approach to nursing care encourages the use of contemporary practices. Massage allows the nurse to utilise the skills of touch and comforting, associated with caring, which can facilitate physical and psychological wellbeing.

Massage allows the nurse to become more comfortable with affective touch, thereby extending the scope of the nurse's ability to communicate with the older person. Massage can also enhance the nurse's feeling of wellbeing, making it possible for both the nurse and the patient to share the benefits of this method of care. Massage techniques can be easy to learn, as they follow normal movements of the hands. The technique of stroking or effleurage is a gentle form of massage that promotes comfort and relaxation in older people. The ability to use touch and massage with older people can be learnt in the same way as other communication skills. It has enormous potential in developing the nurse–patient relationship and can promote positive attitudes towards the older person and their carers. Carers can be taught to explore the use of touch and massage with relative to enhance their communication and the quality of their relationship. Carers should be encouraged to practise this within the health setting and on discharge.

Non-verbal communication should not be viewed in isolation, but should be interpreted within the context in which it appears. If nurses are able to interpret the non-verbal signals of patients as well as to reflect on their own non-verbal skills, the chances of misinterpretations and misunderstandings will be reduced. The importance of non-verbal communication with older people cannot be overemphasised. For many older people the need for non-verbal communication and touch will be even greater than the need for verbal communication.

Verbal communication

Verbal communication represents only a small part of the social meaning of a conversation. Verbal communication consists of spoken or written words. Nurses must become more skilled in both verbal and non-verbal communication as they are an essential prerequisite for effective assessment and care management of older patients. Assessment of a patient requires the nurse to practise and be aware of a number of complex non-verbal and verbal communication skills. The ability to utilise such skills is imperative during the assessment phase of care as this will enable the nurse and patient to identify the initial needs of the patient. The nurse will then be in a position to plan care more effectively, identifying the different types of communication necessary to meet the needs of the older patient.

Questioning

The skill of questioning is extremely important if a patient's needs are to be assessed effectively (Macleod-Clark, 1991). There are a number of different types of question that can be used depending on the situation.

Closed questions

Closed questions enable the questioner to have control over the conversation because there are a fixed and limited number of responses. Closed questions can provide useful factual information and can help if the older person appears anxious, as being able to answer a simple question can reduce tension. However, too many closed questions can cause problems. Nurses who ask patients closed questions in which the older person responds with one word answers find themselves asking more and more questions and paying less attention to the answers. The older person will also sense a lack of interest by the nurse, which may inhibit the nurse–patient relationship. For example: 'You look better today. The medication must be helping to relieve the pain. I understand you've seen the physiotherapist today. When is she coming back to see you?'

Open questions

The use of open questions gives the patient the opportunity to discuss the things they want to or the things they feel relevant. This enables the nurse to adopt an active listening role. For example: 'Tell me how you are feeling today.' 'How can I help you?'

Affective questions

Affective questions relate to feelings and emotions. The nurse can use this type of question to ask how older people felt in the past, how they feel now and the reasons that underlie these feelings. This offers the person the opportunity to reflect on how they feel, and the nurse is able to communicate concern and empathy by asking such questions.

Probing questions

Probing questions can encourage and prompt the older person to talk when they fail to do so spontaneously. Prompts and probes are verbal tactics for helping patients to talk about themselves and to define their situation more clearly. For example: 'You said that some days you feel more anxious than others. Can you tell me about that?'

'You said that you are worried about your daughter having to spend more time with you. Tell me more about how that makes you feel.'

Listening

In interpersonal interaction, the process of listening is of crucial importance. To respond appropriately to the older person it is necessary to pay attention to the messages they are sending and to relate future responses to these messages. Porrit (1984) in her discussion on nurse–patient communication, states that 'most life events including admission to hospital do not require highly skilled counselling but do require skilled listening'. As we listen to older people we evaluate them and what they are saying, we plan our responses, rehearse this response and then respond. The process of planning and rehearsal usually occur subconsciously. They are important because they can interfere with the listening activity.

Reflective listening

Reflective listening involves nurses reporting in their own words what they think the older person is saying, thinking and feeling. Reflective listening is important because it checks understanding and enables the nurse and patient to correct one another if either is wrong. It also lets the older person know that the nurse wants to understand them. For example: 'When you think about your mobility difficulties you feel more anxious.' 'Your daughter having to spend time with you makes you feel guilty.'

Silence

Silence is another powerful form of communicating. Many people feel uncomfortable with silence, and there can be a temptation for the nurse to do something to bridge the gap in the conversation. Silence, when used effectively, allows the older person and the nurse the opportunity to collect and organise their thoughts.

Summarising

Summarising is also an important skill in therapeutic communication. It involves the nurse reflecting on what has been discussed or agreed. It emphasises an understanding of the discussion and allows clarification of any agreed outcomes. It is also useful before moving on to different topic areas. For example: 'It seems to me that what you are saying is that because of your mobility difficulties you feel more dependent on your daughter, and the fact that she has to spend more time with you makes you feel guilty. Is that right?'

Addressing older people

Nurses are aware of the need to treat older people with courtesy and respect, and one way of doing this is by addressing the person by name. It is unfortunate that many nurses address patients by their first names without the courtesy of asking permission. Many older people prefer to be addressed by their first name as it makes them feel warm and welcome and it is more personal. The use of first names may also make the older person feel that the nurse cares for them. On the other hand, the use of first names may lead to contempt by the older person and their carers resulting in a loss of dignity. Such feelings can do much to hinder the nurse–patient relationship. If the nurse addresses older people by their surname when this is not preferred, it may lead to feelings of depersonalisation – which can also hinder the nurse–patient relationship.

There are too many examples of older people being addressed differently by different grades of staff and other health care disciplines. For example, a consultant may address the patient as 'Sir', the physiotherapist as 'Mr Jones', the sister as 'William' and the staff nurse as 'Billy'.

Nursing staff must make a concentrated effort to identify how the older person prefers to be addressed. This can be achieved by skilfully asking the older person what they prefer to be called, being careful not to influence their decision.

Offering information

Offering information to the older person while they are in receipt of health care is an essential role of the nurse, yet patients are often deprived of such information. Uncertainty about diagnosis and treatment can make people vulnerable to stress. Older people should be informed about the nature of their illness, and adequate information and emotional support is vital if older people are to make informed choices about their treatment. Nurses should encourage older people to express their anxieties and emotions; however, many nurses have difficulty in coping with patients' emotions. Nurses must face the challenge of dealing with people's feelings about their diagnosis and treatment. Many older people feel inhibited about asking doctors questions. Nurses are in a good position to help patients to understand their illness and treatment. Open communication or information giving helps to reduce the older person's anxiety and gives them a sense of control over their situation. It may also enhance their feeling of trust in the nurse.

Communication problems of older people

A range of factors can result in problems of communication for older people. Degeneration of neuronal tissue in the central nervous system can occur as a result of ageing or of pathology. Common difficulties arise from reduction in sensory inputs, especially hearing and vision. There may also be changes an older person's ability to express their needs or in understanding others. Such changes obviously have great impact on the person's communication channels and may result in social withdrawal, decline, and loneliness and isolation.

It is essential that nurses make a comprehensive assessment of the individual's communication strengths and weakness in order to plan care that will maximise their ability to communicate. Nurses must also see it as part of their role to share knowledge, skills and methods of enhancing communication with older people and their families and friends.

Visual impairment

Problems involving visual deficiencies are very common as people reach old age. The power of visual accommodation diminishes and there can be difficulty with accommodating to darkness. Farsightedness or presbyopia, is a common problem resulting in the need for many older people to wear spectacles. Because an older person relies on visual stimulation, falls and accidents from poor vision are numerous. As a result of visual impairment, an older person may have very limited interests and hopes to pursue. Living alone without much social contact, they may soon become isolated, withdrawn and depressed because of their visual deficiencies. Visual limitations can make communication problematic because facial expressions and gestures, which are as important as words, may be missed or misinterpreted.

It is important that the nurse includes vision within an assessment. Many older people wear spectacles that are ineffective as they have not had regular eye tests. The nurse should encourage them or their carers to have their eyesight tested again. Eye examination will also find many diseases, for example glaucoma or cataracts.

Nurses and carers can maximise communication with older people who have visual impairment by:

- Introducing themselves before speaking to the person

- Facing the person when speaking (stand or sit in a position that allows the person direct eye contact)
- Ensuring that appropriate lighting is provided and giving carers advice on lighting in the older person's home
- Ensuring that spectacles are clean and well fitted
- Using aids as appropriate, for example large print books, talking books, radio, large numbered clocks and hand magnifiers
- Keeping the older person's environment as familiar as possible to maximise independence and prevent accidents.
- Ensuring nurses, relatives and visitors spend time talking to the older person (explore the possibility of a 'befriending scheme' if the person has limited social contact)
- Using non-verbal communication such as touch essential during interactions
- Exploring with the older person suitable leisure activities.

Hearing impairment

The incidence of hearing impairment also increases with age. There is a gradual loss of ability to hear high pitched sounds, and the perceived quality of sound also changes. Cochlear problems include diminished hearing and tinnitus. It is known that tinnitus can lead to depression in older people and vestibular problems result in disturbance of balance.

Feelings of depression and isolation are frequently associated with hearing loss and in some older people can exacerbate a tendency towards paranoia (Birren and Woods, 1985).

Nurses often assume that the answer to hearing loss is to provide a hearing aid. However, if the older person has a high frequency hearing loss or a hearing loss that misses sounds, a hearing aid will not be very helpful in discriminating sounds as it only amplifies sound. Some older people refuse to wear hearing aids, and some are be unable to tolerate hearing aids because of the amplification of noise. Many older people do not understand how their hearing aids work or have difficulties in operating the volume control.

Nurses must become more skilled at assessing older people's hearing to facilitate planned care to enhance communication.

Nurses and carers can maximise communication with older people who have hearing impairment by:

- Eliminating background noise when conversing with an older person
- Ensuring that their hearing aid, if appropriate, is fitted and working
- Ensuring that their ears are checked regularly for build up of wax
- Facing the person directly, making sure to adopt a position to enable lip reading (do not turn away in the middle of a sentence)

- Speaking slowly and clearly, avoiding shouting and not exaggerating speech
- Using question and answer techniques to check understanding (rephrase the sentence if it is not understood)
- Changing to a new subject by pausing and ensuring that the person follows the new subject
- Using other means of communication as appropriate to enhance the spoken word, for example pictures, writing and call bells.

Speech difficulties

There are numerous factors that cause speech impairment in older people. Speech difficulties may result from hearing loss, ill fitting dentures, confusion and social isolation. Speech problems can also occur as a result of disease or pathology such as cerebrovascular accident, cerebral atrophy or Parkinson's disease. Cerebrovascular accidents are quite common in older people, and they pose special communication challenges to the person, to their families and to nurses.

Speech is a major means of organising and maintaining environmental security. Communication problems are the most disastrous consequences of cerebrovascular accidents (Ebersole and Hess, 1990). Speech and communication difficulties following cerebrovascular accidents are complex. The main terms used to describe these speech problems are aphasia and dysphasia.

Aphasia and dysphasia

Aphasia means 'loss of language'. *Dysphasia* ranges from partial to severe loss of language ability and is commonly associated with a cerebrovascular accident affecting the left (dominant) hemisphere.

The terms aphasia and dysphasia are used interchangeably, although technically aphasia should mean loss of language functioning and dysphasia should refer to a disturbance of language (Hodges, 1994). There are two types of dysphasia: receptive and expressive dysphasia. Receptive dysphasic patients cannot understand language, although they may recognise objects and their uses. Expressive dysphasic patients can understand verbal and written communication but cannot organise concepts into words or meaningful expressions (Ebersole and Hess, 1990).

Skelly (1975) interviewed patients with dysphasia. Patients' responses included: feelings of fear and anguish that they thought could have been reduced if someone had explained what had happened to them; feeling insulted by professionals who talked as if they were children; being sensitive to non-verbal cues of inpatients or annoyance; and feeling that professionals often asked too many questions or spoke too quickly, making it difficult to respond. These responses should be considered carefully by professionals when communicating with patients who have aphasia or dysphasia.

Dysarthria

The older person may experience difficulty in speaking clearly due to muscle weakness, although there is no language loss. This is called dysarthria. Other communication disorders associated with cerebrovascular accident may include impairment of memory, loss of orientation in place and time, and loss of concentration. Emotional states are often heightened, which may cause crying or laughing with very little cause.

Nurses and carers can maximise communication with older people who have speech impairment by:

- Addressing the older person by their preferred name
- Facing the person directly, ensuring that they can see and hear you
- Speaking slowly and clearly using simple sentences
- Giving the older person time to understand and respond (avoid putting words into their mouths)
- Not underestimating the older person's capacity to communicate
- Speaking one person at a time
- Using closed questions if the required response is one word, for example 'yes' or 'no'
- Referring the patient to a speech therapist and follow their advice on promoting communication
- Encouraging the use of gestures, nodding, blinking, etc., if the older person has great difficulties in speaking
- Choosing appropriate communication aids, such as pictures, cue cards and written instructions
- Making every effort to understand the older person (do not be frightened to say that you have difficulty understanding them)
- Asking the person to repeat what they are saying
- Showing interest in people by spending time with them (do not appear to be in a hurry: give the person time to express any anxieties and attempt to help with suggestions of possible solutions)
- Observing the person's non-verbal communication for signs of distress and responding appropriately.

Involve relatives and friends in care and teach them methods to enhance communication. For example:

- Encourage the older person's family to accept their relative as a social member of the family
- Encourage the person to keep their former social contacts, friends, clubs, interests and hobbies
- Ensure that the person has something useful to do in the home
- Encourage the person to say the names of objects around them

- Do not make the older person speak when they are tired or angry and do not push them to do or say things they cannot
- Suggest that the family encouragement and praise for every achievement.

Cognitive impairment

Nursing or caring for an older person suffering from a dementing condition requires great skills, especially in communication. In dementia deterioration is characterised by memory loss, with recent memory loss being commonly affected; however, recall from distant memory may also be impaired. The person may also become disorientated in time, place and person, which may result in increased confusion, wandering, getting lost and difficulty in recognising family and friends. There may also be a decreased ability to solve the problems of day-to-day living, and social skills may become impaired. As the disease progresses the person may exhibit marked behavioural and personality changes. The pattern and rate of deterioration in functioning are variable to each individual. The normal use of language may be affected in people with dementia. Older people may have difficulty in expressing themselves and in understanding others. Along with other functional deficits, this may result in feelings of hopelessness, depression, agitation and humiliation. The person may lose self confidence and self respect and become withdrawn. The process of communication is therefore crucial to the quality of care of the older person with dementia. Communication provides a sense of security to older people, reassuring them that there are people who will listen to them and value them as respected individuals. The nurse and carer must become skilled in using a range of different verbal and non-verbal methods to enhance meaningful communication.

Reality orientation and validation therapy are therapeutic methods of communication with older people who have dementia. Reality orientation may be used in a formal group or as an informal 24 hour approach whereby current information is offered to the person. There may become a stage in dementia when reorientation is impossible because of intellectual deterioration. The older person may not accept orientation information, and may become distressed if they are reminded of the real situation. At this stage, the use of validation techniques becomes more appropriate. Validation therapy is the process of communicating with disorientated older people by validating and respecting their feelings in whatever time or place is real to them at that time, even though it may not correspond with our reality (Feil, 1982). Therefore, a response to the disorientated person who keeps saying he wants to go home is to ask such questions as 'what do you miss about home?' Key questions such as who, what, where and when offer the person the opportunity to describe relevant events of their lives.

The non-verbal communication abilities of the person with dementia may remain intact even as other abilities decline. Positive affective non-verbal messages foster positive responses, whereas negative non-verbal messages elicit withdrawal and discomfort. Touch, facial expression, eye contact, tone of voice and posture all communicate with the older person with dementia (Beck and Heacock, 1988).

Nurses and carers can maximise communication with older people who have dementia by:

- Referring to them by their preferred name
- Looking directly at them and attempting to gain their attention before speaking
- Introducing themselves before speaking
- Maintaining a calm reassuring tone of voice
- Using non-verbal cues to reinforce verbal communication
- Giving the person time to respond (repeat verbal and non-verbal communication if the person fails to respond initially
- Being consistent with the words used to describe things
- Attempting to elicit key words and repeating the words or feelings attached to them if they can't understand the person
- Using reality orientation, validation or reminiscence techniques to promote awareness of environment and self
- Spending time talking to them encouraging them to express their feelings
- Not attempting to force them to co-operate if they don't want to (return when the person is more approachable)
- Eliciting the person's feelings by being sensitive to their non-verbal communication
- Encouraging the person to participate in activities and hobbies that interest them (spend time talking to the person about their interests)
- Promoting the use of touch if the person responds positively
- Ensuring that the person is involved in decisions affecting their care.

Social isolation

Many people enjoy an active lifestyle, pursuing leisure activities throughout old age, and they maintain a positive quality of life. However, many older people are unable to adjust to physical and social losses in their lives and become bored, lonely or depressed. Such symptoms may lead to a complete withdrawal from society, increasing the risk of social deprivation or social isolation, and the older person may view themselves and their lifestyle in a very negative manner. Social isolation is not the same as solitude, which is the voluntary choice to be alone for rest. Patients experiencing social isolation may be observed to be alone much of the time to demonstrate mood or behaviour changes, to have alterations in sleep and eating patterns, and to verbalise feelings of boredom, abandonment, insecurity and poor self concept (Elipoulos, 1993).

Nurses care for older people in a variety of settings. Most older people live in the community and may come into contact with district nurses, health visitors or community psychiatric nurses during their life. Nurses also care for older people in day hospitals and hospital settings, where many older people return to their own home following care. It is important that nurses do not just concern themselves with enhancing the communication of older people while in hospital, but that they assess the older person's home lifestyle. Nurses can offer advice to older people and their carers in methods of enhancing social outlets and promoting interest and activities.

Nurses should assess the person's roles and interests and use this information to help them to develop opportunities for increased socialisation.

Maintaining activities and interests

Attempts should be made to increase meaningful activity for the older person when they are in health care settings and when they are in their own home. Being in hospital can be a traumatic experience for older people: there may be reduced opportunities for choice and they may have little control over the environment. If there is little activity, the person may become isolated and lonely.

The nurse can involve older people and their carers in exploring the older person's past and current lifestyle, highlighting past or present interests, hobbies and social life. Nurses and carers can encourage the older person to reinstate their old hobbies or interests, or to explore new interests which can be facilitated in the health care setting, in the person's home or within the community.

It is wrong for nurses or carers to assume that all older people will respond positively to activities. Many older people are encouraged to attend day clubs where the only activities are tea drinking and bingo. This kind of activity may be appropriate and enjoyable for some, but for others it may provoke anger and resentment, especially if the person has never enjoyed such activities during their life. There are many community resources offering a wide variety of activities and interests for older people, for example history groups, art clubs, pottery classes, craft classes, tea dances, walking clubs and music appreciation.

If the older person is housebound, activities could be chosen that rely on minimal resources, for example music tapes, videos, talking books, reminiscence materials, newspapers, books, gardening and craftwork.

Friends, relatives, children and neighbours may also be encouraged to visit regularly, and if the older person has previously been active within the community or church they may appreciate visits from people with similar interests and the priest or vicar could be a source of comfort.

Reminiscence and life review

One important activity for older people that can be exploited in a number of ways is reminiscence. Reminiscence is a normal activity that comes naturally to everyone, but it has been suggested that reminiscence becomes increasingly important as people grow old. As people grow old they may have to come to terms with physical and mental health problems, and their social circumstances may change dramatically. Reminiscence involves a person looking back and reflecting on their past personal life. The ability to recall the past is an area of functioning that is likely to remain intact well into old age. Studies have linked the ability to reminisce with life satisfaction (Barnat, 1985). The argument is that older people who are capable of going through their past life history and have an understanding of how such life events led to their present situation will have a stronger sense of personal identity. Reminiscence allows the older person the chance to remind themselves of their life achievements and contributions, and therefore it can enhance the person's self esteem and self worth. Reminiscence can play an important role in meeting the older persons emotional, social and psychological needs. It can assist the individual in coming to terms with and adapting to old age, and can aid the life review process. Reminiscence is a communication centred approach, which promotes interpersonal and social interaction. Reminiscence provides an important opportunity to enhance the quality of the nurse–patient relationship. Most importantly, reminiscence therapy offers the opportunity to recognise older people as individuals who have something positive to contribute to life.

Reminiscence with the confused older person

Reminiscence can be particularly effective with older people who suffer from a dementing illness. A common feature in dementia is short term memory impairment, which affects the ability of the individual to recall recent events. This can make the present seem confusing and threatening. Long term memory may remain well preserved, therefore reminiscence can help the individual to concentrate on a period when the memories are much stronger and more certain. This can promote personal identity and enhance individuality.

Reminiscence therapy provides the optimum conditions for verbal and non-verbal communication to take place, and it is normally an enjoyable and stimulating experience. Older people who have memory loss and failing abilities may gain a sense of self esteem by sharing their past life history and memories. Reminiscence therapy offers the opportunity for the older person to feel valued by those caring for them (Woods, Portnoy and Jones, 1992).

Reminiscence can be used on an individual basis to enhance interpersonal communication between the older person and the nurse or carer, or it can be used as a group therapy. Group therapy involves the use of structured sessions in which the older person shares their memories with others. Group therapy encourages interpersonal communication between patients and staff. Reminiscence materials such as photographs, tastes, smells, objects, music, poetry and personal mementos can be used to stimulate memories and discussion.

Nurses undertaking reminiscence therapy need to be very skilled sensitive communicators. It is imperative that the nurse should assess whether the therapy is suitable for the individual. Reminiscence therapy can provoke painful memories as well as joyful memories; for example, many older people enjoy reminiscing about the war years, but some individuals will have lost friends and relatives or have been held as prisoners of war. The nurse needs to be very sensitive and to be skilled at dealing with such situations. Some older people may also avoid reminiscence as it may make them feel unhappy to think of the contrast between the past and present and heighten the experience of loss. Nurses can ensure that carers are given a valuable role in reminiscence. Carers can be encouraged to share their knowledge about the older person's past life. Information such as schooling, relationships, occupations, achievements, hobbies and interests can be shared. Carers can also be encouraged to use at home reminiscence techniques that have proved to be successful while their relative has been in hospital. This offers the opportunity to strengthen the nurse–carer relationship and to heighten meaningful communication between the carer and their relative.

Carers could also help their relative compile a life diary using their past and present life history, including chosen photographs and memorabilia. The diary may then be used to facilitate communication between the older person and their carers or visitors. Formulation of such a diary can be a very interesting and enjoyable experience for the carer and the older person.

Conclusion

This chapter has emphasised the pivotal role of the nurse in maximising the older person's ability to communicate. Nurses must continually examine their non-verbal repertoire and develop skills to enhance communication with the older person. Therapeutic communication has the potential to greatly improve the quality of life of the older person, and nurses who care for older people must address this challenge.

References

Altschul AT (1972) *Patient–Nurse Interaction: A Study of Interaction Patterns in Acute Psychiatric Wards*. Churchill Livingstone, Edinburgh.

Argyle M (1972) Non verbal communication in human interaction. In Hine R (ed.) *Non Verbal Communication*. Cambridge University Press, Cambridge.

Argyle M (1978) *The Psychology of Human Interpersonal Behaviour*. Penguin, Harmondsworth.

Armstrong-Esther CA, Browne KD and McAfee JE (1994) Elderly patients still clean and sitting pretty. *Journal of Advanced Nursing* 19, 264–71.

Barnat J (1985) Exploring living memory: the uses of reminiscence. *Ageing and Society* 5, 333–7.

Barnett K (1972) A survey of the current utilisation of touch by health team personnel with hospitalised patients. *International Journal of Nursing Studies* 9, 195–209.

Beck C and Heacock P (1988) Nursing interventions for patients with Alzheimer's disease. *Nursing Clinics of North America* 23, 95–121.

Birdwhistell R (1970) *Kinesis and Context*. University of Pennsylvania Press, Philadelphia.

Birren JE and Woods AM (1985) Psychology of ageing. In Pathy, MSJ (ed.) *Principles and Practice of Geriatric Medicine*. Wiley, Chichester.

Burnside IM (1973) Touching is talking. *American Journal of Nursing* 73, 2060–3.

Copstead LE (1980) Effect of touch on self appraisal and interaction appraisal for permanently institutionalised older adults. *Journal of Gerontological Nursing* 6, 747–52.

Davies P (1994) Non verbal communication with patients. *British Journal of Nursing* 3, 220–3.

Ebersole P and Hess P (1990) *Towards Health Ageing: Human Needs and Nursing Response*. CV Mosby, Toronto.

Ekman P and Friessen WV (1975) *Unmasking the Face*. Prentice-Hall, Englewood Cliffs, New Jersey.

Elpoilos C (1993) *Gerontological Nursing*. JB Lippincott, Philadelphia.

Feil N (1982) *Validation: The Feil Method*. Edward Feil Productions, Cleveland.

Hodges JR (1994) *Cognitive Assessment for Clinicians*. Oxford University Press, Oxford.

Macleod-Clark J (1983) Nurse–patient communication: an analysis of conversations from surgical wards. In Wilson-Barnett J (ed.) *Nursing Research: Ten Studies in Patient Care*. Wiley, Chichester.

Mason A (1988) Massage. In Rankin-Box D (ed) *Complementary Health Therapies: A Guide for Nurses and the Caring Professions*. Croom Helm, London.

Oliver S and Redfern SJ (ed.) (1991) Interpersonal communcation between nurses and elderly patients: refinement an observation schedule. *Journal of Advanced Nursing* 16, 30–8.

Porrit L (1984) *Communication: Choices for Nurses*. Churchill Livingstone, Melbourne.

Royal College of Nursing (1993) *The Value and Skills of Nurses Working with Older People*. RCN, London.

Skelly M (1975) Aphasic patients talk back. *American Journal of Nursing* 75, 1104–6.

Watson WH (1975) The meaning of touch: geriatric nursing. *Journal of Communication* 25, 104–12.

West B (1993) The essence of aromatherapy. *Elderly Care* 5, 24–5.

Wolfensberger W and Thomas S (1983) *Program Analysis of Service Systems Implementation of Normalisation*. Canadian National Institute on Mental Retardation, Toronto.

Woods B, Portnoy S and Jones G (1992) Reminiscence and life review with persons with dementia: which way forward? In Jones G and Miesen BML (eds) *Caregiving in Dementia*. Routledge, London.

Wright S (1988) *Nursing the Older Patient*. Harper and Row, London.

Further reading

Coleman PG (1986) *Ageing and Reminiscence Processes: Social and Clinical Implications*. Wiley, Chichester.

Jones G and Miesen BML (1992) *Caregiving in Dementia: Research and Applications*. Routledge, London.

Redfern SJ (1991) *Nursing Elderly People*, 2nd edn. Churchill Livingstone, London.

Yurick AG, Spier BE, Robb, SS and Ebert NJ (1989) *The Aged Person and the Nursing Process*. Appleton and Lange, California.

7

Sexuality and sexual health

Pauline Ford

This chapter explores physiological and psychological ageing in relation to sexuality and sexual health. Some well known studies will be referred to, thereby highlighting the sexuality of older people. It will explore the needs of heterosexual and homosexual older people and the nurse's role in meeting those needs, and is underpinned by the following beliefs:

- Older people are sexually active
- Older people have sexual health needs
- Older people need sexual health education
- Older people may be HIV positive
- Older people have the same rights as the rest of us.

What is sexuality?

Most people are interested in sex and sexuality. We live in a society that seems increasingly tolerant of sexual determination for virtually every member of society. However, sexuality has traditionally been considered between puberty and retirement age. This chapter will demonstrate that sexuality is an important issue for those living into their seventh decade and beyond. Let us start by defining sexuality as

> the quality of being human, all that we are as men and women encompassing the most intimate feelings and deepest longings of the heart to find meaningful relationships
>
> Hogan, cited by Redfern, 1992, p.262.

This quote demonstrates that sexuality and sexual health mean different things to different people across all age groups. Sexuality is not solely related to sexual activity or sexual intercourse. It refers to our sexual expression, how we portray ourselves as men and women. Thus our clothing, hairstyle, use of fragrances and make-up, for example, all go to make up the essence of self expression as sexual beings. We may wish to portray ourselves as being overtly feminine or masculine, or to cross-dress or to share sexual experiences with the same sex. All of this affects the presentation of our sexual self.

This is as relevant in old age as it is at any other period of the life span.

What is different for older people?

Sexuality in western societies appears to be tied to youth and physical attractiveness. The images of slender and/or muscular, high-cheek-boned blonde beauties confront us day and night on television, in magazines and on billboards. This bombardment of media values can make any man or woman who does not fit into the stereotype of beauty feel inadequate or unattractive. Older people may be used for advertising (for thermal underwear and laxatives and insurance), but it is unlikely that they will be portrayed as sensual or sexual beings.

In western society it is contended that usefulness is socially constructed (Phillipson and Walker, 1986). For men, social usefulness is defined by productiveness at work, and for women the menopause is widely presumed to herald the beginning of a sexless and therefore reproductively useless phase of life (Kuhn, 1976). Such attitudes discriminate against older people in general and those older people who consider themselves to be gay or lesbian. It perpetuates the myth that all men work until retirement and then become a burden on society and that all women exist purely as reproductive machines. It makes no allowance for the considerable contributions that older people make in society, nor for those who choose less predictable or traditional modes of living.

Victor (1987) suggests that growing old is easier for men because being male is associated with competence and autonomy, valued attributes which can often withstand the ageing process. Women, she argues, are desired for beauty and childbearing abilities. It is possible to see the influence of public relations. Sexually active older men may be labelled as 'dirty old men', but men are supposed to maintain their 'manhood' for longer than women maintain their 'womanhood' (Sontag, 1978). For example, Charlie Chaplin and Picasso are applauded for becoming fathers later in life. But where are the dirty old women? As de Beauvoir (1973) reminds us, old men may be considered handsome but old women are rarely described as beautiful. It is worth noting that the English language has no equivalent term for virility to describe high levels of sexuality in women.

Those who are currently old were likely to have been brought up in a period of strict religious morality (Comfort, 1976) when sex outside marriage or even for pleasure was considered sinful. It is important, however, to remember that older people are not a homogeneous group. The young old (60–70 years) are likely to have been influenced by society's changing attitudes and to have a more liberated view of sexual activity. Despite these different experiences, most members of the human race have a need for relationships, for demonstrations of affection and friendship. According to Colton (1983) humans cannot survive in any degree of comfort without touch, and its complete loss may lead to psychotic breakdown. In all cultures, gently touching each other conveys affection and friendship. For older people who do not have sexual partners or close companions, touch is likely to assume an even greater importance. Love is closely connected with our skin sensation and appearance. How that skin appears affects others' willingness to touch us. Beauty may only be skin deep but that skin is highly significant. The skin of an older person shows the beautiful lines of hard work and experience. Old hands and faces tell us a lot about the owners' capacity for intimacy. But in western society lines of work and experience are frequently viewed negatively, which results in the denial of older people's sexuality by the young. This denial starts early. Can you recall as a teenager finding it repugnant to consider your parents engaging in sexual intercourse? Did it disgust you? How do you feel now? That's what is different for older people – society's attitudes towards sexual expression. Beauty and sex continue to be the reserved territory of the young.

Biological ageing

Some of the normal physical changes associated with old age are likely to affect sexual behaviour. It is not within the remit of this chapter to cover all the physiological changes associated with old age. Many may, however, impact on sexual expression, in terms of both self esteem and physical ability to engage in sexual activity. (See the further reading recommendations at the end of this chapter.) Clearly some older people are susceptible to chronic disease and many of these conditions, such as myocardial infarctions, diabetes, arthritis and depression, may affect sexual function (McCracken, 1988). This chapter concentrates on the normal physiological changes associated with old age and sexual function.

For men, penile erection may take longer, and more direct stimulation is likely to be required. The penis may also be softer than previously in its erect state. Without an understanding of these normal changes, men may become so preoccupied with the slowness of response that impotence may occur. As Broderick (1978) points out, 'There is nothing more recalcitrant than a recalcitrant penis. If you are trying to get it to perform, it seems the harder you try, the more difficult it is.'

The ejaculatory phase is also affected by age. It is less powerful and there will be fewer penile contractions. Ejaculation may occur only every third episode, and a longer refractory period of 12–24 hours between ejaculations may occur. It is important for sexual partners to understand ageing male changes; otherwise, they may assume that they are no longer sexually attractive or competent in the sexual act. Longer penile stimulation either manually or orally will usually enhance lovemaking.

For women the orgasmic phase is shorter. The vagina becomes narrower and shorter, with a thickening of the vaginal mucosa. Vaginal secretions are scarcer and less acidic. The clitoris and uterus decrease in size but the capacity for multiple orgasms remains. Women may experience an increase in sexual desire after the menopause. This is widely attributed to women no longer facing the risk of pregnancy and, disturbingly, the view that there is no risk of contracting sexually transmitted diseases. (This latter point is considered further in the section on sexual health.) Physical changes will undoubtedly impact expressions of sexuality. Reduced sensory responses will render the older person in need of more direct and positive forms of sensory stimulus: more fragrance so it can be smelt, and the use of sensual fabrics such as silk and satin. Finding ways of preserving a positive self image in the face of increasing old age or the onset of a disability will clearly affect sexual identity. Older people face a double challenge – of throwing off the personal effects of ageing and of dealing with the attitudes of society.

Psychological ageing

A number of important psychological factors have been identified that seem to play an important role in determining the extent of sexual activity in advanced age. These include the individual's degree of sexual activity in earlier life, psychological resilience in adapting to altered physiological conditions influencing sexuality, demographic factors and society's attitudes.

Both depression and the treatment of depression with drug therapy may result in decreased libido. Alcohol greatly affects sexual performance, as do all narcotics, tranquillizers, sedatives and anxiolytic drugs. Nurses must be aware of the effects of depression and of medication. Discussion of these factors and possible solutions should be included in any assessment of need conducted. Gibson (1984) notes that studies in several countries show that the main constraints in sexual expression are social rather than biological, and some of these have already been discussed. Demographically there are more older women than men, both because women live longer and because of the two world wars. This demographic imbalance can create considerable problems for ageing women. They have fewer opportunities for heterosexual relations with unmarried men of their own age, and may therefore choose partners from their own sex or from among younger men. They may elect to live a life of celibacy or to seek out male prostitutes, or they may resign themselves to masturbation (Kassell, 1966). One suggested way of resolving women's lack of male sexual partners is polygamy (Kassell, 1966). This is refuted by Gee and Kimball (1987), who argue that it benefits men at the expense of women. It does assume that older women would automatically elect to have a male sexual partner and there is no evidence to suggest that this is necessarily the case. Woods (1978) reports that women who have always been single are more likely to resort to masturbation, whereas widows and divorcees will seek out alternatives.

Some older people face severe prejudice regarding their gay and lesbian preferences. They also face socially constructed ageist propaganda and sexual misinformation. The prejudice is often reinforced by families. It is recognised that children have difficulty viewing their parents as sexual beings. They may also fear the loss of a convenient childminder or household help if a sexual partner is found. The economic motive strengthens ageism, with older people being discouraged from spending family money or forming new loving relationships that may divide an expected inheritance. Central to ageism, then, is the question of sexuality. If older people are not capable of, or entitled to, a proper sex life, they cannot claim their full rights as adult citizens. The situation is even more serious for older people who have same-sex relationships.

Homosexuality

Homosexuality in older people has been little studied, particularly in men, yet the problems faced by older homosexuals are in some ways those of heterosexuals – to find suitable partners. Interestingly, gay men face the same stereotypes as heterosexual women, the burden of youth. It is suggested by Weg (1983) that life may be easier for older lesbians because the number of eligible partners is likely to be larger and because of a commitment to longer term relationships. In the USA it is estimated that approximately 10 per cent of older people are homosexual, but no accurate figures are available according to the work of Berger (1982) and Kehoe (cited by Ebersole and Hess, 1990). There appears to be a scarcity of data pertaining to the UK. Apparently, both gays and lesbians tend to use a self selection process to establish friendship, maintaining few associations with heterosexuals. Could this be related to the attitudes of society towards same-sex relationships and is it perhaps related to the current cohorts of older people? Anecdotal evidence seems to suggest that younger homosexuals have a wider mix of friendships.

According to Kehoe (cited by Ebersole and Hess, 1990), 'older lesbians are hampered by being women, elderly and deviant and tend to keep a low profile'. In an American study of 100 lesbians aged 60–80 years, it was found that most lived alone and were retired from the caring professions; many described themselves as lonely, but did not differentiate between emotional and social loneliness. They were currently celibate and desiring a relationship with a woman aged within ten years of their own age; they also wanted retirement communities for lesbians.

A literature search revealed little pertaining to gay older men, Berger (1982) being a notable exception. After decades of condemnation by society, perhaps older gay men are reticent openly to express sexual preference – it is a rich area for research, as is HIV and AIDS in older people.

In terms of ageing, the gay man has much in common with ageing women in that, according to Lee (1991), 'the homosexual man thinks of himself as middle aged and old before his heterosexual counterpart does'.

In the absence of kinship bonds, gays and lesbians develop homosexual friendship networks (Raphael and Robertson, 1980). It is suggested that homosexual elders adjust more easily to old age because they have already had to adjust to their sexuality. According to Friend (1991), many gay men and lesbian women have historically married heterosexually assuming this to be their only option for some degree of happiness. They may wait for their spouse to die before managing their sexuality in a different way, or they may be bisexual. Not only do older lesbians and gays potentially provide a significant role model for younger lesbians and gays, but they also offer valuable insights for all people regarding what it means to grow old in ways that promote independence, self determination and a sense of engaging in life. This is perhaps epitomised by Quentin Crisp, a prominent member of the gay movement. Over Christmas 1993 the traditional institution of Her Majesty's Christmas message was complemented by an alternative Christmas message delivered by Crisp from New York. It was good to see Channel 4 recognising individual lifestyles and preferences. Traditional institutions, such as the Queen's message on Christmas day, need to strike a balance between preserving the traditions and reflecting and encompassing the wants and needs of individuals. This will always present challenges, and in the case of care provision for older people the challenge is how to preserve all the best traditions of residential care while guarding against ritualistic practice that tends to serve the institution rather than the clients.

Transsexuality

It would seem that transsexuals aged over 65 comprise roughly the same percentage of the transsexual population as older people comprise of the general population. The fight for recognition does, however, become more difficult with age. Many transsexuals have held off from surgery until late in life in an attempt to avoid hurting family members. It would seem that about one third have no contact with siblings, parents and children. Transsexuals are not all sure whether they would be viewed as suitable carers should their partners become ill. At the end of life, families often reappear and prevent partners from grieving properly. Health care workers have many issues to resolve as they strive to meet the individual needs of patients. It is more common now to hear nurses discussing the sexual health needs of patients, particularly married couples. But where and how do you care for the woman who has need for prostate surgery? How do you meet the needs of the transsexual who requires residential care?

For ageing transsexuals it is likely that the issue of ageing assumes lesser priority than the issue of gender.

Blowing away the myths

In studying the literature on studies conducted to explore sexual habits, one thing becomes immediately apparent. Heterosexuals predominate, normally in the form of husbands and wives. Variations on the conventional couple relationship involving gay men and women are seldom dealt with. The literature highlights the emotional and social life of the heterosexual couple and their sexual relationship. The health status of both partners is a major determinant of satisfaction, and satisfactory sex is an important ingredient in later life satisfaction. Clearly patterns of reciprocal caring and sexuality are an area long overdue for research. Despite the bias of the studies they offer some interesting insights into our knowledge of older people and their sexual habits. The key findings of relevance to older people from these studies are set out below.

In 1968, Pfeiffer, Vorwoerdt and Wang published the Duke Longitudinal Studies. The first study commenced in 1955 and was followed in 1968 by a second study; both were completed in 1976. Overall, 254 people of both sexes were studied. The median age for stopping coitus was 68 years in men (range 49–90) and 60 years for women. The eight year difference was attributable to age differentials between spouses. Of the sample, 47 per cent stated that they had regular and frequent intercourse in the 60–71 years age range. After 78 years of age this finding was reduced to 15 per cent. During the five year observational period, 16 per cent of the sample reported a reduction in sexual activity and 14 per cent reported an increase. Substantial proportions of older married persons were found to have continued sexual activity until at least their 80s.

The now famous Masters and Johnson (1966) study used direct observation and physical measurement in a laboratory setting to investigate the anatomy and physiology of human sexual response patterns. A major finding was that there appeared to be no time limit drawn by advancing years to female sexuality. For men there was a slowing down in the reaction pattern, but this did not necessarily diminish satisfactory sexual activity.

The Starr Weiner report (Starr and Weiner, 1981) collected questionnaire data from 520 women and 280 men between the ages of 60 and 91 years and asked 50 open ended questions. They had all reached adulthood long before the 1960s and many were raised with strict Victorian standards. When asked for their views about older people having sexual relationships or cohabiting outside of marriage, 91 per cent of men and 89 per cent of women enthusiastically endorsed such arrangements. It would seem, therefore, that older people's views are similar to those of younger generations. Age was also considered to be irrelevant. Findings demonstrated that:

- 83 per cent approved of older women with younger lovers
- 86 per cent approved of older men with younger lovers
- 64 per cent of women and 74 per cent of men approved of older men and women who had no sexual partners of visiting prostitutes.
- 75 per cent of the respondents said that their sex life was as good as or better than when they were younger.

More recently the Janus report (Janus and Janus, 1993) marked the conclusion of a nine year study in which 800 Americans of all ages were interviewed. It confirmed many of the findings from earlier studies. In the over-65 group, 53 per cent of men and 41 per cent of women reported that they had a reasonably active sex life. All said that sex was at least as gratifying as in earlier years and often more gratifying because they had no fear of pregnancy or AIDS. This latter finding is extremely disturbing, as will be discussed in the section on sexual health. The study also reported that older people masturbate more often than teenagers, and those who had enjoyed sex in early life continued to do so. The report gave little space to homosexual practices, but it found that 22 per cent of men and 17 per cent of women had had at least one gay or lesbian experience. Given this finding, it is time that major studies start to focus on homosexuals as well as heterosexuals. It is refreshing to learn that sex is good for you and that older people still have it! In a study of 70-year-old women and men in Sweden, Persson (1980) found that men who continued to have sexual intercourse slept better, and had better mental activity and a more positive attitude towards sexual activity. Similarly, women who continued to have sexual intercourse retained their former levels of emotional stability, had lower levels of anxiety, had better mental health, felt generally more healthy and had a positive attitude towards sexual activity in old age. Butler and Lewis (1976) found that sexual activity helps arthritis by stimulating the production of cortisone, reducing physical and psychological tension and promoting good physical condition.

Contrary to popular belief, both older men and women can and older clearly do continue to enjoy sexual activity. Some older people believe that sexual activity actually delays the ageing process. There is no evidence to suggest that older people use different techniques to resolve any difficulties. If there is a shortage of vaginal lubrication or difficulty in obtaining an erection, older people can and do use manual and oral methods of stimulation.

Given that all the research studies and anecdotal evidence inform us that older people are interested in sex and many have active sex lives, it does seem feasible to consider this age group's sexual health needs.

Sexual health education

In work by Rogstad and Bignell (1991), the risk of prevalence of HIV (human immunodeficiency virus) and sexually transmitted disease in older adults attending two departments of genitourinary medicine was studied. Historical review of case notes for 1988 and 1989 showed that 69 per cent of men and 53 per cent of women in the sample were sexually active, with casual partners cited by 68 patients and the number of contacts being between 1 and 30. The use of prostitutes overseas was cited by five patients and current or past gay relationships by 16, six men were participating in casual anoreceptive sexual intercourse without condoms, 15 men were sexually participating in both their marital relationship and relationships with other partners concurrently, and two women attended the clinic after rape. Sexually transmitted diseases were diagnosed in 47 men and 11 women. Anxiety regarding HIV infection was the primary reason for attendance in 22 men and six women, although none tested positive.

Although this study was a small one, it serves to illustrate the diversity of older people's sexual health needs. Clearly, if prostitutes and rent boys are likely to be used by some older people, the principles of engaging in safe sex will need to be discussed. Women should be advised to use femidoms – particularly when their male partner is unwilling to use a condom. Men should use condoms with female and male partners. In lesbian sexual acts it is recommended that vibrators and dildos are not shared. However, as an alternative, condoms could be used over the appliance. The study infers that older people who are sexually active should receive the same sexual health services as any other age group. In addition, services will need to be age specific in terms of advice and information on the normal ageing process and on adapting to any chronic illness or disability.

At the time of writing within the UK there are over 2000 people aged 50 years and over who are HIV positive. Although this represents only 7 per cent of the total number infected, each new set of statistics shows an increase in this age group. There is, however, as the research studies reported indicate, a general view held by older people that they are not at risk. This lack of awareness exists among health professionals as well, which is perhaps not surprising given that so many find it difficult to accept that older people are sexual beings who may be sexually active. Recent statistics published by Age Concern (Kaufmann, 1993) claim that 11 per cent of people living with AIDS are over 50 years of age (p. 33). At the end of June 1993, 2 per cent of people living with AIDS were over 60 years of age, as were 2 per cent of those diagnosed as HIV positive (Public Health Laboratory Service, 1993, table 20). In the USA the number of reported cases of AIDS in the over-60 age group has continued to rise with the increasing total number of cases.

There is also some evidence to suggest that these statistics may be higher than reported in older age groups. Wide ranging lack of awareness among health professionals about sexual activity among older people will lead to the general view that HIV is not an issue of concern for the older members of society. For example, the HIV virus may affect the nervous system and present as HIV encephalopathy (dementia). Initial features are subtle: changes in attention span, concentration and personality. AIDS dementia can readily be misdiagnosed as Alzheimer's disease or Parkinson's disease. The lack of sexual health education material aimed at older people may have caused a low awareness of the issues of risk behaviour and the possibility of contracting HIV. The risk of HIV infection and HIV related disease has been statistically most prominent in homosexual groups. Older people often feel uncomfortable about discussing or disclosing their sexual behaviour (Hargreaves, Fuller and Gazzard, 1988) and may live in fear of family reactions.

Gibson (1992) cites three reasons why sexual health education is especially needed by people in later years:

- People in the oldest cohorts lived through a time when it was usual to give young people a great deal of misinformation about sexual matters.

- Older people have been, and still are, likely to be the subject of ageist propaganda which misrepresents the nature of sexuality in late life.
- Older people are entering periods of changing sexual experiences.

The Rogstad and Bignell (1991) study, although it was limited in size, clearly demonstrates sexual activity and sexual health needs in older people. Additionally Kaufmann (1993) refers to the presence of HIV and AIDS in older people. By February 1993 nearly 1000 people aged 50 years and over were known to be infected with HIV, and over 700 of them had AIDS. This represents around 11 per cent of the total population of people with AIDS. However, these figures may under-represent the true scale of the problem, particularly because of frequent misdiagnosis. Clearly there is a need for sexual health services for older people, but there is increasing concern among some professionals that the 'glamour' of HIV and AIDS will overshadow the very real crisis of dementia. The challenge will be to ensure that care workers recognise that older people may be sexually active and as such have the same sexual health needs as everyone else, but we must guard against all our energies being diverted to the subject of diseases that routinely feature in the press and scientific journals.

Living in a home

Lone elders are especially likely to enter residential care, and one aspect of the social control exercised over residents is the prohibition, formal and informal, usually placed on sexual behaviour. The sexual imbalance among older people in institutions is clearly a limiting factor but, where partners are found, staff disapproval creates obstacles. Thus, we may find the sexes segregated into separate sitting rooms. Staff may enter bedrooms freely, without knocking or being told to enter. Additionally, very few older people are able to lock their rooms. Imagine trying to meet your sexual needs when at any minute a member of staff may burst into your room. Staff have also been seen to use humour as a way of overcoming their embarrassment at attempts by older people to express sexual identity. There may therefore be inappropriate attention drawn to demonstrations of affection between residents, and laughter and joking may ensue. Although practice is slowly changing, care staff need to be better informed about sexuality in later life. Gibson's study in 1984, supplemented by numerous smaller local studies, found that only a tiny minority of older people in residential care had the opportunity to express their sexual feelings. There is no indication that this finding has changed significantly in the last ten years. It should not be assumed that all older people wish to have an active sex life, but the combination of the numerical imbalance and social attitudes deprives many a lone woman of choice. Future cohorts are likely to have higher expectations. Older adults, like younger adults, need the kind of lifestyle that facilitates privacy as well as 'social permission' to engage in sexual relationships. Sexuality is still ignored in residential care establishments: sexes are separated, married couples may even be forced to live separately There is often little opportunity for privacy, with closed doors not respected by staff and no locks on doors and cupboards.

Lowenthal's (1965) work has clearly demonstrated the value of a confidant and the association with good morale and mental health. For many people one's closest confidant is the person with whom one is having or has had some sexual relationship. Having a partner with whom one is intimate physically is likely to facilitate positive mental health. Despite this, it would appear that even now there are still formidable obstacles preventing older people from developing intimate relations in care settings. Nurses need to become more informed in all aspects of ageing, including the sexual needs of older people – who need to be free from social and psychological pressures that can inhibit a fulfilling sex life. Sadly, although many nurses enjoy relationships with a wide variety of friends, all of whom have individual preferences sexually, they seem to find it extraordinarily hard to accept these preferences in older people. It is, of course, possible that this is linked to nurses' knowledge and acceptance of sexually active older people in general, but it is (at the very least) unprofessional to bring personal prejudices into professional practice. Even when formal education gives only cursory consideration to the subject of older people and sexual needs, nurses are beholden to ensure that they increase their personal knowledge and understanding – especially given the wide availability of literature on the subject.

The role of the nurse

Nurses cannot intervene to provide sexual partners for older people, but there is much that they can do to ensure that older people are seen as sexual beings who have sexual needs. Nurses are in a unique position to educate older people in respect to sexual relations in general and the effects of ageing and chronic disease on sexual activity and to dispel the myths that surround sexual practice or the lack thereof among older persons.

Nurses can do this work in all settings, but in individual cases should always commence with a sexual assessment. McCracken (1988) refers to the work of Glasgow, who developed a sexual-history taking format. It is recommended that sexual questions should be asked as part of the total history taking process. She further specifies that the questions should not be preceded by an apology or any suggestion that the questions are embarrassing. Sexual problems among older people may arise from lack of education in sexual techniques, lack of adjustment of technique alongside the ageing process and/or as side effects of disease or disease treatment. I have already made reference to the increased susceptibility to chronic disease in old age. This will inevitably have an effect on sexual performance. In her chapter 'Sexuality and the elderly', Laflin suggests alternative sexual positions which may be useful for some. For example, it may be easier to have intercourse lying side by side or using pillows to provide support. If the couple are used to one person doing most of the active movement, this may have to be reconsidered. For example, if the male partner of a heterosexual couple has paralysis caused by a cerebrovascular accident, intercourse may be easier if the woman moves on top in the missionary position. Nurses have multiple roles in the area of sexuality and the aged. They may be employed as trained counsellors on all matters pertaining to sexual health, or they may advise older people who attend special clinics. The vast majority of nurses, however, will not have received any special training and will come across older people who are in need of help and advice in almost all settings where nurses practise. The nurse is a facilitator of an atmosphere conducive to discussions regarding sexual matters. Most important is the provision of privacy and allowing the older person to take control over their sex lives. Clearly, for this to be achieved, the nurse must act as a resource and as an educator. This implies that the nurse must not only be knowledgeable about sexuality and sexual health for older people but also be comfortable with personal sexuality in order to feel confident and relaxed when older people wish to discuss their sexual needs.

Older people are unlikely to initiate such conversations for reasons covered earlier in this chapter. Therefore the nurse will need to develop a method of assessment that reflects the potentially sensitive nature of such discussions. The following suggested questions may be of assistance in helping the nurse to develop an appropriate assessment tool. The questions should be included within the general assessment and should be approached in much the same manner.

1. Are you currently sexually active?
2. With one specific partner or more?
3. Is/are your partner/s male or female?
4. Do you have any illness that affects your sexual function?
5. Has age affected your sexual function?
6. How do you feel about sex?
7. Are there any factors that prevent you from being sexually active?
8. Do you have any difficulties in meeting your sexual needs?
9. Do you experience difficulty with vaginal penetration?
10. Do you have any difficulties achieving or maintaining an erection?
11. Do you have any difficulties in ejaculating or having an orgasm when you want to?
12. How long has this been a problem?

13. Do you feel able to discuss this with your partner?
14. How do you feel about getting some help with this problem?

The nurse must also approach this private and often sensitive area with great sensitivity and tact. It would be unacceptable to conduct a sexual health history in great detail if there was no cause to do so. Clearly, the older person may simply choose not to answer the questions and this should be respected. If the nurse remains concerned, it is possible to give the patient some advice as to who to contact if there ever should be a problem.

Anticipation of difficulties in older people's sexual experiences can ward off anxiety, misconceptions and an arbitrary cessation of sexual pleasure. Validation of the normality of sexual desire and activity in old age may be required. Discussions of the normal physiological changes associated with ageing and how these may affect sexual performance will do much to relieve concern that a dry vagina or softer erection means that sexual intercourse cannot take place. Nurses need to be able to advise their clients on how to maintain sexual interest and activity despite the presence of any chronic illness and disability. Such advice may be relatively simple; for example, the use of alternative positions, taking analgesics and having a warm bath before sexual intercourse, or using pillows to provide support for the body. Vaginal or anal lubricants, vibrators and Cock rings (which will assist in the maintenance of an erection) are frequently in everyday use by younger members of society, so why is it that they are frequently not recommended to older people?

The primary need for older people is for information (Webb, 1992). Myths and stereotypes need to be confronted and replaced with accurate information provided by health professionals who have the relevant knowledge and skills. These professionals must also demonstrate comfort with their own sexuality and the sexuality of their client group. Nurses, wherever they work, have the potential to influence, and should be working to ensure that older people's needs are met. Such needs may range from the provision of sex education (including the maintenance of sexual health) to the provision of aids to assist in sexual activity and of privacy (thus facilitating sexual expression) and to recognising that older people are sexual beings and as such need to express their sexuality. Thus the older man who persists in masturbating in the day room could be redirected to masturbate in a more private place. To suggest that such behaviour is dirty and unacceptable even in private is to deny the sexual needs of older people.

To be effective, nurses must also be aware of their own attitudes towards ageing and sexual health. These attitudes are likely to have been greatly influenced by society's views, and the older person will be affected by them too. It is not enough to have a heading on a care plan under which the nurse writes 'likes to wear make-up' or 'needs a shave every day'. Sadly, this happens all too often – particularly when a nurse is unable to recognise that older people are sexual beings just like the rest of us.

Conclusion

This chapter has considered aspects of sexuality and the implications for health education. It is not meant to imply that all older people are sexually active or that sexuality relates explicitly to sexual behaviour. As the definition of sexuality implies, all that we are as men and women is expressed through our sexuality. Thus, our clothing, hair style, use of fragrances and make-up and so on, all go to make up the very essence of our being.

Some nurses have extensive education in sexuality and are in a position to provide intensive therapy for people with sexual problems. The majority of nurses will not have the knowledge or skills to act as sex therapists. However, every nurse working with older people has a duty to personally educate themselves, thus ensuring that they have a good working knowledge of the sexual health needs of their clients and can assist in the maintenance of sexuality. This chapter is a starting point. The references and further reading recommendations will assist the nurse to gain the required knowledge and skills. This chapter should be viewed as an introduction to the subject: it does not claim to be a conclusive text on all matters to do with old age, sexuality and sexual health.

References

Beauvoir S de (1973) *The Coming of Age*. Warner, New York.

Berger R (1982) *Gay and Gray: the Older Homosexual Man*. University of Illinois Press, Urbana, Illinois.

Broderick C (1978) Sexuality and ageing: an overview. In Solnick R (ed.) *Sexuality and Ageing*. Ethel Perry Andrus Gerontology Center, University of Southern California Press.

Butler R and Lewis M (1976) *Sex After Sixty*. Harper and Row, New York.

Colton H (1983) *The Gift of Touch*. Sea View/Putnam, New York.

Comfort A (1976) *A Good Age*. Crown, New York.

Ebersole P and Hess P (1990) *Towards Healthy Ageing: Human Needs and Nursing Response*, p. 443. CV Mosby, St Louis.

Friend R (1991) Older lesbian and gay people: a theory of successful ageing. In Lee J (ed.) *Gay, Midlife and Maturity*, pp. 99–117. Haworth Press, New York.

Gee E and Kimball M (1987) The double standard of ageing: images and sexuality. In Gee E and Kimball M (eds) *Women and Ageing*. Butterworths, Toronto.

Gibson M (1984) Sexuality in later life. *Ageing International* 11, 8–13.

Gibson H (1992) *The Emotional and Sexual Lives of Older People: A Manual for Professionals*. Chapman and Hall, London.

Hargreaves M, Fuller G and Gazzard B (1988) Occult AIDS: *Pneumocystis carinii* pneumonia in elderly people. *British Medical Journal* 297, 721–2.

Janus S and Janus C (1993) *The Janus Report on Sexual Behaviour*. Wiley, Chichester.

Kassell VC (1966) Polygamy after 60. *Geriatrics* 21, 214–18.

Kaufmann T (1993) *A Crisis of Silence: HIV, AIDS and Older People*. Age Concern, London.

Kuhn M (1976) Sexual myths surrounding the ageing. In Oaks W *et al.* (eds) *Sex and the Life Cycle*. Grune and Stratton, New York.

Lee J (1991) *Gay, Midlife and Maturity*, pp. 66 and 99. Haworth Press, New York.

Lowenthal M (1965) Interaction and adaption: intimacy as a crucial variable. *American Sociological Review* 33, 20–30.

Masters W and Johnson V (1966) *Human Sexual Response*. Little, Brown, Boston.

McCracken A (1988) Sexual practice by elders: the forgotten aspect of functional health. *Gerontological Nursing* 14, 13–17.

Persson G (1980) Sexuality in a 70 year old urban population. *Journal of Psychosomatic Research* 24, 335–42.

Pfeiffer E, Verwoerdt A and Wang H (1968) Duke longitudinal studies: aged men and women. *Archives of General Psychiatry* 19, 753–8.

Phillipson C and Walker A (1986) *Ageing and Social Policy: A Critical Assessment*. Gower, Aldershot.

Public Health Laboratory Service (1993) *AIDS/HIV Quarterly Surveillance Tables No. 20*. Communicable Disease Surveillance Centre, June 1993.

Raphael S and Robertson M (1980) Lesbians and gay men in later life. *Generations* 6, 16.

Redfern SJ (ed.) (1992) *Nursing Elderly People*, 2nd, p. 264. Churchill Livingstone, Edinburgh.

Rogstad K and Bignell C (1991) Age is no bar to sexually acquired infection. *Age and Ageing* 20, 377–8.

Sontag R (1978) The double standard of ageing. In Carver V and Liddiard P (eds) *An Ageing Population*, pp. 72–80. Hodder and Stoughton, London.

Starr B and Weiner M (1981) *The Starr Weiner Report on Sex and Sexuality in the Mature Years*. McGrath, New York.

Victor C (1987) *Old Age in Modern Society*, p. 96. Chapman & Hall, London.

Webb C (1992) Expressing sexuality. In Redfern S (ed.) *Nursing Elderly People*. Churchill Livingstone, Edinburgh.

Weg R (ed.) (1983) *Sexuality in the Later Years: Roles and Behaviour*. Academic Press, New York.

Woods N (1978) Human sexuality and the healthy elderly. In Brown M (ed.) *Readings in Gerontology*. CV Mosby, St Louis.

Further reading

Damrosh S (1984) Graduate nursing students' attitudes towards sexually active older persons. *Gerontologist* 24, 299–302.

Gibson H 1992 *The Emotional and Sexual Lives of Older People: A Manual for Professionals*. Chapman & Hall, London.

Kaas M (1978) Sexual expression of the elderly in nursing homes. *Gerontologist* 16, 39–44.

Laflin M (1985) Sexuality and the elderly. In Lewis C (ed.) *Ageing: The Health Care Challenge*. FA Davies, Philadelphia.

Power Smith O (1992) Encounters with older lesbians in psychiatric practice. *Sex and Marital Therapy* 7, 79–86.

8

Living alone: living with others

Hazel Heath

Generally when people relocate, whether it be from house to house or town to town, there is a sense of future. For elderly people, moving to a nursing home meant the end of the line. They could no longer think in terms of a future. It was as if they were crossing an invisible line: on the one hand they were people who had lives, possessions, identities and futures, and on the other they had none of these and would just live day by day. When people feel that they have lost everything that they have spent their life building, and they know that they have neither the time nor the capacity to 'start again', how can they perceive a future?

(Nay 1995)

The concept of home is central to the lives of most people, wherever and however they live. For older people, the home environment is seen as playing an important contributory role in general wellbeing, and in physical and mental health (Bond, Coleman and Peace, 1993). The notion that older people should be able to live in their own homes as far as possible has been fundamental to health and welfare policies for many years and, when it is no longer 'feasible' or 'sensible' for people to remain in their own homes, a 'homely' or 'home-like' setting is recommended (Department of Health, 1989). But what does the concept of home actually mean to individuals, and what is the nature of the relationship between an individual and his or her home? If older people make the transition from living in their own homes to living in a communal home, how can this process be managed so that it is a positive, rather than a potentially devastating, experience? Finally, in communal homes, what are the key features of a 'home-like' environment, and how can nurses and care staff maximise the quality of life of the older people who live in them?

This chapter will explore the current living circumstances of the UK's older population. It will review the role of social networks in the community and the range of housing options to support older people to remain in their own homes. The concept of 'home' will be analysed and linked to research on relocation and its meaning for older people. Conclusions will be drawn on the role of nurses and care staff in helping older people to make choices and transitions between living in their own homes and living with others.

Where and how older people live

In the UK today, over 95 per cent of people over 60 years of age live in private households (OPCS, 1993). Approximately half of people aged 65 and over own their own homes, and over 90 per cent of these have no mortgage (Institute of Actuaries, 1993). It is estimated that the numbers of older owner-occupiers will increase from the 1985 figure of 2.8 million, to 3.7 million households by 2001 (Leather and Wheeler, 1988). About 6 per cent of the population live in privately rented accommodation. Older people, particularly those aged 70 or over, older women, and those who live alone, are more likely to rent accommodation privately (Smythe and Browne, 1992). Older people living alone are also more likely to live in purpose-built flats or maisonettes.

Older people more commonly live in older housing than younger householders, and particularly if the accommodation is rented (Department of the Environment, 1988). In many areas, the over-representation of people from minority ethnic groups in the poorer socioeconomic classes means that they share with other poorer people the experience of inadequate housing and unhealthy environmental conditions (Fenton, 1991). The homes of older people, and particularly those aged 75 and over, are more commonly in poor condition or even unfit for habitation, lacking in amenities, and with substandard heating. In successive General Household Surveys, only about half of elderly households had central heating (OPCS, 1982, 1988), and Hunt's (1978) survey found that approximately 8 per cent of older people were not warm in bed or in their living room and 12 per cent were not warm in their kitchens. This raises concerns about the effects of poor housing on the health of older people (Byrne *et al.*, 1986). Inadequate housing has been cited as a contributory factor in the admission of older people into residential care (Phillips, 1992).

For many older people, their home is their only asset, but they may be unable or unwilling to undertake maintenance. Various equity release schemes are currently available which help older people to remain in their own homes and to keep the home in good repair. These include remortgages, home reversion schemes (which involve the sale and lease back of the property) and home insurance plans (where a loan against the property is used to purchase an annuity). However, it is suggested that current generations of older people are reluctant to reduce their assets in this way as they wish to pass on their wealth to their families (Institute of Actuaries, 1993). Various schemes are being developed to help older people to remain in their homes. These 'staying-put' options have been reviewed by Tinker (1984).

As people age, they are more likely to move into supportive housing and, particularly during the 1960s and 1970s, the building of warden-controlled sheltered housing was encouraged as a means of assisting older people to remain living in their own homes. Many older people see this as an attractive option (Butler and Tinker, 1983), but the segregation of older people from the remainder of the population, and the creation of what have been called 'geriatric ghettos' is seen by some social commentators as undesirable.

Independent sector organisations, and particularly housing associations, provide a variety of managed housing options for older people. In 1991 there were 7000 housing associations managing over 150 000 sheltered housing units (Fletcher, 1991). Charities, such as the Abbeyfield Society, provide a range of options from supportive housing to extra or extended care.

Family and social networks

More older people now live alone. In 1962, 22 per cent of older people lived alone, 33 per cent with spouse only, and 60 per cent with others. In 1989, 36 per cent lived alone, 46 per cent with spouse, and 18 per cent with others (Dale, Evandrou and Arber, 1987). It is now estimated that 41 per cent of older people, some 3.4 million, live alone (Help the Aged, 1995). There are many reasons for this change, including a reduction in the average number of children and greater geographical mobility. Very few older people move into the households of younger generations, with 95 per cent remaining in their own households (Dale, Evandrou and Arber, 1987).

Studies have identified various types of support network for older people (Wenger, 1995). The two most common types are those described as *family dependent* (which rely primarily on local kin) or *locally integrated* (in which the support derives from family, friends and neighbours). Approximately 50 per cent of older people in the general population have one of these two types of network. It is suggested that these two types of network make it easier for older people to remain in the community if they become frail or dependent. In family dependent networks, problems arise when carer stress leads to inadequate levels of care. Residential care may be resisted, but professional respite in the home may be needed, especially where the older person has dementia. Problems arise in locally integrated networks where an older person lives alone, or where carers break down or become ill. In this group, support from neighbours is common, but this can become stressful. Despite social contacts, older people in this group can feel lonely owing to lack of emotional contact. Maintaining their personal autonomy is also very important to older people living alone.

Only a minority of older people have what are described as *private restricted* networks, but it is this type that is most common in community care case loads. In private restricted networks there is no local kin and minimal contact with the local community. Mental illness and 'difficult' personalities are common among people with this type of network, and carers are often isolated and under increased stress. Individuals in this group may adapt poorly to residential care.

On the basis of this work, it is suggested that community care workers have been able to recognise older people with different types of network and thus have been able to predict more accurately what interventions would be most appropriate (Wenger, 1996). Other studies have sought to investigate relationships between the types of social support available to specific groups of older people, such as those who are visually impaired (Barron *et al.*, 1994) or those with mental health needs (Simmons, 1994).

The charity Help the Aged commissioned a survey of over a thousand adults aged over 65 in over a hundred parliamentary constituencies. The survey found that, although older people chose to live independent lifestyles, thousands had little or no social contact, and many did not receive the help and support they needed to live fulfilling lives. The survey found that:

- 88 per cent wanted to stay in their home, and 35 per cent said that under no circumstances would they move into residential care
- Almost two thirds (2.1 million) received no outside help at home
- 8 per cent (288 000) had been left alone needing help for more than six hours at least once in the last year
- 6 per cent (200 000) had no present on their last birthday
- In the week preceding the survey, on average they spoke with only 4.4 neighbours; 9 per cent (over 300 000) did not speak with any neighbours and 2 per cent (almost 70 000) spoke with no-one at all.

(The figures in brackets represent the number of people who would have been affected if the findings were generalised to the population of 3.4 million people aged 65 and over who live alone.)

The Help the Aged survey was commissioned to mark the fifth anniversary of the death of pensioner John Sheppard, whose body was not discovered until three and a half years after his death in this north London flat, when workmen, trying to trace a water leak, broke in (Help the Aged, 1995).

There are, of course, positive aspects to living alone, and people who live alone do not always perceive themselves to be lonely. Indeed, some individuals who are married and living with a spouse have described themselves as feeling lonely (Barron *et al.*, 1994). However, studies have identified that loneliness may be more than unpleasant – it may be linked to various health problems (Berg *et al.*, 1981; Schultz and Moore, 1984; Holmen *et al.*, 1992). Living alone is also the largest demographic risk factor, after age itself, for admission to hospital or entry into long term care (Laing and Hall, 1991).

The meaning of 'home'

The concept of 'home' is complex in that it encompasses many characteristics of the wider community, the immediate surroundings, the physical environment, the social milieu and the subjective feelings of individuals towards the home. The meaning of home to an individual may also change with age. Concepts of what constitutes a home are influenced by culture and subculture, class and generation.

Home in a community

The concept of home usually links with living within one's community, where people speak with specific languages or accents and behave in traditional ways. Individual perceptions of home will link with a person's experience of communities in which they have lived throughout their lives. Following retirement, most older people continue to live in the community in which they have lived during their working lives, and only about 10 per cent move to another area (Law and Warnes, 1982).

Home allows maintenance of contact with the community, but also the exclusion of strangers or unwanted/uninvited individuals from the home itself. It thus allows some control in maintaining our immediate environment, allowing in those we wish to include and excluding those we do not.

The home environment

The 'homely' environment is comfortable, domestic and suited to various functions. It usually contains various spaces for the different activities of living, one for cooking and eating, one for washing and using the lavatory, one for sleeping.

The environment is seen as facilitating chosen lifestyles and roles, as well as day-to-day domesticity, intimacy, privacy or solitude.

Those who live in the home

A home usually contains a small number of people, usually a family or those who have chosen to live in the same home, or have always done so. The concept of home is often linked to the idea of family (Willcocks, Peace and Kellaher, 1987; Peace 1988, 1993).

The subjective meaning of home

The interrelationship between individual people and the spaces that individuals occupy is complex. Willcocks, Peace and Kellaher (1987) describe the subjective meaning ascribed by individuals to home. Home is a place with which individuals identify, and to which they usually have a positive attitude. It links with the concept of territory. Individuals usually describe feelings of security, and personal control in the living environment.

For older people, home can be particularly significant. It can represent connection with one's life, one's roots and sense of history, either through the memories of what happened in the home or by personal possessions and mementoes. It can also signify one's place and identity within a community.

Home can also be particularly significant to older people when their capacities begin to decline. People with failing sight will be able to move around the home because of their familiarity with the environment. Adaptation of the environment over time can also help to facilitate their activities, for example using the furniture for support when moving around. To be able to retain control over one's activities in the home assists older people to retain control over their lives and to remain independent. Older people can also mask failing capabilities because of the support given to them in, and by, the home. Familiarity of the home environment, and continuity with this, are particularly important for people with mental health needs such as dementia.

Thus, home is a base from which identity, personal power and control can be generated, maintained and reinforced (Willcocks, Peace and Kellaher, 1987). Even if other people are brought into the home to help, the older person can still maintain cognitive control of the environment.

Sixsmith's (1990) study identified three themes which underlie the meaning that older people generally associate with home:

- *The home as the major focus of life.* Sixsmith found that, as people age, they become more orientated towards home. Home is seen as a refuge and, as other social roles in later life are relinquished, becomes increasingly important.

- *The need of older people to remain independent of others.* They appear more concerned with the instrumental aspects of home.
- *The attachment that older people have for their homes.* The importance of memories is significant, with past associations affecting the present experience of home.

Independence was a strong theme of Sixsmith's work. To the older people interviewed, independence meant:

- Being able to look after oneself, without being dependent on other people
- The capacity for self direction – the freedom to choose what they do
- Not having feelings of obligation.

To the older people in Sixsmith's study, the home was a symbol of independence, and was also instrumentally significant in facilitating independence. The interviewees described being 'contented at home', 'doing things for yourself', 'not beholden to anybody', 'not dependent on anybody', 'nobody tells you what to do', 'you can do what you want'. They also described a sense of 'stability and protection'. Sixsmith's work suggests that an older person's home is an integral aspect of his or her independence, and that independence in later life cannot be fully understood without reference to the home. Several of the participants in Sixsmith's study were seriously disabled and he suggested that, for these people to do something for themselves, however small, represented independence to them and also supported their belief in their own physical capabilities and, ultimately, their self esteem.

Supported living and long term care options

Families and informal carers provide the majority of care to older people in their own homes (Warner, 1994; Parker, 1990) and receive a variety of services to support them. Day hospitals and day care facilities play a key role in maintaining older people at home and providing support for carers. Schemes are currently being developed to enhance the homeliness of day hospitals (Bacon and Lambkin, 1994).

Despite the emphasis on care in, and by, the community, it has been suggested that some form of residential provision will always be needed (Henwood, 1992; Department of Health, 1989). Between 4 per cent and 5 per cent of people of pensionable age are living either temporarily or permanently in an institution. In the 1991 Census, 9.7 per cent of people aged 75 and over, and 23.7 per cent of people aged 85 and over were resident in an institution (OPCS, 1993). Supported living and long term care are provided in a variety of homes run by the state, private enterprise or charities.

The NHS provision is gradually decreasing. In 1970 there were something like 75 000 places for physically and mentally frail older people provided by the NHS. By 1992 this had reduced to 65 000 (Laing, 1993). One report suggested that from 1988 to 1993, NHS provided long stay places reduced by 40 per cent (Rickford, 1993).

In 1992, local authorities provided approximately 104 000 residential places, compared with a peak level of 137 000 places in the mid-1980s (Laing, 1993). Local authority provision is gradually reducing, with homes either closing or being sold to the private sector.

The private sector has grown rapidly, with places increasing from 85 000 residential and 38 000 nursing in 1985, to 162 000 and 153 000 respectively, in 1992 (Laing, 1993). Within this sector there is a broad range of provision, with the suggestion that, for the future, the large corporate providers may predominate.

The charity, non-profit, providers are the smallest sector. In 1987 they provided 8000 nursing home places, and they now provide nearly 14 000. Residential care places have remained constant at about 47 000 (Laing, 1993).

What older people want from residential care

Many studies have taken cross-sectional data from samples of older people before and after admission to residential homes.

Counsel and Care (1992) interviewed people attending day centres about what they would expect of a residential home. They also interviewed a group of residents currently in private and voluntary homes. The sample did not include any people from minority ethnic groups. Although both groups said that human contact was essential, whether from staff or from wider social contacts, other results showed that the views of older people before going into a residential home were very different once they were living in the home. It may be possible that the individuals were fearful of what life would be like, or of the reputation of residential homes.

People outside homes were unequivocal in what they wanted from a residential home:

- They wanted to go out when they chose, not to be pushed about, to have no restrictions. One said 'Freedom to be yourself; you wouldn't want to be regimented'.
- They recognised the need for company within a home, and visits from family and friends.
- The quality of care given by the staff was important. People wished to be treated with kindness and respect.
- The importance of private space was recognised, particularly a room of their own.

From respondents within homes there was a change of emphasis. For example:

- 95 per cent said they would want a single room. In reality, about 74 per cent had single rooms but, for those who had to share, there were particular problems, such as the woman who gave a distressing account of a series of room sharers who had died.
- 83 per cent said they would want to lock the door of their room; 40 per cent had bedrooms with lockable doors.
- 90 per cent said they would prefer an ensuite toilet, and 27 per cent had these.
- 73 per cent of those questioned in day centres wanted to take their own bed and wardrobe with them into a home; 42 per cent of residents had been able to take their own large items of furniture into the rooms.
- 62 per cent said they would like to have more than one sitting room, as this would give them choice as to where they could spend their days. Just over half of those in a home had more than one sitting room. One resident said 'I sit in my room all day because I don't like the TV blaring with children's programmes'. Counsel and Care suggested that the absence of an alternative communal area could thus lead to greater isolation.
- 90 per cent of people in day centres said they would want a home to have transport to enable them to go out on trips and visits, but only 23 per cent of residents lived in homes that had this.
- 95 per cent of people in day centres said they would like to be able to go on outings if they were in a home, but only 54 per cent of those in homes had the facility to go on outings. One home offered residents regular opportunities to revisit the areas in which they had lived before they came into care, and this was felt to be very worthwhile.
- 80 per cent of people in day centres said they would positively welcome social activities in the home; 52 per cent lived in homes that provided leisure activities.
- 90 per cent of people in day care centres said they would want to be in charge of their own money, whereas only 38 per cent of the resident group looked after their own financial affairs.
- 67 per cent said they would like a choice at mealtimes, but only 35 per cent of residents had a choice.
- 73 per cent wanted menus in advance, but only 36 per cent received this.
- 81 per cent wanted to choose what time they got up in the morning, but 48 per cent of the residents in homes had to get up when they were told.
- On relationships with staff, 72 per cent wanted staff to treat them as a friend; 61 per cent felt that they actually did. Only 1 per cent of

respondents wanted to be treated as a patient, but 12 per cent felt that this was their experience.

The Counsel and Care survey concluded that the expectations of older people living in homes are severely depressed by the reality of day-to-day provision.

A National Carers' Survey asked people at home what they would choose if they needed 24 hour care. Only 13 per cent chose a residential home. They also asked open-ended questions of older people living in residential homes. What the people in the sample said they liked was the help and care given by staff, the surroundings, the meals, the independence and the security. Overall, what people said they disliked included the poor social environment, loss of independence, inadequate buildings, lack of privacy, poor meals and loneliness. However, some said that there was nothing they disliked.

Allen, Hogg and Peace (1992) explored what older people and their carers felt about residential care, and found that the idea was not as abhorrent to older people living in the community as might have been imagined. 33 per cent said they would consider it, 55 per cent said they would not, and 12 per cent were not sure. Women were more likely to consider residential care than men, of whom just over one fifth said they would. The carers presented a very similar picture, with about one third of the carers saying that the elderly people they were looking after would consider residential care. However, the majority of elderly people who said they would consider residential care added the proviso that they would have to be ill or unable to look after themselves before they did. In the view of most of them they would have to be in very poor shape before they needed residential care. The people who said they would not consider it did so because they wanted to stay in their own homes or wanted to remain independent. There was a very strong undercurrent of what might happen to them in residential care among many of the elderly people interviewed.

Reasons for moving into a care home

Willcocks, Peace and Kellaher (1987) found that the main reason given by residents for admission was a reduced ability to manage in their own homes. Factors contributing to this included a period of poor health, an accident or gradually failing capabilities to perform daily living activities.

Admission is sometimes prompted by families or carers deciding that they can no longer cope. Willcocks, Peace and Kellaher (1987) found that approximately one in five admissions were linked with problems of carers. Breakdown or inability to cope accounted for 20 per cent of male admissions and 15 per cent of female admissions.

Allen, Hogg and Peace (1992) found that older people were sometimes unable to relate why they had moved into residential care, either because they were too upset to discuss their admission or because they could not remember. When carers and heads of homes were asked, the responses given by all types of respondent were similar. There appeared to be five main reasons:

- Following a fall or fracture
- Following an acute illness
- Because of a general deterioration in their health and in their ability to look after themselves
- As a result of increasing pressure on their carer
- Because of loneliness.

In Allen, Hogg and Peace's study, only half the residents said that they had talked to someone about moving into residential care before the final decision was made. More than a third had talked to their main informal carer about going into residential care, around one fifth had talked to a relative, and some had talked to friends or neighbours. There did not appear to be much discussion with professionals. Only a small proportion said that they had had more detailed discussions, such as which home they should move into, what parting with their own home might mean, what residential care would be like, and the financial implications.

The process of relocation

The effects of relocation on older people have been studied extensively. Early work suggested that relocation in itself was detrimental to health, and could increase morbidity and hasten death. Subsequent reviews suggested that relocation in itself was not hazardous, provided that the individual enjoyed an adequate support system (Coffman, 1981).

Willcocks, Peace and Kellaher (1987) discuss the process of becoming a resident, and the gains and losses of residential life for people in need of some level of physical or social support. They emphasise the compounding of factors such as loss of health and, with the loss of home, the severance from tangible connections with one's current life and biography. They found evidence not only of the important of residents' lifestyles before admission but also of how the transition into residential care subtly reduced the power of individuals and undermined their individuality. Nevertheless, their study suggested that a small number, about 10 per cent, organised their own lives in ways that maximised the best that residential life could offer and minimised the worst.

Schultz and Brenner (1977) found that individuals who were relocated involuntarily consistently suffered from some form of setback in personal adjustment, whereas those who moved from choice maintained, or even improved, on some of the indicators they used in their research. They concluded that:

- The greater the choice, the less negative the effects of the relocation
- The more predictable the move, the less negative the effects of the relocation
- Pre-relocation preparation appears to increase the predictability of the new environment, and effectively contributes to improved health.

The literature suggests that involuntary location, especially where there is no preparation, is likely to have adverse effects (Mikhail, 1992). If individuals recognise a legitimate reason for relocation, and are involved in the move, relocation can be a revitalising and beneficial experience. These individuals also reported less homesickness and better relationships (Willcocks, Peace and Kellaher, 1987).

Nay's (1995) work sought to understand the experience of relocation, and produced four key themes:

- *There was no choice*: Many of the respondents recognised that relocation to a home was, at best, a forced choice, with no realistic alternatives. 'An analogous situation would be if a person were told that if he or she did not have a leg amputated, he would die.' Most respondents wanted to be given the opportunity to be involved in the decision making.
- *Everything went*: The experience of relocating to a home was substantially one of loss. 'Everything went: home, possessions, friends, family, affection, pets, freedom, favoured locations, and the environments, roles and lifestyles that were known and predictable.' The respondents spoke of the importance of being able to take treasured possessions into the home, and the perception of loss was not so much for the material objects but rather for what they symbolised and the memories they evoked.
- *Devalued self*: All respondents perceived themselves and their care as a burden. There was a perception of lack of control, loss of identity, loss of self esteem and being devalued. 'Residents felt that the best they had left to offer loved ones was freedom from the burden of their care.'
- *The end of the line*: For many of the respondents, there was a sense that they were leaving themselves behind and that there was no future. 'Life as they had known it was over.'

Adjusting to living with others

Nurses, other professionals, and care staff who work with older people have a key role in helping them to make the transition from living in their own homes to living in a communal home.

A first step is to recognise the potential devastation of the transition, as described in the quote at the beginning of this chapter.

McCormack's (1996) adapted framework suggests that nurses can help older people to make the transition from their own homes to a care home in five ways: creating a total healing environment, supporting the older person, confirming the value and self worth of the individual, helping them to seek meaning, and helping than to participate as fully as possible in their chosen lifestyle.

The healing environment

Much of the research into communal homes has suggested that the culture of what Goffman described as 'total institutions' has predominated. These characteristics include: all activities being conducted in the same place and under the same authority; daily activities being conducted with a large group of others, all treated the same and required to do the same; all activities being designed to meet the aims of the institution; and phases of the day being tightly scheduled, with rules imposed and enforced (Goffman, 1961). McCormack (1996) suggests that the environment should be constructed so that the surroundings and approaches to care recognise the unique journey of each older person, alongside his or her values and priorities. Such an environment promotes individual choice, control, maximum autonomy and personal fulfilment.

Supporting

This encompasses believing in the inherent worth of older people and their strengths and abilities, despite any ill-health or disability. It involves acknowledging and demonstrating understanding of the changes being experienced by the older person, including feelings of loss and grief. Supporting involves helping older people to recognise their values, wishes and priorities in the transition situation, to assess the risks to be undertaken, and to make choices.

Confirming

Confirmation is again underpinned by respect for the self worth of each individual, irrespective of current health state, and treating people as valued adults who retain all adult rights. It is about recognising individual differences in ways of coping, managing or responding in transition situations, and helping the older person, and family if appropriate, to feel comfortable with the decisions they take. It can also be about facilitating continued cohesion of the family unit, and continuity with the pre-relocation lifestyle of the older person. Confirming can also encompass the confirmation of individual abilities and the facilitation of the realisation of these in everyday life in the home.

Seeking meaning

Nurses can help older people to make their own sense of the experiences of relocation by providing ample opportunities for potential relocatees and incoming residents to talk through their feelings, and find personal meaning and understanding in what is significant to them as individuals. Nurses can also help older people to find their own new meaning in the new living situation.

Participating

Much of the research discussed in this chapter emphasises the desire of older people to participate in decisions, to make their own choices, to realise these choices, and to retain their maximum independence. They also want to assume responsibility for the risks they choose to take.

The Department of Health's 1989 document *Caring for People* recognised that some older people will continue to need to enter nursing or residential care homes. It declared that choices should extend to all older individuals in this situation, even those for whom total independence is no longer a possibility. The document states that, for such older people, 'this form of care should be a positive choice'.

References

Allen I, Hogg D and Peace S (1992) *Elderly People: Choice, Participation and Satisfaction*. Policy Studies Institute Publishing, London.

Bacon V and Lambkin C (1994) Mixed messages: day care design. *Health Service Journal* 30, 20–21.

Barron CR, Foxall MJ, Von Dolen K, Jones PA and Shull KA (1994) Marital status, social support and loneliness in visually impaired elderly people. *Journal of Advanced Nursing* 19, 272–80.

Berg S, Mellstrom D, Persson G and Svanorg A (1981) Loneliness in the Swedish aged. *Journal of Gerontology* 36, 342–9.

Bond J, Coleman P and Peace S (1993) *Ageing in Society: An Introduction to Social Gerontology*, 2nd edn. Sage, London.

Butler A and Tinker A (1983) Integration or segregation: housing in later life. In Butler A and Tinker A (eds) *Elderly People in the Community: Their Service Needs*. HMSO, London.

Byrne DS, Harrison SP, Keithley J and McCarthy P (1986) *Housing and Health: The Relationship between Housing Conditions and Health of Council Tenants*. Gower, Aldershot.

Coffman T (1981) Relocation and survival of institutionalised aged: a re-examination of the evidence. *Gerontologist* 21, 483–500.

Counsel and Care (1992) *From Home to a Home*. Counsel and Care, London.

Dale A, Evandrou M and Arber S (1987) The household structure of the elderly population in Britain. *Ageing and Society* 7, 37–56.

Department of the Environment (1988) *English House Condition Survey 1986*. HMSO, London.

Department of Health (1989) *Caring for People: Community Care in the Next Decade and Beyond*, Cmmd 849. HMSO, London.

Fenton S (1991) Ethnic minority populations in the United Kingdom, In Squires AJ (ed.) *Multicultural Health Care and Rehabilitation of Older People*. Edward Arnold/ Age Concern, London.

Fletcher P (1991) *The Future of Sheltered Housing – Who Cares?* Policy report. National Federation of Housing Associations, London.

Goffman E (1961) *Asylums*. Doubleday, New York.

Help the Aged (1995) *Living Alone – Sharing Responsibility*. Help the Aged, London.

Henwood M (1992) *Through a Glass Darkly: Community Care and Elderly People*. Research Report 14 King's Fund, London.

Holmen K, Ericsson K, Andersson L and Winbland B (1992) Loneliness among elderly people living in Stockholm: a population study. *Journal of Advanced Nursing* 17, 43–51.

Hunt A (1978) *The Elderly at Home: A Study of People aged 65 and over Living in the Community in England in 1976*. OPCS, London.

Institute of Actuaries (1993) *Financial Long-term Care in Great Britain*. Institute of Actuaries, London.

Laing W (1993) *The Care of Elderly People Market Survey 1992/3*, 6th edn. Laing and Buisson, London.

Laing W and Hall M (1991) *The Challenges of Ageing: A Review of the Economic, Social and Medical Implications of an Ageing Population*. Association of the British Pharmaceutical Industry, London.

Law CM and Warnes AM (1982) The destination decision in retirement migration. In Warnes AM (ed.) *Geographical Perspectives on the Elderly*. Wiley, Chichester.

Leather P and Wheeler R (1988) *Making Use of Home Equity in Old Age*. Building Societies Association, London.

McCormack B (1996) Life transition. In Ford P and Heath H (eds) *Older People and Nursing: Issues of Living in a Care Home*. Butterworth-Heinemann, London.

Mikhail M (1992) Psychological responses to relocating to a nursing home. *Journal of Gerontological Nursing* March, 35–39.

Nay R (1995) Nursing home residents' perceptions of relocation. *Journal of Clinical Nursing* 4, 319–25.

OPCS (1982) *General Household Survey 1980* HMSO, London.

OPCS (1988) *General Household Survey 1985*. HMSO, London.

OPCS (1993) *The 1991 Census: Persons Aged 60 and Over, Great Britain*. HMSO, London.

Parker G (1990) *With Due Care and Attention: A Review of Research on Informal Care*. Family Policy Studies Centre, London.

Peace S (1988) Living environments for the elderly, 2: promoting the 'right' institutional environment. In Wells N and Freer C (eds) *The Ageing Population: Burden or Challenge*. Macmillan, Basingstoke.

Peace S (1993) The living environments of older women. In Bernard M and Meade K (eds) *Women Come of Age: Understanding the Lives of Older Women.* Edward Arnold, London.

Phillips J (1992) *Private Residential Care: The Admission Process and Reactions of the Public Sector.* Avebury Press, Aldershot.

Rickford F (1993) Longstay beds for elderly cut by 40 per cent. *The Guardian,* 5 August.

Schultz R and Brenner G (1977) Relocation of the aged – a review and theoretical analysis. *Journal of Gerontology* 32, 323.

Schultz NR and Moore D (1984) Loneliness: correlates, attributions, and coping among older adults. *Personality and Social Psychology Bulletin,* 10, 66–7.

Simmons S (1994) Social networks: their relevance to mental health nursing. *Journal of Advanced Nursing,* 19, 281–9.

Sixsmith AJ (1986) Independence and home in later life. In Phillipson C, Bernard M and Strang P (eds) *Dependency and Interdependency in Old Age – Theoretical Perspectives and Policy Alternatives.* Croom Helm, London.

Sixsmith AJ (1990) The meaning and experience of 'home' in later life. In Blytheway B and Johnson J (eds) *Welfare and the Ageing Experience.* Avebury Press, Aldershot.

Smythe M and Browne F (1992) *General Household Survey 1990.* HMSO, London.

Tinker A (1984) *Staying at Home: Helping Elderly People.* HMSO, London.

Warner N (1994) *Community Care: Just a Fairytale?* Carers' National Association, London.

Wenger GC (1995) A comparison of urban with rural support networks: Liverpool and North Wales. *Ageing and Society,* 15, 59–81.

Wenger GC (1996) *Support Networks of Older People and the Demand for Community Care Services.* Centre for Social Policy Research and Development, University of Wales, Bangor.

Willcocks D, Peace S and Kellaher L (1987) *Private Lives in Public Places: A Research-based Critique of Residential Life in Local Authority Old People's Homes.* Tavistock, London.

9

Disease or distress: an exploration of mental health and age

Alan Crump

This chapter delves into the main issues involved in the nursing care of older people with mental health needs. It is not intended to be an all embracing breakdown of the disease processes or a classification of the major mental health illnesses. It is rather an exploration of the issues and underlying principles. The hope is that it will tempt the reader to seek out other writers and ideas from across the spectrum of nursing literature. At this early stage in the chapter is perhaps important to state my personal position so that the general perspective and direction of the chapter is fully understood.

I believe in the value of the therapeutic relationship between nurse and patient. It is this relationship, whether in the hospital, home or nursing home, that has the most significant effect on the lives of (older) people who have mental health needs. This is not to underestimate the action of our colleagues in medicine, occupational therapy, social work or the other disciplines but to make clear that the efforts of these teams of people can work only where there is first a therapeutic (and perhaps that only means a 'working') relationship.

An example of this would be the reliance and faith of some medical practitioners solely on drug therapies without appropriate psychological support. This form of care is tunnel visioned and does not offer the patient the best opportunity of long term recovery or rehabilitation. Wattis and Church (1988) have pointed out the need for a broader base of skills and interventions when supporting the older person with mental health needs. The over-use of medication in mental health care has been explored by Lader (1977), who suggested that there is a 'worthwhile improvement' in most patients with the use of drugs, but that these drugs 'do not necessarily cure'. He also points out the major side effects of most drugs. Peplau (1994), in reviewing some of the current challenges to mental health nursing, suggests that medical practice 'seems primarily interested in reconstruction of biochemical imbalances' through the giving of medication and that regrettably 'giving pills' has become 'the only treatment'. Peplau goes on to argue for nursing to reclaim the therapeutic nature of practices 'based upon social and interpersonal theories'.

The use of medication in mental health care complements the relationship-forming processes, but it is relationships that form the very core of mental health nursing. Medication alone creates neither lasting stability for the individual nor the sense of wellbeing that relationships provide. If this chapter is about anything, it is about relationships and how best to use them in the support of older people with mental health needs. In trying to explore the nature of mental health nursing with older people it is possible that the nature of care itself will be explored.

Negative images

I believe that the negative image of old age and mental health is the biggest factor holding back a quality mental health service for older people. Contact with negative attitudes and opinions both inside and outside nursing only reinforces this belief.

Some years ago I elected to have a short spell on a general surgical ward, mainly to test my own feelings towards caring for older people. I am not a surgical nurse (as my colleagues would all have readily agreed!);

however, I gained a great deal of insight into the distress caused by physical illness. Despite my shortcomings I enjoyed the experience. However, after a 12 month period I realised that surgery was not the area for me and I hankered to return to the nursing care of older people. On leaving the ward I received the compulsory good luck gift, which was a football signed by the staff on the ward. The ball had been signed by all those with whom I had worked. The comments on the ball were a range of the stereotyped attitudes that describe older people and, although none were truly malicious, they indicated that they believed I was signing my own professional death warrant. This cameo reflects the professional stereotyping that occurs and I believe gives us an insight into the attitudes of the wider community.

It appears that all branches of caring highlight the dangers of ageism. Stevenson (1989) offers a view from social care where she describes 'the extreme and ugly negativism' of our own attitudes to ageing. The psychologist Stokes (1992), in reviewing some of the literature on ageism, suggests that the main image of the older person is largely negative. The nurse theorist and writer Cormack (1985) devotes a chapter to it, suggesting that although nurses did not 'create' ageism they are its perpetuators. Lookinland and Anson (1995) have gone further by suggesting that the qualified nurse of the future (i.e. in education now) may have an even more negative image of working with older people than previous nurses. They propose changing the emphasis within the nursing curriculum to promote more positive attitudes and beliefs.

Negative images are everywhere. Midwinter (1991) points out that the images of old age in broadcasting and the media tend to stereotype and label. He suggests that, where older people are portrayed, they are 'rigid, less productive, had a decline in intelligence, sexless and had marked decrepitude'. This image is reinforced by other media, such as advertising and the papers. Advertisements to sell cars do not use older people; it is more likely to see an older person advertising a solid and dependable life assurance scheme. These images are subtle, but reinforce the stereotypes that exist and make it more difficult to create lasting positive images. The images that persist are those of older people as a race apart: a race stripped of status, stripped of choice, labelled inappropriately, but above all stripped of the simple dignity of being an individual.

Minority groups

Mental health in old age receives the same labelling treatment. The words 'senile' and 'geriatric' have moved into everyday conversation to describe the vulnerability of old age to potential to mental illness. Norman (1982) suggests that 'with regard to mental illness in old age we are (slowly) emerging from the dark ages' and she condemns the negative terms that are used to convey the 'limbo existence' which is the common experience for an older person with a mental health need.

Perhaps the most worrying aspect of this labelling is that much of it comes from those who work with older people. Political correctness can be taken to extremes, but there is a point where it is absolutely essential to use language that is not just neutral but that offers an accurate, almost positive, image. The language we use to describe events and people reflects the value that we place on those events and people. When nursing staff use derogatory remarks to discuss the mental health of older people, it should not be a surprise that others also use negative terms.

Discrimination in our society is an ever present restriction to full citizenship for many individuals. Norman (1987) ably illustrates the nature of ageism and the impact it has on the lives of older people. Norman (1985) has also looked at the issues for older people who have settled here from other countries and the degree to which they suffer not only from age discrimination but also as a result of their nationality, colour or religion. To limit the effects of discrimination, legislation now attempts to coerce us into treating everyone as equals. There appears, however, to be a natural tendency to discriminate; it is 'minority' groups who shoulder the burden of discrimination even if their numbers would indicate that they are not a minority!

Women are a clear example of a section of society that holds minority group status and yet is far from being a minority. Oakley (1985) illustrates this, suggesting that as a social group women are invisible within society at large and even within the academic literature. Groups being discriminated against have certain characteristics: they are perceived and treated as weaker, they have fewer opportunities to redress the balance, the status quo favours those who discriminate, the laws are created by those who discriminate, and the system is self fulfilling. Those who are discriminated against are believed to have less value, and the system creates the conditions in which failure is expected. The assumptions concerning women are that they are weaker and cannot do the same work or carry out the same roles as men (men make the rules and the conditions). As the system works against them there are fewer opportunities to succeed and more opportunities to fail, which only reinforces the stereotype.

Stereotypes and prejudice

The same kind of self fulfilling stereotypes are created for those who are old and have mental health needs. Norman (1982) believes that a negative image of geriatric medicine (and as a result geriatric nursing) persists, but that this poor image is multiplied three times over for those who work in psychogeriatric care. Cormack (1985) suggests that 'contemporary youth-orientated societies value being young, looking young and being econom-ically productive and independent'. With youth there is beauty, strength, sexuality, productivity, sociability, flexibility and speed. These qualities are so valued that youth itself is valued and as a consequence the accepted antithesis, old age, is not. The truth is, of course, that this picture of youth is no more accurate a picture than the opposite is for older people.

Many images of mental health persist, often bolstered by inappropriate coverage in the media, like that of the dangerous madman, the eccentric loner or the obsessive and introspective teenager; mental illness is always something that happens to somebody else. The very presence of mental illness indicates weakness and failure. To have 'it' in the family can be the ultimate shame, causing the hushed whisper in conversation to avoid saying the words 'mental illness'. To work with mentally ill people is still misunderstood; to work with older people with mental illness is con-sidered positively unusual. Mental health care remains the very poor second cousin of the more glamorous surgical and medical areas.

It is important to understand the background against which nursing older people with mental health needs is placed. Our attitudes and values towards it cannot be taken in isolation from wider attitudes and beliefs. Norman (1987) has posed the question of whether any of us can be truly positive towards those who are older. She argues that none of us are unaffected by the issues of mortality and morbidity that old age repre-sents and, despite our efforts to respect those who are old, our actions display our true feelings. These actions include the language that is used in everyday conversation, the representations of older people in the media, and the absence of legislation to curb ageist work practice and the policy changes which have discriminated against older people.

If these prejudices towards old age are set alongside the fear that surrounds mental illness, one can begin to see the true extent of the influences on nursing practice.

Positive forces

Despite this negative picture, much has been accomplished in recent years to move the image of caring for older people with mental health needs forward. This is all the more impressive given the very negative starting point within the wider community and all the caring disciplines. Goff-man's (1961) description of institutional care for vulnerable groups reflected perfectly the custodial care offered to all those with mental illness. Older people with mental health needs received the same deper-sonalised service as other age groups. In a study by Hall and Buckwalter (1990) into the changes in care for older people with dementia in America, it was suggested conditions there were no better. People with dementia received no specific care and often all those with mental health needs, young and old, were cared for in the same environment. They go on to point out the part played by mental health nurses and social policy planners in making the care of the older person with dementia more humane.

It appears that when services for older people with mental health needs moved forward it was as a result of energetic and positive individuals who wanted to improve the services provided. These individuals created new therapeutic environments where previously there was only the despair and greyness of institutional care. They forged relationships with older people: the same older people who were previously considered to be beyond relationships and beyond care. These relationships created warmth and normality in the lives of people where before there was only emptiness. These are the individuals who applied thought and believed that the service had to change. Those of us who now work with mentally ill older people need to continue the positive work started by those who were committed to improving the care of older people.

These individuals were ably supported by larger organisations like the World Health Organization and, in the UK, organisations such as Counsel and Care, the Centre for Policy on Ageing, the Royal College of Nursing and many others. These positive forces continue to offer a backdrop against which good practice in mental health nursing and care can flourish, but good practice is down to individuals. Both the individuals who lead and those who offer the practical everyday contact with people need to ensure good practice. This is a constant process of development and re-assessment. It is my belief that to stand still, in other words to stop thinking and developing, in any climate is to start sliding backwards. If individuals begin to think they have achieved the best service (for older people with mental health needs) the care they offer has already begun to move backwards. If thought is part of the forward movement of care, absence of thought creates stagnation and ultimate backward movement in care.

Institutionalisation: the absence of thought

Goffman (1961) spoke at length about institutional care within mental health asylums, and we have all experienced some forms of this institutionalisation. It is characterised by a lack of thought and a lack of energy aimed at the provision of care. It is also characterised by the provision of uniform care that is uninspired and monotonous. It will be geared to the needs of the system that supports the care and, where there is application of thought, it is concerned only with maintaining the system.

This is not only an issue of the early nineteenth century or a reflection of the scandals of the last twenty years. It is an issue for us all now.

Bennet and Kingston (1993) report both on the extent to which the needs of the organisations are still put above the needs of the people who receive care and on the extent to which this constitutes abuse of older people. Eaton (1993) discussed the implications of the increasing number of cases of suspected poor practice within nursing homes being reported to the UKCC. Nursing homes are increasingly the continuing care facility for older people with mental health needs. Nursing homes face the same potential for institutionalised care as other larger hospitals. Where the mental health care of older people becomes institutionalised it is not because of the environment or the size of the institution but because those who are carrying out or leading the care have stopped thinking.

Institutionalised care can happen in the brightest newest building. Bennett (1994) writing in *The Guardian* wrote a feature on nursing homes that reflected the potential for bland and unthinking care even in the most up-to-date establishments. In the same weekend I listened to a news report about a nursing home where the care, attitudes and environment could not have been better. The positive force of this latter report was all the more impressive as it was the spoken words of those who were receiving 'institutional' care.

In any nursing workplace, where development is essential, staff who think and question should be seen as essential. In conventional institutions, however, they were seen as endangering the system and were ignored or pushed 'out of harm's way'. These strong willed individuals are still within the health care system now. They are the ones who continue to ask awkward questions and to challenge conventional practice. Some of the scandals of today are more complex and less visible: they involve the provision of services and resources without any thought.

Despite a drive for openness within the Health Service with the Patient's Charter (Department of Health, 1992), there is a danger that current modes of thinking within some trusts will result in a return to the closed systems of practice that were characteristic of old institutions. Mallick and McHale (1995) discussed some of the issues of highlighting poor practice and the feeling that many employers were increasingly trying to 'muzzle' complaints. There appears to be a new controlling culture within NHS trusts, dominated by secrecy, and this has already created dilemmas for practitioners who speak out. I have a grave concern that this will again create the conditions where the once motivated and thinking individual becomes merely an unthinking trustee.

The positive impact of theory

In the preceding paragraphs there has been a great deal of emphasis on individuals in practice, but there have of course been other major influences on the nursing care of older people with mental health needs. A good deal of this was related to the growing body of nursing theory and the move away from a reliance on medical and biological modes of practice. One might even suggest that part of the institutionalisation of previous nursing care of mentally ill older people was a result of adhering to a cure based model of nursing. With the advent of philosophies that supported the individual in a more holistic sense, there was the opportunity for more individualised approaches and these, by their very nature, were not institutional. Nursing is still in the process of creating its own models and philosophies, but already this activity has affected the care of older people and older people with mental health needs.

The right model for mental health nursing

The nursing care of older people with mental health needs is moving away from a model strictly defined by medical nursing. Nolan (1991), in discussing the history of training within mental health nursing around the middle of the nineteenth century, suggests that there was no body of knowledge and that 'care' was offered by attendants who were paid less than half the weekly wage of a farm labourer. The first training was almost all offered by medical staff to help in the provision of medical regimens. It was based around the medical thought of the time and emphasised obedience, order and cleanliness. Breaking away from such powerful influences has been very difficult for both mental health nurses and all other areas of nursing.

The medical model of care has emphasised the disease nature of illness and, although this may work well in areas such as surgery where a single problem area can be defined and eliminated, it becomes increasingly difficult to justify this approach with mental health care. Dawson (1994) has suggested that the nature of mental health is still poorly understood but that medicine continues to attempt to explain it in scientific terms that produce rational scientific answers. This leads to the belief that all mental 'illness' can be cured if only the answer can be found. Nursing has long worked with similar doctrines, but is now defining itself in more complementary ways.

A continuum of mental health

The title of this chapter should lead the reader to reappraise their standpoint on mental health nursing. There are some who would look to the 'disease' of mental illness and look for cures and explanations. I feel more comfortable with a model that accepts a continuum of mental health and mental distress: one on which we all move back and forth, attempting to strike the right balance. Barker (1990) believes that the language and models we use to describe mental health nursing reflect the degree to which it is person centred or professional centred. He suggests that 'to treat patients as people is bound to be difficult', especially if 'it is claimed that patients are fundamentally different from those who are not'. If there is an accepted split between patients and people, we are on the path to accepting the concept of mental illness as a disease process.

Instead of seeing the issue of mental health as all or nothing, it is perhaps useful to see it as a continuum: we all have both wellness and illness. One might then accept that people who have moved along the mental health continuum away from health are still the same people but are now distressed and in need of support and understanding. The difference is not merely political correctness: it is crucial to how we perceive mental health nursing and, more importantly, how we perceive those who find themselves requiring mental health support. Disease or distress is not just a snappy title, but the beginning of the debate over what is at the core of mental health care.

CASE STUDY 1

A 70-year-old man arrived at the day hospital with a 'diagnosis' of depression. He had been visited at home by his GP and had been referred to the hospital based services. He appeared as a well read man with a wealth of experience to relate. He spoke about his feelings of low confidence, anxiety on leaving his flat and a loss of interest in his beloved music. He had lost his wife some years before and had been living alone since. He developed a relationship with his primary nurse that appeared to work, and his trust in the nurse grew over the weeks, despite only coming to the day hospital twice a week. They discussed his feelings and he explored his doubts. He started to teach his nurse about his music, and he was able to relive some of his past glories in the field of engineering and to share stories of his deceased wife. With some structured activities to build up his confidence it did not take long for this man to regain his self esteem and confidence and rejoin the mainstream of life.

Nothing unusual here. That is exactly the point: there was nothing unusual about it at all. This man was like us all. In seeking the balance of good health, something had moved him towards the feeling of mental distress. He did not have some strange disease that marked him out as different – he was just like us. Perhaps that is why mental illness creates such an uncomfortable feeling. It is too close for comfort and far enough away to ignore; for given a similar set of circumstances, we too might be feeling the same level of distress.

Nursing models tend to emphasise the complexity of the human system and the interrelationships that exist between the different components of the individual. Pearson and Vaughan (1986) suggest that nursing models 'perceive health as a much wider concept relating to wellness and the achievement of potential'. Where medicine reduces in order to predict and explain, mental health nursing has moved towards understanding the whole. In making efforts to understand the whole rather than explain it, the emphasis within care shifts towards building relationships with individuals rather than just treating them. The pioneering theories of Hildgard Peplau over 30 years ago set the agenda for mental health nurses to move into relationship building as the major therapeutic influence in nursing care. These assumptions about the nature of nursing and of health have helped to shape current practice. Peplau (1994) returned to her belief in the potential of relationships within nursing care, saying that 'of greater significance and therapeutic benefit are the interpersonal interactions which nurses have with patients'. The development of relationships is now at the core of good mental health nursing. If nursing is seeking to define its activity, it should seize this area as its own.

The potential of relationships

The formation of relationships is perhaps the most underestimated area within nursing care. Kitson (1987) suggested that 'we cannot deny that nursing is all about developing and sustaining relationships with people . . .'. Fosbinder (1994) showed that patients' perceptions of good care were related to the nature of the interpersonal relationship with staff. Part of the problem for nurses is how to measure good relationships. In an era where everything needs measurement, how do we measure good relationships? What are the qualities that lead to the formation of a working relationship? This is not easy, but perhaps it starts with an assumption that the older people who come into our services are like us only more distressed, more confused or in more disarray. If we cannot accept these people as individuals, we will not be able to form relationships that are based on genuineness and understanding. Barker (1990) also believes that we first need to consider patients as people before we can offer an appropriate service. Benner (1984) points to the intuitive nature of some 'expert' nurses to say and do the right things at the right time. This is about knowing people and knowing their needs and comes from having a close relationship. This ability does not arrive without practice, education or experience, but it does imply that there are underlying personal qualities within a nurse who is able to form relationships. I suggest that these qualities are the same qualities that you would expect of good practitioners in other fields of work where relationships are central to practice. These qualities would include:

- Tolerance
- Understanding
- Humour
- Patience
- Self awareness
- Respect
- Empathy
- Integrity.

Kitwood and Bredin (1993) have also suggested that in the care of people with dementia the most effective carer needs to be 'adequately resourced' personally as well as practically. They point to a set of positive characteristics in the carer that help to promote the wellbeing of those for whom they are caring:

- Inner quietness
- Lowered psychological defences
- Empathy
- Ease in making contact
- Stability and resourcefulness.

These checklists are not intended to imply that once these qualities are identified a nurse is able to form working relationships, but that they form a good starting point. These qualities need to be combined with the application of thought and the need to experience and learn from other skilled practitioners. There is no single simple way to feeling comfortable in relationships.

To believe that by the act of nursing someone you will have formed a meaningful relationship is to ignore the great potential that lies within the process of real understanding and mutual development that a working relationship can offer. Add to that the individual chemistry of each relationship and the true potential and extent of relationships starts to become apparent. The mental health nursing of older people is working with people in perhaps their time of greatest distress. Dealing with the physical limitations of age is something that we all eventually come to expect; however, developing a mental illness in old age is the unexpected and certainly the unwanted. When the combination of physical decline and memory loss or lowered mood or altered perception is considered, the distress that this might cause can be fully understood. A person in such a situation requires not just a cursory acknowledgement of their name but an understanding of them as a person: one with a life full of triumphs and disasters, weddings and funerals, beginnings and ends. To know this, one has to know the person behind the name – and, to do this, one has to have a relationship which is more than merely nursing them.

The empathy factor

A further aspect to achieving the full potential of relationships is that one has to step into the experience of the other person. Rogers (1951) has called this kind of process empathy, and he coupled it with warmth, genuineness and unconditional positive regard. Stevenson (1989) suggests that 'a prerequisite in forming relationships with other (older) people is empathy', but she also realises the difficulties that this may create by pointing out that, as younger people caring for those who are older, we have not yet experienced old age. She accepts that this might be a barrier.

These qualities are crucial if valuable relationships are to be formed. However, it is not good enough to know the definitions of these words in order to form therapeutic relationships. Benner and Wrubel (1989) have talked about the 'being with' or presencing that some expert nurses are able to achieve. These nurses have a wealth of theoretical knowledge, but also an understanding about themselves, and are able to feel comfortable with people in their distress. Feeling comfortable with the distress and anguish of others is never easy and we have all, at times, felt unable to bear the pain expressed by an individual in our care as a result of their physical or mental distress.

Coping with these times of emotional conflict marks out the skilled and experienced nurse from the novice. It is sometimes difficult to pinpoint the exact skills that expert nurses utilise in these situations, but they are able to move in and out of apparently stressful situations with ease. The relationship forming skills of these nurses rely on a combination of sound theoretical knowledge, self awareness and intuitive experience. Benner and Wrubel (1989) believe that this intuitive sense within some nurses can be considered the very essence of care.

In these times, when for knowledge be truly accepted it needs to be generated from a scientific research-based source, it is probable that the ability to be at ease with someone and have an intuitive understanding of their distress is a vastly underestimated process. Whatever the exact nature of the skills of the expert nurse, it is evident that the relationship formed can be both the vehicle for all therapeutic activity and part of the healing process itself.

Supervision and support

Sharing the distress of another is never easy, and as nurses part of our learning is the experience of feeling and sharing the pain and distress of someone for whom we are caring. It is to be hoped that these early experiences do not desensitise but rather start the process of learning about the potential of supporting an individual through the extremes of illness. Learners (and we should all count ourselves learners) working with older people who are perhaps experiencing the bleakness of despair and self doubt as a result of severe depression, or the anguish of bereavement after years of living with the same person, may find the sharing of these times particularly stressful – and it is to be hoped that the frequency of these events is not great. The experience can, however, be tremendously rewarding, and if appropriately supported by a clinical supervisor or personal tutor the experience may be one that shapes the future caring of the nurse.

These kinds of experience need the benefit of reflection and shared discussion for the full potential to be derived. Bishop (1994) points out how clinical supervision should now be a part of all our practice, both as students and beyond, aiming to enhance the care that we offer. It offers opportunities to explore our feelings in relation to care that were previously locked away. The culture is changing with respect to how care makes us feel, and this in return can make us stronger in offering the right kind of care at the right times.

The danger of relationships

More experienced staff who avoid forming meaningful relationships with those in their care are perhaps wary of committing the degree of emotional energy that is required. Stevenson (1989) has pointed out that 'everyone puts limits on their emotional involvement with others' and she goes on to accept that 'comprehensive engagement would be intolerable'. Within all relationships there is a balance of how much we feel we can expose of ourselves; and within the professional relationship the same is true. The degree to which a given nurse holds back in a relationship may be a completely appropriative response if that nurses is still building up a repertoire of skills and moving towards greater expertise. It may, however, be the response of a nurse unable to share in the world of patients. As a result, those patients do not have access to a relationship that would complement and enhance other forms of care.

It is likely that this nurse would not have had the benefit of truly supportive peers or managers who were able to offer real support. It is crucial that, if strong relationships are to be formed with patients, the nursing staff involved need to feel nurtured and valued. The nurse who is unable to commit to relationships may have worked in an environment where being close to patients was unacceptable and the display of genuine emotion was seen as a weakness. However fast the culture is changing in some places, it should never be assumed that these changes are universal.

Whether a patient has a physical or mental illness, whether they are in the community or in hospital, they benefit from relationships that are more than just 'the doing for'; the real benefit for the patient and the nurse comes from 'the being with'. There is no doubt that being with people at times of distress is one of the most demanding areas of nursing.

The limitation of relationships

The application of these ideas when working with older people directly affects the quality of care offered. If it is the quality of relationships that marks out good nursing care, then in working with older people with mental health needs it is crucial to create meaningful and appropriate relationships. At this point it is important to recognise the tensions that limit our ability to form these 'working' relationships.

If there is a degree of both explicit and implicit ageism expressed within nursing and in the wider community, as earlier discussed, there are some serious issues that need to be addressed. If Norman's (1987) analysis of ageism, that it is related to a fear or reminder of our own mortality, is a possible reason for our ageist attitudes, this will be a constant limiting factor in the ability to form relationships with older people. It is therefore valuable to study our attitudes towards older people and how this may be a product of the wider scene.

CASE STUDY 2

After returning to the nursing care of older people I nursed a man who did not conform to any of the 'normal' characteristics of a patient. He was constantly angry at people and seldom allowed care to be performed despite requiring support for a series of physical illnesses. At times he was charming and at others he was frankly without charm at all! Despite my belief that I knew about older people I was an absolute beginner as far as this particular man was concerned. As I look back I sense that I never knew what he wanted – what caused him such anger and pain or any of his life events. The care offered considered him solely as a patient with a chest infection to be offered the same care that other patients which chest infections received.

I reflect now on the care I tried to offer, and realise that I had not taken into account my own attitudes and experiences of old age. I had a fixed idea of what the average older person wanted and tried to put him into that category. He did not fit. My ageist attitudes (I now see them as such) had coloured my approach, and my enthusiasm and lack of thought had led to a very poor relationship. I hope I could now form a better relationship with that man, but only because my mistake of grouping all older people together and assuming that there is an average kind of older person has now been acknowledged and altered. There is not an average older person, just as there is not an average younger person. Some lessons are learnt the hard way, and however skilled we may be in one field there is always another in which we are still learning.

If we can never really feel at ease with older people, will we ever be able to really support them and live their experiences with them? The answer is that there are people who feel at ease with older people, both nurses and others. Empathy is one of the qualities that helps us share the experiences with others. When we are close to others, we can share their triumphs and disasters, their joy and pain, even if we have not had those exact experiences ourselves. There are good examples of nurses who do feel at ease with older people and can build relationships that are truly meaningful. The issue of ageism adds another dimension to relationship formation and can only be worked on with the application of thought. To combat our ageism it needs to be acknowledged and a degree of self awareness concerning our attitudes accepted.

Relationships and dementia

The formation of relationships is of no greater importance than in the care of people experiencing dementia. This is the kind of mental distress that requires the greatest degree of understanding. The varied explanations for dementia rest only in the domain of the purely scientific, and yet this science has not come up with any real answers. Understanding the distress of the individual with dementia is at the core of good nursing practice. Kitwood (1993) has contested the certainty of those who claim that the cause of dementia lies solely in the destruction of nerve structures as a result of physical changes. At the core of his thinking is that people with dementia are initially labelled as 'demented' and subsequently treated in such a way as to cause a loss of their very selves, their very 'personhood'. This process, in which there is a loss of personhood, creates the conditions in which individuals progressively lose their own identity and self, leading to the extremes of severe dementia. Kitwood suggests that the way people living with dementia are treated adds to the known physical changes within dementia. The process of depersonalisation is exemplified by the medical approach to care, which attempts to solve problems rather than to understand the personal distress and offer care.

Goodwin and Mangan (1985) have ably described the conventional nursing care of the person experiencing dementia. This was to offer a regimen that was clean, comfortable and safe. The safety could be observed in terms of both the physical environment and the psychological risks in that the patients were never put in a position that would have stretched them to their full potential. It did not offer excitement, opportunity or variation, and as a consequence the nursing care offered only encouraged further dependency. There was no attempt made to offer any fulfilment, and as a result this form of care could be described as a process of institutional disempowerment.

Kitwood and Bredin (1992) would suggest that this scenario only forces the person to lose their identity and self still further, moving them down 'desolation lane'. It was also safe for nursing staff because they could hide behind an array of tasks and 'get the work done'. They would not have had the risk of becoming emotionally involved at more than a superficial level because that was not part of the care. Relationships can be unpredictable, stressful and risky. They might even cause an individual nurse some distress, and the best way to avoid this is to avoid the relationships. Conventional nursing of people experiencing dementia can be seen as a very safe and predictable form of care. One might argue that this model of care is reflected not only in the nursing care of people with dementia but in many other areas outside dementia care.

Kitwood and Bredin (1992), in developing their ideas on assessing dementia care through a process of mapping care environments, argue that in dementia care the most important aspect is the interpersonal process: the dynamic interaction that goes on between people. Their work points to a strong belief that we are social beings and thrive through interaction. People living with dementia are no different and also need the warmth and nourishment of relationships. Kitwood and Bredin suggest that all the actions and behaviours of the person with dementia are forms of communication to be understood: even inaction is a message that needs to be interpreted.

Feil (1993) has also taken an alternative look at the care that people with dementia receive, and has rejected conventional views. The assumption that she makes about dementia is that efforts need to be made to understand and validate the experience of the person experiencing dementia from their standpoint. Although largely untested, her theories with respect to individuality, creating an understanding relationship, using the time reference of the person with dementia and 'walking in step' with that person all have a certain resonance.

Stokes and Goudie (1989) have also responded to the accepted culture of dementia care. They promote the need to understand feelings within the person with dementia and to help them to achieve a resolution of their immediate distress. They encourage the use of a Rogerian type approach to interaction with confused older people. The use of counselling skills with people who experience dementia breaks with conventional practice, but it reinforces the idea that there is distress that needs to be understood and explored. The person with dementia may not explore their distress in the same ways as other people, but this should not prevent us from using similar techniques.

Neal (1994) takes this process a stage further when he uses the process of transactional analysis to explain how relationships might be improved still further. This is the process described by Eric Berne (1964), which concerns the interactions between individuals. Berne suggests that there are different parts to our being, which he called ego states. In interacting with others, if communication is to be smooth and effective, the two individuals involved need to operate in the same ego state. Neal (1994) describes how in conventional practice the communication with older people with dementia is of a critical or 'over-caring' nature and often given in such a way as to resemble that of a parent to a child. This kind of communication has the effect of closing down channels rather than opening them up, and the person with dementia needs to keep open all the channels of communication possible. Neal has argued that this process serves only to create barriers between nurses and older people living with dementia, and by maintaining a barrier nurses are able to work without having relationships with those in their care. As a result, people with dementia could be viewed as objects and not individuals. He advocates using the appropriate complementary ego state to achieve the maximum potential from any communication.

All too often the nursing care of older people with dementia is characterised by a need to get things done before the end of the shift. Manthey (1992) has described this kind of process and suggests that 'what is assigned is not patient care, but tasks'. She goes on to criticise nurses for assuming that, if the tasks have all been completed, patients will have received good care. This summarises succinctly the essence of the dis-empowering and depersonalised nature of conventional dementia nursing. In achieving all the separate tasks, a nurse is able to break down the older person into a series of different functions: the individual no longer remains.

The real master stroke is the reverse process: the skilled operator is the nurse who can knit all the tasks together without there being a seam and create twice the cloth. That nurse will be the one offering real care.

This also reinforces another idea of Kitwood (1993) about the nature of the relationship between the individual and the nurse. In a genuinely supportive relationship there are no ulterior motives. In a conventional caring situation the motive is getting through the work, and the person with dementia is the task to be completed. According to Kitwood the premise of the 'working' relationship is based on no other criteria than genuineness.

Relationships and the older depressed person

Working with older people who are depressed, one is struck by the similarities and not the differences of working with any other group of depressed people. Pitt (1988) suggests that one of the differences may be the propensity to blame the features of a depressive illness on physical attributes rather than accepting that they may be caused by mental distress. Indeed, this may be related to the twin perceptions of acceptability of physical illness and the unacceptable stigma of mental illness.

We have all worked with older people who live with the effects of low mood. The experience of each of these individuals is very different. They may display a series of behaviours that are considered to indicate depressive illness: poor appetite, sleep disturbance, loss of pleasure in activities that once stimulated, feelings of low worth and low esteem, fatigue and withdrawal. In some situations these feelings can become extreme, and these individuals may start to believe that they are evil, that there is a conspiracy against them, that they are rotting or possessed. They may report hearing voices that disparage and insult them. They may feel that they are so worthless and their distress may be so great that they want to end their life.

With such a range of possible presentations, part of the care of older people with low mood is to work out whether these experiences and reaction are 'normal'. It may be that they have lost a life-long partner and are working through the grief reaction. It may be that they are coming to terms with a change in their own self image following serious or chronic illness. Perhaps a major life event, moving house or retiring has caused greater isolation leading to a period of lower mood that is only a transition. Using a continuum of mental health, it may be possible to explore these experiences as part of a normal reaction to events, a normal reaction to stress. By labelling negative experiences as part of a disease that needs to be cured, we are making assumptions before completing an accurate assessment. The need for a full assessment of all individuals is crucial when any mental health need is suspected. Darby *et al.* (1993) have promoted the value of a full and dynamic assessment in order to enhance the effective care of the older person with a mental health need. If a period of distress is related to a stressful event, there is real potential for using relationships and understanding to help people to come to terms with these changes; labelling people as 'ill' may not be the appropriate response.

The issue, then, has to be whether the individual is responding within normal boundaries or outside them. If a response is 'out of character' or perhaps lasting longer than one would ordinarily expect, there would be a strong case for more structured support in a hospital ward or day hospital or through the growing number of specialist community mental health nurses working with older people. This support would lead to a full assessment and care from a multidisciplinary team working solely in the field of the mental health needs of older people. In all of these situations, knowing the person becomes of paramount importance.

Information from loved ones and carers, friends and professionals is crucial to work out the nature of an individual's distress.

Where there appears to be no outside cause to the low mood, where it appears to be from 'within' or a stress reaction seems extreme, more formal support is likely to be an option. This support should be the result of a full individual assessment in combination with all other disciplines. This would set the scene for effective and appropriate nursing interventions. It also lays the foundation to commence working relationships.

Despite the range of experiences in the older depressed person, nursing care should centre on the formation of an understanding relationship whether in the community, in a nursing or residential home or in hospital. Understanding the mechanism of certain medication is important, as with all medication, but it is critical that this is seen as complementing the effects of a supportive relationship. Giving medication is the least complex part of caring for a depressed older person: being with them in despair and helping them to see through the darkness is the really complex and skilled activity of care. Peplau (1994) remarks that nurses must see themselves as the change agents in people's lives and that 'patients transform themselves'. The interaction with older people is the process by which that change can occur; the working relationship creates the conditions in which that interaction has most potential.

Nurses are a little like wound dressings – dressings can help wounds to heal, but the body heals the wound. Older people who are depressed are not made well by relationships or by medication, but they can be helped to move through the distress of depression within strong relationships.

Making relationships really work

Fosbinder (1994) showed that when patients reflect on nursing care, either in hospital or in the community, it is the relationships with the individuals who offered the care that are remembered. This work developed the idea that interpersonal relationships are what patients most value. Illness in older people has a tendency to be multifactorial and more complex. Periods of incapacity are longer and thus the potential for relationship building is greater. This is the case both in mental health nursing and in general nursing. Theorising about relationship building is one thing, but there are practical steps that can be taken to enhance the process of relationship formation.

Nursing taken to task

The system used for the delivery of nursing care drastically affects how patients and nurses interact. Earlier it was suggested that some nursing staff go out of their way to prevent relationships forming because these might be seen as causing emotional ties that might make the nurse feel at risk. Conventional nursing delivery systems were created in such a way as to minimise the risk of forming strong relationships with patients. Pearson and Vaughan (1986) described systems of task allocation in which one nurse had a responsibility for a specific activity for every patient within a given ward or unit and how this allowed for the care of a patient to be broken down into a series of separate tasks. In this way the patient would not be in a position to form strong links with any one nurse. This helped to regiment care, making it more controlled and predictable.

This model for the delivery of care reflected the reduction of the individual into different systems to be treated separately in much the same way that Henry Ford broke down the building of motor cars into a production line. This is a very efficient way of producing goods and a very efficient way of 'doing' nursing. However, it is a very poor way of 'being with' people who are in distress. People in distress are not predictable; they cannot be cared for at an hourly rate and there is no such person as the standard patient. If older people with mental health needs could be uniformly packaged, the complexity of nursing care would be a thing of the past. The tasks of care may have some uniformity and they can be assigned to the time-and-motion clipboard, but the real spanner in the production line of care is the nature of the relationship between nurse and patient. Benner (1984) suggests that 'the nurse–patient relationship is not a uniform, professionalised blueprint, but rather a kaleidoscope of intimacy and distance in some of the most poignant and mundane moments of life'. It is not surprising that some nurses find the unpredictable nature of relationships so stressful that they avoid them at all costs.

Primary nursing can help

The delivery of nursing has gradually changed towards care centred around fewer individuals. This has meant that one nurse would be responsible for the delivery of care to a defined numbers of patients. (Car manufacturing has also changed to incorporate more personal responsibility for the completion of the overall product.) The endpoint of this care is where one nurse is responsible for the prescription and delivery of nursing care to a defined set of patients. That nurse is responsible and accountable for the care offered to those individuals and, as a practitioner, will be asked to justify the nursing care offered. Most understand this form of practice to be primary nursing. Manthey (1992) suggests that it can facilitate good care by empowering nurses to work at their maximum potential; it does not in itself improve care. Once again, it is the responsibility of individuals to provide quality nursing care. Wright (1989) and

Ford and Walsh (1994) have provided good descriptions and critiques of primary nursing.

Taking into consideration the need for strong relationships between the older person and the nurse and the relatively longer stay in hospital (or the prolonged contact in the community), primary nursing should be considered to be the most appropriate system to deliver care for older people with mental health needs. Community nurses would of course argue that they operated forms of nursing care approximated to primary nursing long before hospital based nurses. There is some truth in this; however, primary nursing is not only about one nurse delivering care. It is also about accepting absolute responsibility for prescribing care so that in your absence someone else will follow your prescription. In caring for older people this professional accountability for care crosses all boundaries, hospital, home and nursing home, and in all environments primary nursing has the potential to improve care.

Primary nursing offers the nurse the opportunity to build meaningful, or at the very least knowledgeable, relationships with patients. As a consequence, the primary nurse can personally deliver and prescribe nursing care that is appropriate and consistent. Relationships are stressful and primary nursing deliberately aims at reaching the full potential of this process. McCormack (1992) has clearly identified the stresses that some primary nurses feel, and this should be considered to be a more exacting system for the delivery of care. It also requires a change in terms of the power structures that exist on wards. Good primary nursing can exist only in a supportive environment, and the role of the team leader, charge nurse or supervisor is crucial if primary nursing is not to become as 'institutional' and task orientated as other forms of care. Primary nursing changes the rules of engagement, and it is more stressful and more demanding, but what it offers patients is the opportunity for real support and real relationships. If nursing older people with mental health needs has at its core the requirement for meaningful relationships, primary nursing affords an opportunity to create the right conditions for that to happen.

CASE STUDY 3

A man in his 80s was dying slowly from chronic respiratory disease. He had suffered several previous admissions to the ward and was thought to be 'difficult', and as a result he had been given his own side room to help keep him 'settled'. He was not a model patient; he was not compliant with medication; he complained about poor food and argued with all members of staff, especially the nursing staff. He returned to the ward this time a little worse than last time, but the treatment offered again gave him new life and energy. With the returning energy came the renewed outbursts against certain members of the nursing staff.

As an inexperienced nurse under the direction of more senior staff, I was allocated to work with this unpopular patient; others seemed content and relieved that he was part of my allocation. This 'difficult' man had played and sang at Leeds City Varieties, had outlived two women with whom he had lived but whom he had never married, had composed songs and was proud of his achievements on the radio. I was lucky to have drawn 'the short straw'. We forged a relationship and spoke at length about his fears and about his life. He was a brave man facing up to his death and had not had the chance to reflect on his defeats or glories. His energy for life and passion for independence has lived with me since. I am pleased that I was given the opportunity to nurse the problem patient.

Everyday good practice

The difficulty in writing about the mental health needs of older people is finding the right approach. Some will want a breakdown of figures and conditions, some will want the coaching manual of 'how to do it' and some don't want it at all! I feel happier discussing the large issues, the principles, and leaving practitioners to use their own professional judgement to think about those ideas and then reject them, modify them and use them, or use them as they are. Even in rejection there is value, as it shows that people are thinking about what they are doing.

This section draws heavily on the work of the Social Services Inspectorate (1993), who have produced some excellent documents detailing good practice in the care of the older people with mental health needs. The strength of the ideas is the degree to which they can be used in all environments and are appropriate to every individual. There are six core values that underpin the ideas:

- Privacy
- Dignity
- Independence
- Choice
- Rights
- Fulfilment

Privacy and *dignity* are closely linked. How they are made possible within care environments depends largely on the attitudes and imagination of the staff. Older people with mental health needs can be dignified, given the opportunities. It may be that staff need to make this possible by creating appropriate conditions. In hospital, this may mean ensuring that there are facilities for washing, dressing and ironing personal clothes. There is nothing quite as undignified as wearing the baggy cast-offs of a previous patient when for the sake of the right attitude personal clothes could be worn. The Disabled Living Foundation (1990) has discussed these issues more fully and suggest that 'a change in attitude works wonders'.

Sometimes it appears that all hospital life happens behind curtains. Have you ever felt the embarrassment of trying not to make a noise while using the toilet in a restaurant? At least in a restaurant there are solid partitions; in hospital you are often expected to perform behind a thin curtain, with your feet dangling out at the bottom. I think of the person recently admitted for the first time into hospital having only ever 'shared' with their partner and only separated by a war: a person with such anxiety and distress that they believe people are plotting against them; a person who has the insight to know that they are unwell and the insight to know that they are embarrassed by their circumstances. How the loss of privacy affects them is a factor in their overall wellbeing and recovery. Privacy for all would appear to be a value quickly lost in the rush of hospital and nursing or residential home life. It is replaced by embarrassment and a requirement for the stiff upper lip.

Independence, choice and *rights* cannot be disentangled. If the rights of prisoners were ignored to the same degree to which the rights of older people with mental health needs are ignored there would be an outcry of public anger. For the older person with mental health needs, independence, choice and rights are regulated, even imposed, by those who provide the care. Their choice is what we allow, their independence is within the limits we set, and as a consequence there is a steady erosion of rights.

Fulfilment is the value that stands out from the rest. It would be possible to argue that the previous five values should provide the foundation of all care. Fulfilment is the sensation that should come as a result of putting all the other values into practice. There is a strong link here to the work of Maslow (1954) in stretching out to do more than just exist but to really achieve a sense of being alive. Fulfilment may simply be the experience of pleasure. There is also a sense that this cannot be achieved without the interaction of others. Perhaps fulfilment comes with the sharing of time with other people, giving us the zest and unpredictability that make life worth living. Kitwood and Bredin (1992) would strongly agree with this analysis in relation to the care of older people with dementia. They suggest that relative wellbeing comes within a positive relationship.

It seems that this chapter has come full circle. The potential of relationships within the mental health nursing of older people is as yet not fully realised. It may never be fully realised if our attitudes towards both mental health and older people do not change. Perhaps I have idealised the potential, but there are different cultures that have a much more positive approach to both mental distress and older people. Very few of the ideas contained within these lines are fresh, but they are important if the mental health nursing care of older people is to move forward.

References

Barker P (1990) The philosophy of psychiatric nursing. *Nursing Standard* 5, 28–33.
Benner P (1984) *From Novice to Expert: Excellence and Power in Clinical Nursing Practice.* Addison Wesley, Menlo Park, California.
Benner P and Wrubel J (1989) *The Primacy of Caring: Stress and Coping in Health and Illness.* Addison Wesley, Menlo Park, California.
Bennett C (1994) Ending up. *The Guardian Weekend* 8 October, 12–20.
Bennet G and Kingston P (1993) *Elder Abuse: Concepts, Theories and Interventions.* Chapman & Hall, London.
Berne E (1964) *Games People Play.* Penguin, Harmondsworth.
Bishop V (1994) Clinical supervision for an accountable profession. *Nursing Times* 90, 5–7.
Cormack D (ed.) (1985) *Geriatric Nursing: A Conceptual Approach.* Blackwell Scientific, Oxford.
Darby S *et al.* (1993) *Guidelines for Assessing Mental Health Needs in Old Age.* Royal College of Nursing, London.
Dawson PJ (1994) Philosophy, biology and mental disorder. *Journal of Advanced Nursing* 16, 587–96.
Department of Health (1992) *The Patient's Charter.* HMSO, London.
Disabled Living Foundation (1990) *Clothing: A Quality Issue.* Disabled Living Foundation, Harrow.
Feil N (1993) *The Validation Breakthrough.* Health Professions Press, Baltimore
Ford P and Walsh M (1994) *New Rituals for Old: Nursing Through the Looking Glass.* Butterworth-Heinemann, Oxford.
Fosbinder D (1994) Patient perceptions of nursing care: an emerging theory of interpersonal competence. *Journal of Advanced Nursing* 20, 1085–93.
Goffman E (1961) *Asylums.* Doubleday, New York.
Goodwin S and Mangan P (1985) Cosmic nursing: solitude and sanity. *Nursing Times* 7 August, 45–6.
Hall GR and Buckwalter KC (1990) From almshouse to dedicated unit: care of institutionalized elderly with behavioural problems. *Archives of Psychiatric Nursing* 4, 3–11.
Kitson AL (1987) Raising standards of clinical practice: the fundamental issue of effective nursing care. *Journal of Advanced Nursing* 12, 321–9.
Kitwood T (1993) Towards a theory of dementia care: the interpersonal process. *Ageing and Society* 13, 51–67.
Kitwood T and Bredin K (1992) *Person to Person: A Guide to the Care of those with Failing Mental Powers.* Gale Centre Publications, Loughton.
Kitwood T and Bredin K (1993) *Evaluating Dementia Care: The DCM Method.* Bradford Dementia Research Group, Bradford.

Lader M (1977) *Psychiatry on Trial*. Penguin, Harmondsworth.

Lookinland S and Anson K (1995) Perpetuation of ageist attitudes among present and future health care personnel: implications for elder care. *Journal of Advanced Nursing* 21, 47–56.

Mallick M and McHale J (1995) Support for advocacy. *Nursing Times* 91, 28–30.

Manthey M (1992) *The Practice of Primary Nursing*. King's Fund, London.

Maslow A (1954) *Motivation and Personality*. Harper and Row, New York.

McCormack B (1992) A case study identifying nursing staff's perception of the delivery of method of care in practice on a particular ward. *Journal of Advanced Nursing* 17, 187–97.

Midwinter E (1991) *Out of Focus: Old Age, the Press and Broadcasting*. Centre for Policy on Ageing, London.

Neal M (1994) An ethnographic study into the experience of five nurses importing the communication technique known as validation into their work with clients experiencing dementia. Thesis, Leeds Metropolitan University.

Nolan P (1991) Looking at the first 100 years. *Senior Nurse* 11, 22–5.

Norman A (1982) *Mental Illness in Old Age: Meeting the Challenge*. Centre for Policy on Ageing, London.

Norman A (1985) *Triple Jeopardy: Growing Old in a Second Homeland*. Centre for Policy on Ageing, London.

Norman A (1987) *Aspects of Ageism: A Discussion Paper*. Centre for Policy on Ageing, London.

Oakley A (1985) *The Sociology of Housework*. Blackwell, Oxford.

Pearson A and Vaughan B (1986) *Nursing Models for Practice*. Heinemann Nursing, Oxford.

Peplau H (1994) Challenge and change. *Journal of Psychiatric and Mental Health Nursing* 1, 3–7.

Pitt B (1988) Characteristics of depression in the elderly. In Gearing B *et al.* (eds) *Mental Health Problems in Old Age*. Open University/Wiley, Milton Keynes.

Rogers C (1951) *Client-centred Therapy: Its Current Practice, Implications and Theory*. Constable, London.

Stevenson O (1989) *Age and Vulnerability: A Guide to Better Care*. Arnold, London.

Social Services Inspectorate (1993) *Standards for the Residential Care of Elderly People with Mental Disorders*. Department of Health, London.

Stokes G (1992) *On Being Old: The Psychology of Later Life*. Falmer Press, London.

Stokes G and Goudie F (1989) Dealing with confusion. *Nursing Times* 85, 36–7.

Wattis J and Church M (1988) Psychiatric and physical assessment. In Gearing B *et al.* (eds) *Mental Health Problems in Old Age: A Reader*. Open University/Wiley, Chichester.

Wright S (1989) *Changing Nursing Practice*. Edward Arnold, London.

Further reading

Counsel and Care (1993) *The Right to Take Risks*. Counsel and Care, London.

Little J (1986) *Mental Disorder: Its Care and Treatment*. Baillière Tindall, London.

Norman AJ (1980) *Rights and Risk*. Centre for Policy on Ageing, London.

10

Social responsibility: an issue of age

Andrew F.J. Yates

The question of who has the social responsibility for the elderly population is a contentious one. Some may feel that it is the responsibility of
youthful society; whilst others may feel that it is a self directed, self
governing process whereby people take responsibility for themselves. If
one looks to organised religion for the answer, it may be apt to say that
there is a collegiate responsibility between the family and the community
to look after older members. Perhaps it is more alien to us in the western
world, however, whereas in other countries this would be a natural
model. For example, in Asia and other eastern countries, older people are
regarded as repositories of knowledge and skills and may even be revered
and afforded a sage-like status. However, in the UK, the question still
remains: who has this responsibility for the maintenance of this increasing
group of people who have age on their side? If we take the notion that
older people take responsibility for themselves, it is important to examine
the infrastructure that would be needed for this to occur. The concepts
that would require scrutiny are advocacy, self direction, social integration
and finally – the most current and important issue of today – ageism.
Regardless of how self directed the older adult is, it must always be

remembered that generally our society is very biased to a youth orientated model – whether that be ageism practised by the general population or whether it be the concepts of new ageism, which is the ageist beliefs held by health care professionals, who through a lack of education and professional reflection should know better and strive to practice under a model of anti-ageism.

Ageism

It is without doubt true that chronological age alone explains nothing about human ageing (Kastenbaum, 1987; Moody, 1988). Indeed, since time began, humans have dreamed with a Canute mentality of being able to turn back the tides of biological ageing, and find the fountains and elixirs of youth that grant immortality and unblemished beauty. However, it would seem that this is something which can only be dreamt of. With this in mind, it would seem more apt to consider what ageing may bring in a positive sense, and how it may be possible to harness this process to society's advantage.

Danger! Toxic society

Before considering the notion that ageing can be a positive process whereby people can continue to enjoy emancipation and draw on the benefits of a lifetime's exposure to new experiences, it is imperative that we explore how society's attitudes towards its older members can cause them harm. Comfort (1977) believes that the school of gerontology will be able to bring about a positive change in society's attitudes only when its members are not viewed as old first and a person second, but as people who are by chance old. The medical sciences increasingly believe that they have the power to manipulate age and ageing – to intervene directly in for example prevention of disease, treatment of maladies and rehabilitation from debility. However, this does not foster the attitude that to age is an acceptable or natural process which should be allowed to occur visibly and not disguised for fear of being viewed as different or alien.

It is a truism to say that all older people reside in a society governed by preordained rules. Rules are generally set by those who are younger and deemed to maintain economic productivity and stability, thus enabling society to continue its dynamic forward thrust. The reliance on the younger generation to set the tone is something that may ultimately require challenging and may be embodied in the contentious disengagement theory discussed below. The challenge, however, requires an investigation of how society intervenes negatively in the social, cultural, economic and personal lifestyles of the old. The UK, like many other industrialised nations, now has a greater proportion of older people than ever before in its history (Tinker *et al.*, 1994). In 1991, 15.7 per cent of the UK's population was 65 years of age or older (OPCS, 1992), and it is anticipated that by the year 2030 the proportion will be 20 per cent (OECD, 1988).

With the growing numbers of older people it is inevitable that much debate has centred on the task of supporting such a supposedly uneconomical group. This discourse has, not unsurprisingly, opened the floodgates for society to vent its spleen in a supposedly justified forum. The social malignancy that we now know as ageism was originally so called in 1969 by the American gerontologist Robert Butler (1969):

> Ageism can be seen as a systematic stereotyping of and discrimination against people because they are old, just as racism and sexism accomplish this with skin colour and gender. Old people are categorised as senile, rigid in thought and manner, old-fashioned in morality and skills . . . . Ageism allows the younger generation to see older people as different from themselves, thus they subtly cease to identify with their elders as human beings.

Butler saw ageism as a disease that infected all aspects of the society in which the older person lives, i.e. at individual and institutional levels, and included widely held beliefs that the older population is slow, irritable, feeble, unclean and boring. What Butler observed was the widespread subscription to negative stereotyping and damaging myths, i.e. an unashamed horror of ageing and of the old, and the emergence of behaviours that allow younger people to avoid contact with people considerably older than themselves. This phenomenon inevitably, as posited by Butler (1969) and Slevin (1991), culminates in discrimination in the allocation of housing, provision of hospital and community services, and the application of legal and moral codes of all kinds.

Levin and Levin (1980) discuss how the concept of ageism, with its negative set of stereotypes, has become deeply institutionalised within society. When ageism features at an institutional level, they note, it becomes more acceptable to express these beliefs overtly because they are inextricably interwoven with social, cultural and societal norms. The culmination of such a deep rooted institutionalized ageist attitude is inevitably to instill highly negative beliefs in the impressionable minds of our younger adults, thereby tainting the very people who may ultimately enter the health arena in the form of nurses (Slevin, 1991), doctors and other vital health care professionals.

There are various ways in which ageist values are spread. One such route is through the beliefs and values transmitted from parent to child as part of the socialisation process within the family. One extraordinary paradox of this process of discrimination is that within the family there must be some opportunity for an intergenerational mix. Because the number of people over the age of 65 is dramatically increasing, there are more likely to be sexagenarians and over within any family group. What does defy explanation is the extent of the labelling process, particularly as it can be shown that a large number of these older people do remain fit, healthy, active and engaged in the family group well into extreme old age (Abrahams, 1978; Hunt, 1978, 1980; Bond, Coleman and Peace, 1992).

Malignant social psychology

Following on from the concepts of ageism and labelling, it seems opportune to consider the enormous trust that society places on those whose responsibility it is to nurture, care and enable older people when receiving care – particularly when that role can easily become contaminated in various ways. The process by which corruption in the care relationship may occur is through the care provider exploiting the intellectual power and role invested in them.

In attempting to make this phenomenon clear, Kitwood (1992) describes the process of malignant social psychology. This was originally used to assist carers to re-examine their practices and to assist family and sufferers to maintain some control over their lives, and here it is of great value in clarifying the nature of responsibility. The relationship I am drawing on in this case is aimed at maintaining the older person's individuality, autonomy and personal integrity when in varying degrees of dependence. This state of dependence may be actual in that it is due to illness, or by proxy, i.e. imposed on the older person by the society which they are attempting to hold their own in. For Kitwood (1992), malignant social psychology is the dissolution of the individual in the caring partnership owing to carers intervening with over-paternalistic and competency laden notions to care. By way of illustrating the ten facets of malignancy which Kitwood describes, I have added to the following list vignettes from my own clinical practice, which I am sure any reader will be able to identify with:

- Treachery (trickery or deception). Mrs Jones was brought into hospital by her daughter to attend an orthopaedic outpatient appointment. She was admitted to the ward for two week's respite while the family went on holiday.
- Disempowerment: (deskilling; doing for). Elizabeth's husband died and her son became her signatory to ease her worry about balancing her household accounts. Elizabeth never managed her finances again.
- Infantilisation (inferences of the person having the characteristics and mentality of a child). I worked with one nurse who called all the older people in her care 'poppet'. They were clearly her babies and I wondered whether she actually knew their real names.
- Intimidation (threats, impersonal approaches, abuse of power). I heard one health care worker say to an older man that if he did not stop

bothering her she would have to give him some medication to make him sleepy.

- Labelling (diagnoses and self fulfilling prophecies). Albert, who is 66, firmly believed that after his myocardial infarction he was rendered impotent and that this sex life had come to an end. In fact, it was little more than the side effect of the β-blockers. After a review of his medications and some reassurance, his relationship disharmony subsided.
- Stigmatisation (exclusion, becoming an outcast). Martha is only deaf; however, she is treated as an imbecile by those she lives with. She is kept on the periphery of the community's life because she cannot follow the stream of conversations easily and it is a trial to have to repeat everything to her.
- Outpacing (care givers continue at their normal pace). Two nurses were assisting a lady to walk to the lavatory. They walked at their own pace, she was at 45° to the floor and was practically being dragged.
- Invalidation (failure to have feelings and emotions understood or even acknowledged). Agnes is distressed about not being able to find her mother. She is asked how old she is and then asked to consider how old her mother would therefore be; the conclusion is that her mother must be dead. Agnes's distress is not recognised and she is left feeling dreadful and grieving again for her mother.
- Banishment (being sent to Coventry). John had a testicular hydrocele. The other people in the residential care home would not associate with him because of their embarrassment, caused by the visual impact of his greatly enlarged scrotum.
- Objectification (failure to be treated as a person). This can only be summed up as '. . . if you do the feeders, I'll do the toileters'.

It is paradoxical for society overtly to subscribe to the belief that older people require care and protection based on a vulnerability that comes with age when, as Kitwood (1992) can all too clearly demonstrate, this may not be so. This would strongly suggest that society purportedly speaks a language of care and duty to its older members when in fact there may be a covert hostility and resentment directed to them for surviving so long in states of health and fitness.

Ageism in the medical profession

Another professional agency that could be argued to be responsible for keeping ageism alive and well is the medical professions. Butler (1985), when discussing medical ageism, notes how medical schools assist in spreading this disease by the manner in which they introduce medical students to anatomy and physiology. He suggests that the first aged person that new medical students are exposed to on the commencement of their course of training is a cadaver in the dissecting room. This, Butler believes, confronts the 'fresh out of college medical student' with the image of advancing age resulting in little more than a gradual process of biological decline and ultimate death, plus provoking their own anxieties and fears relating to their own mortality. To be presented with such a powerful image of ageing and the seemingly reduced value of the older adult at such an important and influential time in the student's training can do nothing more than transmit the fatalistic message that death is preordained and inevitable consequence of growing old and therefore does not require proactive measures. It would be more valuable to consider ageing as a biographical journey, and hence to recognise that a wealth of past and present experiences will be influential in shaping a person's future and that of those around them. As it stands, to promote the belief that rigorous medical intervention would be inappropriate, because the ends do not justify the means when the patient is of advanced age, ultimately makes people want to project what they as outsiders consider the quality of that person's future life to be. Although medical training has been criticised for how it portrays growing old, nurse education must also receive some adverse comment. In a study undertaken by Treharne (1990), it was found that student nurses who were engaged in caring for older people on their 'elderly' placement developed more negative attitudes towards this client group. It was suggested that this could be the result of inadequate or inappropriate teaching within the institutions providing nurse preparation. A further possibility could be that these negative attitudes were reinforced and further developed from the role models of their mentors within the clinical areas.

When providers of health care are in the possession of such beliefs, it is not difficult to see how ageism can manifest itself detrimentally in the hospital or health care setting. It would be easy to regard older adults as representing an economic burden, and their treatment to result in the haemorrhaging of financial budgets. The sentiment of increased age being equated with high health care cost is vividly illustrated in the writings of Callahan (1987), who regards older people '. . . as a new social threat . . . that could ultimately do great harm'. The cost of maintaining older adults' health are high and when one regards the multiple pathologies that this group may experience this is not surprising. However, this does not mean to say that active or palliative treatment should be compromised in any way. In financial terms the cost of care for this age group is great, but this should be considered alongside the number of older adults within the population. Between the years 1979–1980 and 1989–1990, the expenditure in England and Wales on health services for older people increased by 43 per cent, with £6697 million spent in England in 1990–1991 on community and hospital care for people 65 years and over (HM Treasury, 1991). The National Institute on Ageing has vividly illustrated the relationship between the cost of treating an older patient and the quality and extent of treatment offered. It is suggested that, in a study of 246 patients admitted with cardiac problems, those over the age of 60 years received less information than their younger counterparts relating to services available to them and the management of their condition, and less health promotion. It would appear that wherever one looks there is the feeling that ageing is inextricably linked with poor health and a general physical and psychological decline. This belief is dangerous and dreadfully condemning when held by the general population; however, when this is regarded as being true by those in charge of health care provision, there is a high risk of the older adult remaining in a vulnerable state with no intervention or intervention that is initiated too late. Comfort (1977) noted that there may be a trend for physicians to ridicule and belittle older adults, whom they view as insulting their medical skills and demanding too much consultation time. This, of course, may be indicative of the attitude that older people are less worthy of high-tech resources and interventions, based on the perception of their quality of life and reduced life expectancy.

The language of ageism

It has been noted earlier that ageist beliefs are subtly transmitted culturally, i.e. from one generation to the next. How this process works may be through the use of language loaded with negative stereotypes and mythical beliefs about the older adult. Certainly, the degree to which a commentator subscribes to these beliefs can be seen when the language they choose to describe people of age is analysed (Feezel, 1987; Nuessel, 1982).

As members of a health care profession, nurses and other health care workers need to be aware of how their choice of language may betray their inner thoughts and attitudes, and thereby communicate to others their own opinion of them and the esteem in which they are held. The eminent ethicist Herbert Spencer observed 'how often misused words generate misleading thoughts'. This is true because the power of language as a mechanism of oppression and a way of disadvantaging certain groups of people cannot be underestimated.

The recognition of language as an oppressive tool has led to the inception of the lobby for political correctness, whose aim is to strive to create a form of language which does not encourage discrimination and the oppression of certain groups of people. Certainly, the positive impact which this movement has had cannot be disputed for certain groups of people, such as women, those of ethnic or cultural minorities, those who experience a disability or learning difficulty, or members of the lesbian and gay population. However, it is certainly time for its powers to be extended to the difficulties that older people experience, particularly as an inappropriate use of language may drastically affect the quality of our interactions with this group of people and put them into a depowered secondary social role. Knowles (1987) noted that it was a common occurrence for health care workers to be heard referring to older people in terms which, although meant as endearments, were nevertheless potentially degrading and infantilising.

Sugarisms identified by Knowles included 'darling', 'love', 'poppet' and 'sweetie'. On first impression it would be easy for the reader to disregard a cry for these and many more terms to be avoided, and to fall into the trap of thinking that they are purely innocent and intended to create a warm, cosy, informal and personalised approach to nursing the 'elderly'. In my own clinical practice I have witnessed many examples of ageist language. One particular nurse called every patient 'poppet' and 'sweetie'. On reflection I wondered whether or not this nurse took the time to learn anything about the person, for example their name, personal qualities or individual care needs. This behaviour, I am sure, was nothing more than naive ageism, but nevertheless the consequence was patronising in the extreme. Interestingly, this style of social interaction was evident only when interacting with older people and never when working with younger acutely ill people.

It is certainly an arrogance on our part to think that we can side-step the important social rituals associated with meeting a person for the first time and feel that we do not have to invest too much time and energy in beginning to understand the person's individuality, idiosyncrasies and cultural make-up. Butler (1975) would argue that we do not feel the need to spend time investigating older people because they are 'old' and therefore society has told us all we need to know about them already. Older people, as we have already discussed, do not form a homogeneous group and, although they may share some similar qualities, they are not absolute clones of each other. Although advancing chronological age is something which should be prized, we should be in the business of paying tribute to the experiences invested in reaching those advanced years. Older people's past experiences and exposure to life are an invaluable resource waiting to be tapped. Developing assessment tools, including life biographies and value histories, will provide an in depth understanding into the person and guide the interventions that may be necessary. Such an enquiry, which will emphasise the diversity of older people, may, as Kimmell (1988) suggests, begin to redefine some major ageist assumptions.

There is perhaps not one of us who has not been placed in an emotionally vulnerable or embarrassing position when at family gatherings or the first introduction of a partner to parents the photograph on the sheepskin rug or the school tales have been publically aired. Although this is usually done with great parental pride, our feelings are nevertheless of awkwardness because a private part of our life is being exposed in a matter of fact and public way. While this process does not only happen from the older to the younger; it can and frequently does happen in reverse. The use of 'sugarisms' may for many older people be a source of embarrassment, particularly if they have not been called them from an early age, and may represent an infantilisation. Knowles (1987) suggests why we as health care workers may inadvertently infantilise older people:

> . . . perhaps for many of us putting the patient in a childlike role fits best our ideal of how he should be, that is submissive, vulnerable, in need of protection and dependent . . . . Perhaps for many of us the infant is the ideal patient.

The ability to tap into the correct way to address older people is not difficult: it simply means using their preferred name, avoiding being overly familiar and presuming no prior knowledge of them. In our attempt to make people feel at ease immediately, there is a tendency to assume that we as nurses automatically have the right to call people by their first names. It must be said that this is not so. There are countless numbers of older adults who have resided in a static community for many years, yet still address friends as Mr or Mrs. My grandmother, for instance, was always referred to as Mrs Yates and addressed her neighbours in the same vein. Although she was not opposed to being called Jane or Jinny by friends or family, she was brought up in an era when a formality in address was expected. I remember her attending an outpatient appointment at her local general hospital and being shocked when the clinic receptionist and nursing staff without a second thought automatically called her by her first name. Sadly, she did not feel empowered enough to assert herself in this situation and was upset by their informality. She felt that her own personal identity and privacy were being eroded by people who were over-familiar and also because she was seen as old and frail. Her lack of assertion was typical for her age group, and her immediate feelings of powerlessness meant that her consultation was not beneficial to her. She expressed feelings of being put in her place, as if the hospital and its staff had a one way window into her personal life; they could delve into her private and intimate self, but she could not do the same with them. This is an instance of how some incorrect assumptions and a wrongful choice of language vividly illustrate how a power asymmetry between the users and providers of health care services can develop.

The seven myths of ageing

The Search Organization (1983) in the report *Welfare Rights for the Elderly* and many other commentators have outlined some general myths of ageing (Byethway, 1996; Comfort, 1976; Perry, 1974). However, these broad statements are not a modern concept, as they can be seen to have emerged in early literature and beyond, for example in the writings of Simone de Beauvoir, whose portrayal of ageing was a true but unhelpful one. Cicero, an essayist and lawyer writing during the reign of Julius Ceasar, encapsulates four charges against ageing in the poem *'de senectute'* ('About old age'). Cicero declares that old age first, prohibits great accomplishment; second, weakens the body; third, withholds enjoyment of life; and fourth, stands near death (Hayslip and Paneck, 1992). The general tenets of Cicero's views of ageing can clearly be seen in those which are popular today, and which will be deconstructed shortly. It should be considered that, if these statements are to be accepted as mythical, it is important to begin to understand that they are grounded in nothing more than abject ageism. So prevalent and powerful are the myths that there is a real danger that older people begin to believe in them themselves, and allow them to impede adaptive responses to ageing (Kausler, 1991; Bennett and Eckman, 1973).

Although the myths of ageing which I present next could be argued to be nothing more than gerontological scare mongering, and may not appear to be grounded in our comfortable society, it is worth considering them. From what I have observed in practice and on reading the literature, I would exhort that they are given the consideration which they so richly deserve and not conveniently brushed under the youth orientated carpet because they call into question our brainwashed belief that we do offer people with age equity and equality within our society.

The myth of chronology

The easiest way that I can find to sum up this myth in a understandable way is to quote Chili Bouchier, screen star of the silent and talkie movies, who was applauded after her age of 85 years was revealed by a chat show host. As the applause reached its climax, she gave the most poignant reminder that she was a person who had lived rather than just survived: she replied 'I did nothing, I only lived'. This rather echoes de Beauvoir: when asked about her life goals, she retorts 'My life would be a beautiful story come true, a story I would make up as I went along'. Thus again a plea for a greater biographical approach to the care of older people.

The myth of chronology presumes that the number of years lived equals the extent to which biological, psychological and sociological factors affect the person, and that this is consistent with all people of that age. What this is again presuming is that older adults are a homogeneous group. The truth of the matter is that being able to cross off the passing years, like the tally chart of the prison cell wall, does not mean that we understand anything about what it is like to grow old. Back in 1987, Kastenbaum summarised this myth beautifully when asking us to remember that *'we know that chronological age alone explains nothing about human ageing'*. Certainly, it was Bouchier's life events and achievements which were to be applauded, and not her passive collection of years.

The importance of the life events contributing to the older person's present and future interaction with society can be and often is all too easily forgotten. The bizarre belief in chronological age and anticipated biological vulnerability endangers the very autonomy of the person. From this notion, it is too easy for paternalistic care practices to emerge and smother the life out of the older person. This need to care for those whom we regard as vulnerable has the potential to extinguish the flame of life. The desire to protect from harm, and maybe life itself, reduces exposure to the rigors and stresses of living and brings about an avoidance of the unpalatable, thus cocooning the person in a sterile endurance deprived of the life blood of emotion that human beings survive and thrive on.

It therefore seems a strange practice to assume unquestioned protection of those who may be very well equipped to hold their own and to assert their desires simply because we deem them to be old. If protection is needed, let its intensity, boundaries and duration be defined less by us and more by the recipient. However, to do this we need to listen and be guided, relinquishing our well meaning but invasive desire to intervene in the older person's life unquestionably.

The myth of ill health

This myth is grounded in the mis-assumption that ageing inevitably results in a biological catastrophe that renders the older person incapable of anything more than the involuntary action of breathing. Thereby permitting those who are healthy to define the continued ability of those whom they deem to be unhealthy for whatever reason.

Without exception, as we age there are some ensuing physiological and medical sticking points (as discussed elsewhere in this book). The presumption that being young equals good health and growing older equals poor health is not necessarily as straightforward as it first appears: poor health is not the sole prerogative of the old as good health is not always to be found in the young. There are various medical conditions which are more likely to affect older adults than their younger counterparts, but this does not mean that there is not an adaptive response which will buffer or minimise the extent to which disability or lifestyle is compromised.

There are two areas of tremendous concern with this readily abounding myth. The lesser is that of the development of the self fulfilling prophecy, which will be discussed later in this chapter. However, the most concerning ramification of this myth is that health care providers may presume that old age naturally leads on to ill health and an insidious deterioration into chronicity and inactivity. Unfortunately, when this belief becomes translated into clinical practice, medical and psychological conditions which are eminently treatable remain undetected, leaving the older adult in an unnecessary state of illness and debility. A good example of this is current concern about underdiagnosed cardiac failure due to medicine's preoccupation with age related changes explaining any biological illness.

One great danger when working with older adults in any clinical setting is that it is all too easy to become seduced by the belief that ageing equates with poor health and dependency, and is a time of great sorrow and a yearning for those halcyon days of youth. Day (1988) and Whitaker (1991) among others acknowledge how health care professionals, when exposed regularly to a relatively small and unrepresentative sample of the older population, can begin to generalise the problems of their patients to the entire older population, thus fostering what many now term 'New Ageism'.

The myth that all older adults develop senile dementia

Although the incidence of Alzheimer's type dementia does increase with age, it is a fallacy to think that all older adults will develop it. Undoubtedly the occurrence of dementia is a problem for the older population, particularly as it can be seen that the probability of developing it does increase with age (Table 10.1). Although dementia does appear to abound, depression is the most common mental health problem faced by older people. Aitken (1995) suggests that depressive symptoms have been estimated in 15 per cent of non-institutionalised people over the age of 65 years. When one considers Comfort's (1977) thesis that 'old age is the season of losses' it becomes clear to see why this manifestation of mental ill heath is so prevalent when it is so directly linked to life events. Issues of bereavement, retirement, loss of economic stability, a changing self esteem and the movement into new accommodation are all precipitant of a reactive illness (LaRue, Dessonville and Jarvik, 1985; Phifer and Murrell,

Table 10.1 Incidence of dementia in the UK

Age (years)	Incidence
40–60	1 in 1000
60–65	1 in 100
65–70	1 in 50
70–75	1 in 25
75–80	1 in 17
80–85	1 in 8
85–90	1 in 5
Over 90	1 in 3

Source: NHS Management Executive (1995).

1986). All too frequently, depression is regarded as a natural consequence of ageing, and something to be tolerated. In fact, depression is not to be endured, it is not to be expected and it is not to be left untreated. Early detection is essential if the older person is to be unlocked from the unnecessary suffering of this potentially life threatening yet eminently treatable condition. It is essential for older people with depression to be treated as early as possible; however, detection is not as straightforward as it would first appear. Depression is not ascribed the prominence it deserves, particularly in the minds of many nurses and family doctors, who may be in the best position to detect it (Macdonald, 1986; Barsa *et al.*, 1987). This may be because its detection is greatly dependent on the clinician's assessment skills, as so often older people have a tendency not to volunteer crucial information because low mood is so often inappropriately linked with ageing. Nevertheless, speedy detection and treatment are essential, especially as it is widely recognised that suicide and attempted suicide is a major problem with this age group (NCHS, 1977; Butler, Lewis and Sunderland, 1991; Carney *et al.*, 1994; Grootenhuis *et al.*, 1994; La Vecchia, Lucchini and Levi, 1994).

The myth of rejection and isolation

Old age is not a time when people hibernate because of failing intellectual, interpersonal or psychopathological changes. Nor is old age a time for a quiet retreat into the memories of past achievements. Those who live alone, choose to stay unmarried, or enjoy their privacy and independence may do so through personal choice.

There are, however, older people who live in some sort of shared accommodation, whether it is with their family or in nursing homes (Table 10.2). There is a trap here that many younger and middle aged professional health care workers fall into: the presumption of loneliness. The *British Gas Report on Attitudes to the Ageing* (Midwinter, 1991) showed that 90 per cent of the population in the UK believed loneliness to be a major problem in old age. This somewhat distorted presumption was put into context when Midwinter asked older people themselves whether or

Table 10.2 Residential accommodation in England, Wales and Scotland in 1991

Type of home	Number of people
Local authority	100 210
Voluntary	37 499
Private	142 114
Total	279 823

Source: Department of Health (1992).

not they felt alone. In fact, only 22 per cent of older people over 65 surveyed noted that it was a problem for them; interestingly, this figure was the same for the general population. However, it tends to be assumed that all older people, if alone, are lonely. For some older people this may be true, many enjoy their own company, or prefer to be on their own, but seek companionship when they desire it. Nor should we fall into the trap of believing that older people have degenerated into asexual and solitary beings. The misconception that warmth, humanity and sexual partnerships are relegated to memories is wrongful. Yates (1996) explores the sexuality of the older person and concludes that only two things compromise the continued sexual expression of older people and these are the attitudes of the young, and the opportunity to find available partners.

The myth that older adults are unproductive

The myth that older people are unproductive and that the middle 50s are the watershed may be a direct consequence of what is summed up in the work of Cumming and Henry's (1961) disengagement theory. This myth incorrectly assumes that older people are no longer productive or producers of anything socially viable, and do not wish to carry on being creative and engaged in later life.

However, older adults do generally want to remain active and creative in later life, and many people of note have proved this point by achieving even higher potential with advancing age. There are many examples of older people who have continued to have an impact on society and have illustrated that creativity and older age are not diametrically opposed. (Consider, for example, Betty Friedan, Winston Churchill, Charlie Chaplin, Pablo Picasso, Bertrand Russell and Sigmund Freud.)

I would like at this point to draw on the work of Betty Friedan, whom I have cited as a testament to creativity and intellectualism with age. Friedan (1993) prefaces her exquisite challenge to the specialism of gerontology, *The Fountain of Age*, with a personal and painful experience on her 60th birthday. It is this paragraph which I want to share with you because it cannot be delivered in a more poignant way:

> ... When my friends threw a surprise party on my sixtieth birthday, I could have killed them all. Their toasts seemed hostile, insisting as they did that I publicly acknowledge reaching sixty, pushing me out of life, as it seemed, out of the race. Professionally, politically, personally, sexually. Distancing me from their fifty-, forty-, thirty-year-old selves. Even my own kids, though they loved me, seemed determined to be part of the torture. I was almost taunting in my response, assuring my friends that they, too, would soon be sixty if they lived that long. But I was depressed for weeks after that birthday party, felt removed from them all. I could not face being sixty.

What Friedan is illustrating is that she forgot to grow old. It was something which just crept up on her over many years until one day someone, namely her friends and family, reminded her that she had a long shadow and was now thought to be on the wrong side of the sun's warmth.

For many older people retirement may represent a turning point when lifelong dreams and ambitions can be realised. Academic institutions, the Open University for example, are not unfamiliar with mature students enrolling on degree courses. Nor should older people avoid pursuing courses of new learning. The sooner people begin to reconsider the view that older people are incapable of learning new material and keeping a retentive memory, the greater the opportunity will be to develop new pursuits and to tap into the capacious skills of older people. Commentators such as Salthouse (1991) suggest that myths of intellectual and cognitive decline with ensuing years is not as widespread as is generally thought. Many people revisit past hobbies put aside in younger years or develop new ones, and the pursuit of work related interests may still feature as important (Butler, Lewis and Sunderland, 1991).

The self fulfilling prophecy will be described later; however, it is worthy of note at this point that when older people are subjected to this myth and others, there may be a tendency to feel that other people, particularly those younger, have greater skills. Langer (1982) and Weisz (1983) propose that, when older people are exposed to such thinking, they fall into the trap of denigrating their own skills and abilities. These factors, according to the two commentators, are:

- Being labelled as old, i.e. colluding with how society feels they should conform
- Being prevented from engaging in tasks or pursuing activities that were formally theirs, because they are now being undertaken by others deemed more competent
- Being helped, i.e. permitting others to intervene without question, and assuming that they cannot help themselves, thus fostering a state of dependence.

The myth that all older adults have inflexible personalities

There is really nothing to suggest that growing old creates any significant change in personality, as there is no typical 'aged' personality (Pratt, Diessner and Hunsberg, 1991). The presence of some rigidity may stem from personality traits developed in youth, or may be the direct manifestation of social, political or economic pressures, which are loaded against the older person. What may be misleading is the trend for older people to develop behaviours that provide some structure and purpose to the day. This, in my opinion, is not the result of an inflexible personality, but an adaptation to being forcibly placed in a role which is antithetical to that developed in the so called productive years of their life, and may illustrate the yearning for activity and engagement with life.

The myth of rigidity and resistance to change and adaption in older age may be a defence reaction (Harper, 1991) to society's covert aggression to ageing. The defence may be as simple as a blatant reminder that 'I'm still here, still getting on with life and still able to hold my own'.

The myth that older people are miserable

The myth that older people are miserable may be more to do with the manner in which they are perceived by others than with how they actually are. Being miserable and morose has little to do with chronological ageing as a process, and may say more about the way in which older people are thus projected. The media caricature of the older person tends to be greatly magnified and highly stylised, with stereotypical traits, such as being 'comical, stubborn, eccentric and foolish', accentuated (Davis and Davis, 1986). The negative and unjust portrayal of older people in the media has been widely commented on (Bennett and Eckman, 1973; Palmore, 1971; Greenberg, Korezenny and Atken, 1979; Jubey, 1980; Dail, 1988; Bell, 1992), and is generally regarded as being destructive to the self esteem of the older person and as creating misconceptions in the minds of the young about the experience of growing old.

Recently, there has been much debate about the impact of television viewing on children and young adults. It has been suggested that portrayals of violence and other antisocial imagery seep into the psyche and influence the germination of unwanted attitudes and aberrant outward behaviours directed at the innocent and vulnerable. Inaccurate characterisations of older people by such an omnipotent medium does assist in the continuance of ageist beliefs (Atchley, 1996; Bell, 1992), and may be another means of nourishing the self fulfilling prophecy, and may be particularly so when the exposure to this medium is increased. Davis and Davis (1986) suggest that older people spend a considerable time viewing television (40 hours per week on average), and the treatment they receive for their loyalty is unjust. I remember a recent student of mine named Francis Voyce who was reflecting on the power of media images, and how such negative attributes of ageing are internalised. In a profound and thoughtful way, she lifted her head, and speaking mainly rhetorically, but to the rest of the group said: 'for the housebound older person, the television is the window to their world'. How right Francis is, and how people need to realise this quickly and act upon it.

The typical likeness of the screen older person is seldom one of a person who has not been ravaged by the passage of time. Simone de Beauvoir, writing in *The Coming of Age*, believes that western society is responsible for devaluing and belittling the old. She asserts that occasionally the old feature as being venerated as a sage, but more frequently they are ridiculed, seen as doddering old fools who are mocked by the young.

There is some good news in this saga, however. It would seem that these images are slowly beginning to change with the emergence of some positive role models (Bell, 1992). Dianna in *Waiting for God* is not perfect, but certainly illustrates that older people have an opinion and a voice with which to express it. Also it appears that the opportunity to particip- ate in debates and talk shows are growing, and this inevitably enables the typical older person to expel some of the fantasies that surround them. In summary, perhaps older people are not miserable; maybe we are just told that they are. The best way to find out for ourselves it to take the time to talk to a few and decide for ourselves!

Disengagement theory

From the moment that the sociologists Cumming and Henry (1991) published their work on the disengagement theory it received comment and criticism from the sociological world. Cumming and Henry (1961) offered disengagement theory as a way of illustrating how older people's place and role in society change with age. The process of ageing was viewed as natural and inevitable; thus, along with the usual age related changes, there was the understanding that the individual disengaged from any major roles or duties. In a reciprocal way, society would begin to relinquish its dependence or expectation of the old to perform these duties and seek to replace them with its younger members. It can be seen that this theory is dependent on a repository of youth for the replacement principle to become complete, and Cumming and Henry (1961) would argue that this would be mutually beneficial to both. However, the removal of older people from positions of prominence and influence, whether from parliament or the parlour, would only appear to be beneficial to those who are younger and upwardly mobile. For the older person the benefits may not be as easily noticeable, and they could become detrimental in the long term.

There are many problems with this theory. It presumes that older people desire to let go of certain occupational and social roles. This may be true for some, but not for all, and to generalise its principles to this heterogeneous group would be wrong, for many people who elect to retire early seldom do so without a strategic plan for future action and a patent network in place to support this change. The choice to begin to withdraw when convenient to the individual is one thing, but when that choice is not given, and the disengagement is forced by the society in which the person resides it is quite a different thing. Attempting to decide whether or not older people choose to remove themselves, as the disen- gagement theory suggests, or are forced to do so through the pressure of peers and society is like trying to disentangle the chicken and the egg riddle. Notwithstanding, the theory can be argued to be potentially dangerous, as it does seem to feed into the difficulties older people experience with the self fulfilling prophecy phenomenon and the potential for isolation.

A further criticism is made by Estes, Swan and Gerard (1988), who regard the theory as fuelling negativism and discrimination in social planning (i.e. the location of and services to housing schemes, access to inner cities and availability of transportation) and promoting the impression that occupational and professional skills have a limited shelf life.

One other negative consequence of this theory is that it provides a readily accessible window into some of the misconceptions which have been discussed above, namely the seven myths of ageing. The theory very much validates the belief that older people are dormant and in need of rest, tranquillity and a low key lifestyle. This myth is synonymous with the vignette of the white-haired bespectacled old lady who sits comfortably by the fire stroking her lap cat. Bond and Coleman (1992), like Estes, Swan and Gerard (1988), argue that the principle may also be responsible for a tendency to plan housing schemes in the quiet and soporific periphery of towns, away from the hustle and bustle of the city and with grossly inadequate transportation and leisure systems in place to support a retired population.

Self-fulfilling prophecy

Living within a society that possesses a very rigid opinion of how older adults are desired to act and behave, and a subtlety of sanctions to ensure their compliance, can have dramatic consequences for the older person. There is a great tendency for the older person to become self oppressing through the internalisation of negative stereotypes and mythical beliefs, and to begin to believe that they are true, and thus they become a reality. Inevitably, this can dramatically affect the behaviours and quality of lifestyles of these people.

Beginning to act in a way which is expected of the old, colluding with society's social construction of what to be 'old' is, begins to facilitate the notion that to age represents a feeling of differentness. The impact of this process encourages older people to see themselves as quite apart from the rest of society and requiring special understanding. In terms of the provision of health care, there may be a tendency for medical and nursing systems to compound this problem, through failing to recognise that the pathology of ageing has been traditionally portrayed in a negative light, thus fuelling the multitude of misconceptions that surround this group of people.

There are many examples of how older people either fall into or are placed in the position whereby they take up this externally imposed self oppression. One such malignant example is that they begin to believe that all adverse health is a direct consequence of ageing, and therefore refrain from seeking medical or nursing assistance. Equally, they are reluctant to develop new hobbies and interests, particularly if these involve new learning or the need to formulate new social groups and networks. Part of the reason why older people are inhibited from the acquisition of the new, and in particular younger populated social groups as they traverse the lifespan continuum can be explained by analysing the early but nevertheless informative work of Khan and Antonucci (1984). What they suggested was a lifespan process akin to a convoy in which at different times in one's life there was a peer group that offered support and assisted in coping with change. A typical convoy would be regarded as including supportive relationships with others who are intimate, for example specific family members, including parents, children, spouse/partner and close friends. This theory is like the astral system, whereby planets revolve around a central axis, with some nearer and more accessible while others are distant and remote. When older age is reached, the opportunity to access such a supportive network becomes limited due to movement, migration and death, and there is inevitably the potential for a sense of isolation and loneliness to develop. However, some systems do remain generally constant. It would be easy to assume that when older people are grouped together, or ghetoised, the difficulties of networking would be overcome. However, this does not appear to be the case as there seems to be a block to developing new friendships, and perhaps this may be attributable to the feeling that to invest the energy in formulating new friendships with people of a similar age is wasteful when death lurks around the corner. The potential for friendships to diminish with advancing age is something that needs to be challenged by those working alongside older people. Encouraging a reinvestment in living and the personal satisfaction of regarding themselves as still having a valuable contribution to make is something that should underpin our nursing practice. The process by which this is achieved will centre around continued adaptation which will be discussed in another chapter, but suffice it to say, intergenerational mixing is possible, and the generations are far from incompatible.

Interventions to counteract ageism

Butler (1975) has suggested ways in which ageism can be counteracted and the older adult assisted in maintaining a greater self esteem and being ascribed the regard and respect which they richly deserve. If the fight to eradicate ageism from our society is to be achieved, and the older adult valued, we must take a universal stance of challenging and confronting ageist attitudes and stereotypes. Each and everyone of us needs to re-evaluate our practice, and reflect on the question Do we advertently or inadvertently propagate ageism through our decision making processes or attitudes towards older people in our care? Are we guilty of assuming that the clients whom we see in the clinics, long stay care areas or general wards are representative of all older people, and are we using a youth model to care for older people? Do we perhaps secretly regard older people as a burden or as having no skills? If any of these apply, that does not mean that we should throw in the towel: it means that we need to begin to move on and use our skills and talents in a productive way. Regardless of who we are, there is something that we can do. Ageism is something which can be tackled at many levels, from challenging loaded and negative language to demanding greater parliamentary acceptance of the specific needs of older people.

Ways in which we can begin to mould the future are many. We all have a vested interest in ensuring that the future is better and more cheerful because in the blink of an eye it shall be ours. Some of the solutions listed below are discussed by the founding father, Robert Butler (1975); others are derived from the analysis of the problem. They are as follows:

- Older people have marketable qualities and skills which are valuable; they should regard themselves as a positive commodity.
- Like so many other oppressed groups in the past, older people need to be assisted to set their own benchmark and to develop a philosophy of what they expect from the community in which they live and interact.
- Enablement and not disablement is required – older people need to be in the driving seat and to begin to re-educate society by dispelling the myths and negative stereotypes that surround them.
- Increased financing in biomedical, behavioural and social research plus disease prevention, and increased research into the factors accounting for the differences in life expectancy between men and women are necessary (Butler, Lewis and Sunderland, 1991).
- There is the need to push forward gerontology and gerontological nursing as a specialist field and a means of understanding people who have *aged* and not just survived. This should consider older people from a health perspective as opposed to offering only pathological enquiries.
- The development of a body of knowledge needs to be established. Medical and nursing research should investigate specialist issues of age and ageing, and not assume by generalisation from a youth orientated model.
- Exposure to the well older person as users of services needs to be encouraged within training programmes. Only then will health care workers begin to realise that there is an invisible army of older people who are not ill, outdated and outmoded.

- Nursing education programmes need to challenge ageism from the very moment the students enter the institution, and to promote a positive feeling towards working with older people.
- Older people need to develop a forum whereby they can properly voice their opinions, needs and suggestions for the future. This may be through the development of action groups or associations.
- The generations are not incompatible, and therefore greater consideration needs to be given to how this intermixing can be accomplished.

References

Abrahams M (1978) *Beyond Three-score and Ten: A First Report on a Survey of the Elderly.* Age Concern, London.

Abrahams M (1978) *Beyond Three-score and Ten: A Second Report on a Survey of the Elderly.* Age Concern, London.

Aitken LA (1995) *Ageing: an introduction to gerontology.* Sage, London.

Atchley RC (1992) *Social Forces and Ageing*, 8th edn. Wadsworth, Belmont, California, pp. 181–6.

Barsa J, Jones J, Lantigua R and Gurland B (1987) Ability of internists to recognise and manage depression in the elderly. *International Journal of Geriatric Psychiatry.* 1, 57–62.

de Beauvoir S (1973). *The Coming of Age.* Warnes, New York.

Bell J (1992) In search of a discourse on ageing: the elderly on the TV. *Gerontologist* 32, 305–11.

Bennett R and Eckman J (1973) Attitudes towards ageing: a critical examination of recent literature and implications for future research. In Eisdorfer C. and Lawton, MP (eds) *Psychology of Adult Development and Ageing.* American Psychological Association, Washington DC.

Bond J, Coleman P and Peace S (eds) (1992) *Ageing in Society: An Introduction to Social Gerontology.* Sage, London.

Bouchier C (1995) *Barrymore.* Granada TV. 12 March 1995.

Butler RN (1969) Ageism: another form of bigotry. *Gerontologist* 9, 243–6.

Butler RN (1975) *Why Survive? Being Old in America.* Harper and Row, New York.

Butler RN (1985) *Productive Ageing: Enhancing Vitality in Later Life.* Springer, New York.

Butler RN, Lewis M and Sunderland T (1991) *Ageing and Mental Health: Psychological and Biomedical Approaches.* Springer, New York.

Byethway B (1996) *Ageism.* Open University Press, Milton Keynes.

Callahan D (1987) *Setting Limits: Medical Goals in an Ageing Society.* Simon and Schuster, New York.

Carney S, Rich CL, Burke PA and Fowler, RC (1994). Suicide over 60: the San Diego Study. *American Geriatrics.* 42, 174–80.

Comfort A (1977) *A Good Age.* Crown, New York.

Cumming E and Henry W (1961). *Growing Old: The Process of Disengagement.* Basic Books, New York.

Dail PW (1988). Prime time TV portrayals of older adults in the context of family life. *Gerontologist* 28, 700–6.

Davis RH and Davis A (1986). *Television's Image of the Elderly: A Practical Guide for Change*. Lexington Books, Lexington, Massachusetts.

Day L (1988) How ageism impoverishes elderly care and how to combat it. *Geriatric Medicine*. February, 14–15.

Department of Health (1992) *Residential Accommodation for Elderly and Younger Physically Handicapped People: Year Ending 31 May 1991*. Government Statistical Office, London.

Estes CL, Swan, JS and Gerard LE (1982) Dominant and competing paradigms in gerontology. *Ageing and Society* 2, 151–64.

Feezel D (1987) The language of ageing in different groups. *Gerontologist* 22, 272–6.

Friedan B (1993) *The Fountain of Age*. Jonathan Cape, London.

Greenberg BS, Korezenny F and Atken CK (1979) The portrayal of ageing: trends on commercial TV. *Research on Ageing* 1, 319–34.

Grootenhuis C, Hawton, K, van Rooigen L and Fagg J (1994) Attempted suicide in Oxford and Utrecht. *British Journal of Psychiatry* 165, 73–8.

Harper MS (ed.) (1991) *Management and Care of the Elderly: Psychological Perspectives*. Sage, London.

Hayslip B and Paneck PE (eds) (1992) *Adult Development and Ageing*, 2nd edn. Harper Collins, New York.

HM Treasury (1991) *The Government's Expenditure Plans 1991–1992 to 1993–1994*. Department of Social Security, Cm 1514. HMSO, London.

Hunt A (1978). *The Elderly at Home: A Study of People Aged 65 and over Living in the Community in England in 1976*. OPCS, London.

Jubey RW (1980) Television and ageing: past, present and future. *The Gerontologist* 29, 16–35.

Kausler DH (1991) *Experimental Psychology and Human Ageing*, 2nd edn. Springer-Verlag, New York.

Kastenbaum R (1987) Gerontology's search for understanding. *Gerontologist* 18, 59–63.

Khan RL and Antonucci TC (1984) *Social Supports of the Elderly: Family/Friends/Professionals*. Final Report to the National Institute on Ageing, Hyattsville, Maryland.

Kimmell DC (1988) Ageism, psychology and public policy. *American Psychologist* 43, 175–8.

Kitwood T (1992) Towards a theory of dementia care: the interpersonal process. *Ageing and Society* 13, 51–67.

Knowles R (1987) Who's a pretty girl then? *Nursing Times* 23, 58–9.

LaRue A, Dessonville C and Jarvik LF (1985) Ageing and mental disorders. In Birren JE and Schaie KW (eds) *Handbook of Ageing and the Social Sciences*, 2nd edn. Van Nostrand, New York.

La Vecchia C, Lucchini F and Levi F (1994) Worldwide trends in suicide mortality 1955–1989. *Acta Psychiatrica Scandinavica* 90, 53–64.

Langer E (1982) Old age: an artifact? In Kiesler S and McGaugh J (eds) *Biology, Behaviour and Ageing*. National Research Council, New York.

Levin J and Levin W (1980) *Ageism: Prejudice and Discrimination about the Elderly*. Wadsworth, Belmont, California.

Macdonald AJD, (1986) Do general practitioners 'miss' depression in elderly patients? *British Medical Journal* 292, 1365–7.

Midwinter E (1991) *British Gas Report on Attitudes to the Ageing*. Centre for Policy on Ageing, London.

Moody RH (1988) Towards a critical gerontology: the contribution of the humanities to the thoughts of ageing. Cited in Birren JE and Schaie KW (eds) *Emergent Theories of Ageing*. Springer-Verlag, New York.

Neugarten BL (1977) Personality and ageing. In Birren JE and Schaie KW (eds) *Handbook of the Psychology of Ageing*. Reinhold, New York.

Nuessel F (1982) The language of ageism. *Gerontologist* 27, 527–31.

OPCS (1992) *Population Trends Autumn 1992*. HMSO, London.

OECD (1988) *Ageing Populations. The Ageing Policy Implications*. OECD, Paris.

Palmore E (1971) Attitudes towards ageing as shown by humour. *Gerontologist* 11, 81–187.

Perry PW (1974) The night of ageism. *Mental Health*. 58, 13–20.

Phifer J and Murrell S (1986) Etiological factors in the late onset of depressive symptoms in older adults. *Journal of Abnormal Psychology* 95, 282–91.

Pratt MW, Diessner R, Hunsberg B *et al.* (1991) Four pathways in the analysis of adult development and ageing: comparing analyses of reasoning about personal-life dilemmas. *Psychology and Ageing* 6, 666–75.

Salthouse TA (1991) *Theoretical Perspectives on Cognitive Ageing*. Erlbaum, Hillsdale, New Jersey.

Slevin OD (1991) Ageist attitudes amongst young adults: implications for a caring profession. *Journal of Advanced Nursing* 16, 1197–205.

Tinker A, McCreadie C, Wright F and Salvage AV (1994) *The Care of Frail Elderly People in the United Kingdom*. HMSO, London.

Treharne G (1990) Attitudes towards the care of elderly people: are they getting better? *Journal of Advanced Nursing* 15, 777–81.

Verwoerdt A (1976) *Clinical Gerontology*. Williams and Wilkins. Baltimore.

NCHS (1977) Vital Statistics of the United States. *Suicide rates in the USA by Age, Sex and Colour 1975*. National Centre for Health Statistics, Washington DC.

Weisz JR (1983) Can I control it? The pursuit of veridical answers across the life-span. In Baltes PE and Brim O (eds) *Life-span Development and Behavior*. Academic Press, New York.

Whitaker P (1991) The dangers of ageism in clinical decision-making. *Geriatric Medicine* October 51–5.

Yates A (1996) Sexuality and the older adult. In Matthew L (ed.) *Professional Care for the Elderly Mentally Ill*. Chapman & Hall, London.

11

Community perspectives

Marilyn Cartwright

This chapter examines the ways in which health and independence may be maximised for elderly people living in the community and during any period of transition from home to hospital or vice versa. If care is to be truly holistic, there must not only be a continuity of care giving, but also an integrated co-ordination of care directed towards fully meeting people's health needs. Health is multifaceted and requires a multi-dimensional approach in its promotion. Education for health is a vital aspect of this, and nurses have a significant contribution to make.

The concepts of the individual, autonomy and empowerment are discussed in relation to promoting the health of older people and the ways in which community care seeks to utilise these. Recent political changes have attempted to create a more co-ordinated system of providing care, in which specific people are responsible for creating packages of care for individuals. Nurses possess the required skills to function effectively within this role and should seek to develop their contribution in this arena.

Older people in the UK

The proportion of older people in relation to other age groups has steadily increased during this century. In 1990, 13 per cent of men and 18 per cent of women were over the age of 65 (Department of Health, 1989a), and statistical analysis reveals that this trend will continue (Social Trends, 1994). It is predicted that by the year 2031 over 16 million people in the UK will be over the age of 65, with an increase in the older age bands.

A significant number of the over-65s use the health services, so this has considerable implications for nurses. Old age is frequently associated with a decline in financial, social and health status. Nurses and other health care workers may have a pessimistic view of old age, because most of their professional contact with this age group is with those who have health problems. Research has indicated that negative attitudes towards older people exist (Fielding, 1986; Snape, 1986; Bowling and Formby, 1991). In examining statistical evidence, it is very difficult to estimate morbidity levels: the use of hospital and GP services can be misleading because ill health may be unreported (Williams, 1989). However, a functional ability study of the over-75s in one general practice reveals that 60 per cent were fully independent, 36 per cent had some incapacity but were able to manage, and only 4 per cent were bedfast and dependent.

Ninety per cent of older people live in their own homes (Wheeler, 1986). Institutional care, which is often considered to be an 'inevitable consequence of frailty in later life' (Bond, 1990) is thankfully limited. The number of people in institutional care is set to reduce further in the light of recent government policy (Department of Health, 1989a), which strongly favours community based care. It has been argued that many people living in local authority homes could be cared for at home with adequate resources (Townsend, 1986); the crucial point is that of appropriate and adequate funding. It is a false assumption that care in the community is cheaper than institutional care. For the very dependent person, requiring multiple agency visiting several times a day, care in the community is a more expensive option (Wright, 1979). However, few would dispute that, given the option, most people would choose to be cared for in their own home.

Studies have indicated that institutional care of older people is unsatisfactory, particularly in terms of meeting psychosocial needs (Baker, 1978; Wells, 1980; Evers, 1981). The introduction of an individualised problem-solving approach to care together with the emergence of nursing development units (NDUs), notably those at Oxford (Pearson, 1988) and Tameside (Wright, 1990), have done much to raise the profile and status of caring for the older person and have publicised positive attitudes in care. A prominent feature of NDUs is that they are as uninstitutionalised and home-like as possible. Although home nursing does not automatically eliminate negative attitudes or a task orientated approach to care, it is conducive to a holistic assessment and personalised care of individuals and their significant others.

The elderly carer

There are over six million carers in the UK, two thirds of whom are over the age of 55. Three million are looking after a person over the age of 75 (Fry, 1992). Caring is a strenuous activity, not only with regard to physical activities such as lifting, bending and coping with laundry; it requires physical and mental stamina to deal with the caring situation 24 hours a day, seven days a week, often with the prospect of the person's worsening condition and death to cope with in the future. It is hardly surprising that as many as 65 per cent of carers report that their health has suffered as a consequence (Fry, 1992). Research has shown higher levels of anxiety, depression, low morale, anaemia, arthritis and diabetes in carers than in the non-caring population (Kennie, 1993). Caring also imposes financial costs, directly as a result of increased heating and laundry bills and indirectly through foregoing employment (Equal Opportunities Commission, 1980). Social contact also becomes affected, whether through strained relationships within families or in the restriction of social contact through the unremitting need of the older person not to be left unattended for any length of time.

Carers fulfil an important and essential role and have the right to be supported in this. Community nurses provide support, not only though the provision of direct patient care but through referral to other agencies for social care and through psychological support for the carer. The contact that nurses have with older people offers considerable potential for the promotion of the health of carers through opportunistic case finding. The inability of carers to cope results in patients being admitted to institutional care or requiring a greater amount of community services. Caring for carers is not only beneficial in human terms with regard to the potential problems it may prevent, but has cost saving implications for health and social service providers.

A carer's charter has been adopted in some areas in Scotland (Kennie, 1993). Although it has not yet been evaluated, it has been useful in the prioritisation of resources and 'will serve as a basis for future audit and quality control'. The aim of the charter is to focus attention on the needs of carers and to inform them of their rights and the services available. A further measure which is of benefit is the provision of a co-ordinated package of care to reduce the burden of caring. This involves placing responsibility with one individual to oversee services provided by statutory and voluntary agencies. Case management and keyworking, and their implications for community nurses, are discussed below.

Health and health promotion

The concept of health has been widely discussed in the literature. It is apparent that there are many different perspectives, ranging from the medicalised view of an absence of disease or social difficulties (World Health Organization, 1946) to the humanistic philosophy that health is a highly individualistic fulfilment of emotional and spiritual potential (Mansfield, 1971). A discussion of these perspectives is outside the scope of this chapter, but has been excellently pursued by Seedhouse (1986) and McBean (1991). A definition of health that encompasses medical, functionalist and humanistic perspectives is offered by Seedhouse (1986: 72): 'a person's health is equivalent to the state of the set of conditions which fulfil or enable a person to work to fulfil his or her realistic, chosen and biological potentials'. This theory of health acknowledges the wide range of potential that people have, those which are internal and lie within individuals and also the external potentials under national and international control of governments. It is important to discriminate between these in order to avoid a 'victim blaming' attitude towards those who are 'unhealthy' – an attitude which seems to be increasingly prevalent in society today, and which conveniently absolves anyone else of responsibility. Giving people greater control and choice is a popular political and social concept, but it must be acknowledged that the autonomy of individuals is constrained by the limitations put on them by external factors. Seedhouse's definition does not confine itself to physical health alone: it includes those subjective elements which an individual believes are important. Because health has so many facets it follows, therefore, that to facilitate health a multidimensional approach to health promotion is required.

The plentiful definitions of health promotion (Tannahill, 1985; World Health Organization, 1986a, 1986b; Tones *et al.*, 1990; Downie, Fyfe and Tannahil, 1990) underline this and in varying detail acknowledge the internal–individual and external–organisational factors required in promotional strategies. In discussing the elements of health education French (1990) identifies four aspects of health promotion: disease management, disease prevention, health education and the politics of health control. Public health policies, creating social and ecologically supportive environments, empowering individual community action and a reorientation of health services are the means to achieve this (World Health Organization, 1986a).

Promotion of health among older people is a multi-organisational and multidisciplinary responsibility. The strategy document *Health for all by the year 2000* (World Health Organization, 1979) identifies health promotion as a major component of primary health care (PHC). This includes preventive care and 'education concerning prevailing health problems and methods of ... controlling them'. Greater public awareness of the need for more information regarding health matters has led to an increased demand for knowledge. This has been recognised in one of the points of *The Patient's Charter* (Department of Health, 1992b) regarding the provision of information about treatment. Unfortunately, this appears to relate only to medical treatment and does not fully extend to providing information to help people to achieve their full health potential. Health knowledge is 'a basic human right' (World Health Organization, 1978) and should be given as high a priority in the UK as in the USA, where patient education is a legal requirement of care (Redman, 1984).

The government has declared that 'promoting choice and independence underlies all the Government's proposals' (Department of Health, 1989a). The World Health Organization (1986b) describes health promotion as 'the process of enabling people to increase control over, and improve their health'. This draws on the concept of enablement by increasing the ability of people person to control their health and thus improve it. Yeo (1993) sees the promotion of health as 'a helping relationship', which does not attribute blame but gives control. Nursing as a profession has enormous potential to influence health. Enablement, advocacy and mediation (World Health Organization, 1986b) are the three main aims of health promotion. The role of the nurse as an enabler or facilitator has been a popular theme in nursing literature. Nightingale (1859) describes the nurse's function in manipulating the environment to allow nature to heal the patient. One of the principal ways of empowering people to enable them to take greater control over their lives is to educate them, so that they are able to manipulate their own environment as much as possible.

Nursing theory and the promotion of health

Many nursing models include the teaching function of the nurse within them (Henderson, 1966; Roy, 1984; Orem, 1980; Roper, Logan and Tierney, 1985). In her definition of the role of the nurse, Henderson identifies the contribution to be made to health by helping individuals in the activities that they would perform if they had the 'necessary knowledge'. With the aim of achieving independence, Orem (1980) considers that 'nursing's role is the provision of help to maintain self care, either totally or in part, to assist others to provide that care and to guide individuals towards self care'. The goal of self care is achieved by means of five helping behaviours. Four of these are facilitative: guiding, supporting, providing an environment that promotes personal development, and teaching. In this sense, nursing is perceived as being a health promoting set of behaviours. Its energies are directed towards the empowerment of the individual, by placing control with the patient and facilitating increased knowledge and greater control and independence. Therefore, empowerment maximises a person's capacity for independence and minimises dependence (Malin and Teasdale, 1991). Tester and Meredith (1987) have shown that appropriate health education can assist elderly people living at home and positively influence their wellbeing. They believe that the most effective method of education within this age group is person to person contact. Nurses are ideally placed within the community to meet the health education needs of older people. They not only have contact with unwell older people in surgeries, clinics and domiciliary settings, but also have contact with well older people who may be carers, neighbours or acquaintances of patients. The Cumberledge Report (Department of Health and Social Security, 1986) points out that community nurses could broaden their roles to be more proactive in relation to health. Practice nurses are now heavily involved in screening clinics, and district nurses and health visitors have the skills required to develop and manage older people's screening (Ross, 1990) and health promotion initiatives.

Roper, Logan and Tierney (1985) identify teaching as a specific nursing activity. It is through the process of learning that adaptation to illness is possible (Roy, 1984). Coutts and Hardy (1985) have discussed this aspect of teaching for health 'since learning is an essential part of adapting it can be argued that all nursing is teaching'. This viewpoint of nursing is shared by Benner (1984), who explores what she calls the 'teaching–coaching' function of the nurse in relation to guiding and supporting patients through episodes of illness. Teaching is an essential part of nursing and its value in the provision of competent quality care is acknowledged by Macleod-Clark and Webb (1985) and McGinnis (1987). The contribution of patient education in care has been recognised for many years. Schweer and Dayani (1973) call for it to be approached as a therapeutic tool in patient care and consider 'thoughtful and appropriate' education to be the 'essence of rehabilitation'. Teaching is an important part of nursing, but it is particularly so in community nursing because contact time with clients, patients and carers is very limited. District nurses need to be skilled in 'distance caring', which they define as helping clients, patients and carers to cope effectively during the time when they are not physically present giving care. Much of the emphasis in care is directed towards enabling people to manage effectively as independently as possible, rather than on the 'present' provision of patient care.

Humanism in nursing

The increasing emphasis in the literature on the nurse's role as teacher or educator has coincided with the developing philosophy of humanistic care in nursing. Over the last three decades nurse writers have increasingly discussed the concept of holistic care. The management of the delivery of care has moved from task allocation to team nursing, patient allocation and primary nursing. There has been a shift in emphasis from the needs and wishes of the organisation to those of the client/patient and from the nurse as a carer caring for patients to one who also cares about the person and the fulfilment of their health needs and potential. With the emergence in the literature of the patient as a person has come the perspective of enablement towards self care or partial self care where the patient and family are partners in care rather than passive recipients. These developments have reflected international perspectives regarding health and its promotion. The World Health Organization (1978) has declared the importance of participation in decision making between communities, individuals and health care workers. This movement towards humanistic and holistic care of individuals and communities has been paralleled by changes in nurse education (English National Board, 1985; UKCC, 1986), which has far greater emphasis on nursing in non-institutional settings.

The individual, autonomy and empowerment

The concept of empowerment is considered to be central in health promotion in order to develop an individual's autonomy and potential (Downie, Fyfe and Tannahil, 1990). Autonomy encompasses the values of 'self determination, self government, sense of responsibility and self development'. It is viewed as a 'value', an ideal state, and the individual is impeded from achieving it by social and economic forces. The importance of empowering people is also emphasised by Yeo (1993), who considers it to be 'the primary goal and guiding value of health promotion'. In promoting health, the nurse assists people to overcome some of the barriers to achieving autonomy by teaching–coaching (Benner, 1984) them in health issues. This partnership in care acknowledges the value of the person. It is respectful of the individual, by being a partnership of equals rather than a paternalistic relationship. Humanistic nursing, or 'new nursing' as termed by Salvage (1990), respects and values the person as an individual, and increases their self esteem and consequently their personal capacity to adapt to illness. Nightingale (1859) writes of nurses manipulating external factors so that healing can occur. By empowering the person, the nurse enables individuals to manipulate or influence external factors to promote healing and/or prevent ill-health. This facilitative role of the district nurse is described by Turton (1984) as 'enabling patients and carers to co-operate effectively in sharing information and maximising their potential in a more egalitarian relationship'.

In his discussion on the relationship between empowerment and health, Rissell (1994) points out that there is no specific research evidence to prove that those who consider themselves to have greater control are healthier. However, there is evidence that groups who feel powerless experience worse health (Smith, 1990). This viewpoint is supported by a working group set up by Age Concern and the King's Fund Institute, who have identified that studies in the UK 'frequently emphasise the importance to individuals of such qualities as autonomy, morale, independence and self esteem, and the relationships of these to health' (King's Fund, 1988). The group also considers that increasing the autonomy of elderly people will probably result in a 'significant improvement in their health'. Health promotion has the potential to benefit all age groups. Demographic changes are resulting in increased numbers of older people, particularly the over-75s, and this trend is set to continue (Social Trends, 1994). The over-65s make more demands on the health services than any other age group, and 74 per cent of the district nurse's time is spent with people of this age (Dunnell and Dobbs, 1982). The implications of this for community nurses is discussed below. Health promotion is essential if older people of the future, who will have fewer family and social carers, are to be equipped for self care to a greater degree than at present.

Nurses' perceptions of health promotion

Research into this topic reveals interesting findings of how community nurses perceive educating for health in their work. Turton (1983) discovered that district nurses' perception of health education was either medically or behaviourally orientated. It was seen as telling people about the health services available to them, or a 'don't do' activity. She suggests that the reason for this is the 'conceptual separation of health education and nursing care'. Health visitors have traditionally been seen to be involved in the area of health promotion, whereas district nurses undertake the nursing care of patients at home or in the doctor's surgery.

Four years later Slater (1987) had similar findings. The majority of respondents saw health education in terms of a behaviour change or medical approach. They did not mention the educative client centred or social change approaches. The holistic view of nursing care that nurses have does not appear to extend to the concept of health promotion. A qualitative investigation by Gott and O'Brien (1990) into the attitudes of district nurses, health visitors and practice nurses clearly confirms the conceptual separation between nursing and health promotion. Nursing was seen in terms of motor skills, being medically directed, whereas health promotion used interpersonal skills of giving advice and lifestyle counselling. These results reveal a disturbing reductionist approach to nursing, by viewing it in terms of practical motor skills rather than the higher cognitive skills of educating, facilitating and 'political' activity. In the current social and political climate this is particularly worrying. Such a reductionism of nursing by members of the profession itself may ultimately hasten the demise of many nursing positions. If nurses do not seize the opportunity to adopt and expand their roles as health promoters in its broadest sense, nursing may not be able to defend itself from unsympathetic forces from outside the discipline, with the various facets of nursing being adopted by other groups of health and social workers. It has been suggested that this has already occurred (Vaughan, 1989).

Promoting health in general practice

There has been much debate regarding the usefulness of routine health screening of older people. The discussions centre on the benefits of widespread screening compared with the demands made on resources. Kennie (1993) reviews the options available to primary health care teams (PHCTs): to use systematic screening or opportunistic case finding. Studies have revealed improvements in quality of life and reductions in morbidity and mortality rates for those undergoing screening (Williams, 1989; Kennie, 1993). There have also been several pertinent arguments against screening and the possible medicalisation of old age by viewing the elderly population as having unmet needs until proven otherwise (Macdonald and Rich, 1983). Screening to identify certain health problems may generate levels of anxiety in people which outweigh the benefits of having those problems identified. Research suggests that the vast majority of older people contact their GP each year (Williams, 1984). Freer (1985) advocates a case finding approach for those who consult their GP, because those who do not seek medical advice are not considered to be a high risk group (Ebrahim, Hedley and Sheldon, 1984).

Community nurses have been involved in screening and case finding in the past, but this has not been a widespread formal policy. Where nurses have been involved in strategies to improve health they have proved successful. In recent years district nurses and health visitors have begun to reappraise their work and broaden their roles to meet current challenges in care. Health visitors have increased their contact with older age groups and become involved in case finding with positive results (Luker, 1981; Vetter, Jones and Victor, 1984). An encouraging point which has arisen from research by Vetter, Jones and Victor (1984) is that health visitors are better at evaluating home circumstances than their medical colleagues. Health visitors and district nurses are particularly skilled in assessing people in the home environment, and have considerable knowledge of the practice neighbourhood and its resources. District nurses have considerable contact with older age groups, many of whom may be at high risk of health problems – for example, the very old and recently discharged from hospital (Taylor, Ford and Barber, 1983). Community nurses have a significant contribution to make in local health promotional strategies and the anticipatory care of older people. By adopting a multidisciplinary approach, health monitoring can become part of routine health care and remove 'the artificial dichotomy between preventive and traditional health care' (Kennie, 1993). As the research indicates, such a dichotomy also exists between health promotion and traditional nursing care.

Anticipatory care is one of the characteristics of good primary health care (Fry, 1984). Interdisciplinary co-operation between GPs, practice nurses, health visitors and district nurses is essential if the health needs of practice populations are to be met.

Home to hospital to home

The problems of transfer between hospital and community have generated concern for decades (Hockey, 1968), and have been discussed at length. In comparison, the transfer from home to hospital has received relatively little attention. There appears to be a conceptual barrier surrounding the institutional environment, which has led to a lack of appreciation of what happens in the homes of patients. Jowett and Armitage (1988) note that the 'community awareness' of hospital staff, in addition to their commitment to continuity of care, influenced the effectiveness of transfer home. This is not only confined to nurses: a principal complaint of GPs is that they receive either insufficient or late information from hospital medical staff and that this adversely affects the quality of care that they are able to give people at a particularly crucial time (Victor *et al.*, 1993).

Discharge

Documentation

Nursing documentation suggests that discharge planning is not a priority for nurses (Bowling and Betts, 1984; Waters, 1987a), and medical records reflect a similar attitude in doctors. Tierney *et al.* (1994) have shown that, at times when nurses have many demands placed on them and staffing levels are low, the prioritisation of work frequently interferes with information giving for discharge.

The transfer or discharge process is not generally well documented (Waters, 1987a; Tierney *et al.*, 1994). Accurate records can not only clarify 'the complexities of co-ordinating services for patients with multiple needs', but also serve to demonstrate accountability in organising arrangements. Although the nurses on the wards that Waters (1987a) studied had some knowledge of a person's social circumstances, much of this knowledge remained unrecorded and therefore its usefulness is 'doubtful'. If such details are lacking in patient records, decision making and multidisciplinary communication are impaired. This in turn affects the formulation of 'realistic plans' (King and Macmillan, 1994) for individual patients. Documentation should be accurate, comprehensive and available to all team members. Specific forms that invite staff to document social histories could help to alleviate the problem.

Focus of care

Many of the problems of patient discharge or transfer arise from the fact that the focus has been on care givers and the organisation delivering care, rather than on care receivers and their significant others. Recent trends in health and social care attempt to place the emphasis with the care recipient and 'promote choice and independence' (Department of Health, 1989a). Health authorities have the responsibility to 'ensure that discharge procedures are in place and agreed with the local authority so that people can return home with the support they need or move to appropriate care' (Department of Health, 1989a: 34). The government has instructed health service managers to establish clear discharge policies and evaluation strategies (Department of Health, 1989b) so that the transfer of patients is dealt with in an organised, rather than a haphazard, manner. The commitment to firming up discharge procedures is further emphasised in *The Patient's Charter* (Department of Health, 1992b), where it is one of the national charter standards. This standard incorporates decision making with patients and carers, and agreeing needs and 'arrangements for meeting these needs' with care agencies before discharge.

There is a concern that, if there were difficulties in achieving continuity of care before the recent policy changes, these will only be magnified by the expansion in the number of agencies involved in care. Problems in the liaison between hospitals and local authority social service departments have already been identified by the Audit Commission (1992). This finding is echoed by the Social Services Inspectorate (1992), which notes that, in a survey of five social service departments, only one had implemented a joint discharge policy.

If the focus of care remains with the person and their carers, discharge from hospital to home is seen as part of a continuous process of care.The word 'transfer' has been used in the literature, rather than 'discharge', to signify this concept. We do not say that a person has been discharged from the community into hospital, but transferred. It seems logical to use the term when referring to moving out of the hospital environment. The literature refers to the move from hospital as discharge so, to avoid confusion, discussion of the issues will use common terminology.

Planning

Discharge planning should be carried out from admission onwards (Age Concern, 1985; Department of Health, 1989b; Tierney *et al.*, 1994), not from the time when it is decided to send the patient home (Waters, 1987a). A holistic view of the person accepts that hospitalisation is a transitory and artificial phase of an individual's life. One of its purposes is to facilitate the person's adaptation to illness or the regaining of various degrees of independence before they return home or move to another care setting. Holistic nursing involves nursing the patient not only 'here and now' in hospital but also in the temporal context of 'before and after' in the community. The literature suggests that this has not been the case (Roberts, 1975; Bowling and Betts, 1984; Victor and Vetter, 1984; Waters, 1987a). Nursing models such as those of Roper, Logan and Tierney (1985) and Orem (1980) do incorporate changes from the normal pattern of behaviour, but standard hospital nursing assessment forms do not encourage nurses to document this aspect of people's lives fully.

Who should be involved?

It is widely acknowledged that there should be a multidisciplinary approach to discharge planning (Department of Health, 1989a; Waters and Booth, 1991). There is also a consensus of opinion that, to facilitate communication, a single named person of the health care team should be responsible for co-ordinating discharge arrangements (Waters and Booth, 1991; Tierney *et al.*, 1994). Several authors have suggested that because nursing staff spend more time with the patient than any other member of the team they should record 'more information relevant to the social diagnosis' (Waters, 1987a) and are better placed to co-ordinate arrangements for transfer (Rorden and Taft, 1990; Victor *et al.*, 1993). With the development and implementation of primary nursing by nurses and the concept of 'the named nurse' in *The Patient's Charter* (Department of Health, 1992b), it would seem appropriate for this individual to oversee the process of transfer.

The liaison nurse role has developed during the last two decades, the principal aim being to improve detailed communication between home and hospital nursing teams and to promote planned transfers of patients. O'Leary (1991) suggests that the liaison nurse could act as the discharge planning co-ordinator. The difficulty with this is that the large numbers of older patients may reduce the feasibility of the co-ordinating role for the few liaison nurses currently employed. Perhaps a more realistic model of care would be that of the liaison nurse acting as a resource for ward staff, helping them to incorporate effective transfer planning into their care.

Patient/carer negotiation

Despite government intentions that discharge plans must be agreed with patients and carers (Department of Health, 1989a, 1992a, 1992b; Social Services Inspectorate, 1992), research suggests that this remains a sadly neglected area of practice. In examining the hospital admission and discharge of older people, Victor *et al.* (1993) believe that patients and their carers 'continue to be peripheral to the process', with little active involvement, instead of having a central participative role. This is unsatisfactory, and research has identified dissatisfaction among patients and carers, who had been 'told of, rather than asked about, their discharge' (Tierney *et al.*, 1994). Several said that, although they had been invited to speak during the ward round when decisions were taken, they felt too intimidated to discuss areas of concern. Patient/carer participation is a crucial element of discharge planning (Jewell, 1993) and its contribution should not be underestimated.

The discharge process appears to be paternalistic and denies the individuality and autonomy of the person. Partnership in care is a recurring concept in nursing. It is essential that nurses examine their role in discharge planning and seek to facilitate the active involvement of patients and carers. The nurse clearly has an advocacy role here in ensuring that people's views are clearly represented – for example, during ward rounds when discussions concerning discharge usually take place. An assessment of home conditions and social circumstances cannot be accurate if people are not consulted and involved in the decision making process. As in the counselling or helping process, when it is the client who is best able to make decisions concerning appropriate courses of action, the patient and carer are the people who are best able to judge the suitability of discharge plans, and it is arrogant of health professionals to deny this.

Education for discharge

The period of time that precedes transfer from hospital is not only one of impaired health for the patient, it is often an emotional and worrying time. There is also likely to be much information to be remembered by the older person and their carers, in order for the transfer to be successful. The provision of written information to supplement verbal teaching has been advocated for more than twenty years (Skeet, 1970; Department of Health, 1989b; Waters and Booth, 1991; Tierney *et al.*, 1994). This is particularly needed in relation to medication, where increased knowledge could improve compliance (Waters, 1987a). Other topics that could be supported by written information include contacting community services, dietary advice, levels of activity and advice on lifting or moving the patient for the carer. It would be useful for Trusts to compile a range of patient information on computer, with the facility for staff to compile an individual information sheet for each patient. Knowledge is power, and health knowledge is a basic human right (World Health Organization, 1978). By educating people in this way, nurses are empowering them to have greater control over their lives and helping them to achieve their optimum health potential. It may also reduce the incidence of problems and avoid urgent re-admission to hospital because of medication difficulties or the inability of carers to cope (Williams and Fritton, 1988).

Early discharge

Current trends in hospital discharge have led to patients being sent home 'quicker and sicker' (Naylor, 1990). This has considerable implications for informal carers, who carry the majority of the burden of supporting frail older people. It also greatly affects community nursing services. Research indicates that the need for nursing care of older people increases three-fold after discharge (Victor and Vetter, 1984). Their investigation used a random sample of almost three thousand over-65s in Wales. Because of the size of of the sample involved, the findings cannot be ignored. The utilisation of the district nursing service increased proportionally in relation to the patient's age. Bearing in mind demographic trends, which will result in a large increase in the over-85s, a substantial augmentation of the need for community nursing can be predicted.

Hasty discharge

As we have seen, the preferred pattern of transfer is one where plans have been made from admission onwards, in conjunction with patient and carer. Unfortunately, pressure on beds often precipitates discharge (Waters, 1987b; Victor et al., 1993; Tierney et al., 1994). This has several consequences. Short notice can lead to difficulties for informal carers in making suitable arrangements at home (Roberts, 1975; Bowling and Betts, 1984). Hasty discharge can also result in the 'Friday afternoon discharge syndrome' familiar to district nurses, where patients arrive home without social service support, leading to a gap in care at a critical and vulnerable time in their illness. This can result in placing the health and welfare of older people at risk (Victor et al., 1993). There is evidence that poorly managed hospital discharge can result in re-admission (Williams and Fritton, 1988). It could be argued that inadequate planning could result in increased financial costs to the National Health Service in addition to the emotional and health costs to patients and carers. Nurses have a responsibility to act as advocate and emphasise the difficulties that may be encountered if a patient is transferred to an unsuitable environment. Failure to do so could be considered to be a neglect of the duty to care (UKCC, 1984).

The effectiveness of discharge planning becomes apparent when the older person is at home (Waters, 1987a) and when it may be too late for remedial action: 24 or 48 hours is a long time alone without support (Jackson, 1994). It depletes carers' emotional and physical resources and is stressful for the patient. The criterion against which transfer effectiveness may be measured is the extent to which it counteracts any deficit in the self care ability of the person (Roberts, 1975).

Improving transfer

Strategies that may improve the quality of transfer between care settings centre on improving communication between the staff and agencies involved in care. A principal cause of difficulty in the discharge process has been the emphasis on the organisation and disciplines delivering care, rather than on the recipient(s) of care. If care is to be holistic and patient centred, it needs to be acknowledged by giving the person more power and responsibility. A recognition of such a philosophy would be to provide patient held records. If people held a duplicate copy of their medical, nursing and social care notes and carried them between care settings, this would enhance communication between staff and promote continuity of care. In her research of discharge planning Waters (1987a, 1987b) reveals a discrepancy between nursing care plans and referral information to community nurses. Existing patient problems were not always reported to district nurses. Provision of such information would reduce time spent in duplicating patient assessment.

An investigation by Jowett and Armitage (1988) identifies that a major factor influencing the quality of the discharge arrangements made by nurses is their 'community awareness'. They advocate 'directories' of local social service, voluntary agency and community nursing resources for ward staff. The contribution of liaison nurses in informally educating staff about home care is also recognised. Nurses' appreciation of home care is also enhanced if they have undertaken post-registration courses in community care. Jowett and Armitage (1988) suggest that such courses could enhance the continuity of care. Changes in preregistration education, with its increased emphasis on non-institutional care (UKCC, 1986), has the potential to improve the community awareness of nurses and the continuity of care of patients.

Case management

Case management is a recent development in the organisation of care, which has considerable implications for nurses working with older people. This method of practice has been developed in the USA during the last two decades, motivated by a desire to co-ordinate services and contain costs (Beardshaw and Trowell, 1990). Current social policy in the UK is strongly in favour of non-institutional care. The service led provision, with its gaps and duplications of care, which existed prior to the recent community care reforms, is clearly unsatisfactory. In the latter part of the 1980s, the government and other organisations such as the King's Fund and the Nuffield Institute provided funds for several research studies to examine the value of case management or keyworker models of assessing and administering 'packages' of care. The results were favourable and this method of care delivery is firmly enshrined in government policy, with 'proper assessment and good case management' being the 'cornerstone of high quality care' (Department of Health, 1989a).

There is no single way of administering care under this system. Three models of case management have been identified (Beardshaw and Towell, 1990): the social entrepreneurship model, the service brokerage model and the keyworker system. The social entrepreneurship model is one in which case managers hold a budget and buy 'services' from various formal and informal sources. Most schemes in the UK follow this pattern of working; one example is the Kent Community Care Scheme (Challis and Davis, 1986). In the service brokerage model, case co-ordinators are separate from service provider organisations and act as client representatives in co-ordinating packages of care to meet client needs. The Camden and Islington community care project (Pilling, 1988) is based on this. Experience in the USA suggests that this model is unable to achieve co-ordinated care because the case manager has little control over availability of services and funding and services are therefore fragmented (Arnold, 1987). It does work in instances where services are integrated – for example, the On Lok scheme for dependent adults in San Francisco (Eng, 1987). A keyworker system has a single person who liaises between client and multidisciplinary team and devises a package of care. The Gloucester Care for Elderly People at Home Project (CEPH) is a well documented example of this type of organisation of care (Johnson *et al.*, 1987).

Case management is considered to have several components: case finding and screening, assessment, case planning, monitoring and evaluation (Steinberg and Carter, 1983). This has been simplified by Dant *et al.* (1989) into assessment, planning, investigating services and monitoring. This structure closely follows the problem solving framework of the process of nursing. Nurses possess the skills required to function in a case manager or keyworker role. In fact, some of the community care schemes have utilised nurses in working as case managers or keyworkers, e.g. in Gloucestershire (Johnson *et al.*, 1987), Darlington (Challis and Davis, 1986), and Gateshead (Challis *et al.*, 1990). Research has indicated that, particularly in cases where there are medical problems such as incontinence, deteriorating health status or mental health problems, nursing input favourably affects the outcome of maintaining patients at home who would otherwise appear unsuitable to remain there (Challis *et al.*, 1990).

Evaluation of research indicates that this approach to the management of care (particularly the social entrepreneurship model) can 'significantly improve the effectiveness of social care for very frail elderly people' (Challis *et al.*, 1990). Demographic trends predict a large increase in the numbers of the over-85s during the next few decades, and one can therefore assume that the numbers of people who could benefit from this type of care delivery will increase. This method of organising care also appears to result in lower rates of institutionalisation and improved quality of life for carers (Challis *et al.*, 1990). These findings are supported by a King's Fund report (Salvage, 1984), which considers that the case management approach has many benefits: increased morale, improved mobility and social contact, better health status, greater capacity to cope, a reduced number of hospital admissions, and longer survival rates. Case management will play a large part in community care for the foreseeable future and offers considerable potential to improve the quality of care for older people. This is dependent on a satisfactory level of funding from the government.

In the current climate of cost consciousness, it is tempting to believe that community care is a cheap way of providing care. Evidence from the Gateshead scheme does reveal that the annual cost to social services was less under the case management system of care. This was due to lower admission rates to residential homes (Challis *et al.*, 1990). However, in terms of total costs to society (carers, the NHS and social services), there is no significant difference in the amount between standard provision and the case management scheme (Challis *et al.*, 1990). Experience in the USA also affirms that long term costs are not reduced (Kemper, Applebaum and Harrigan, 1987). In the long term community care could, in fact, be more expensive, because of the increased length of survival of clients (Challis and Davis, 1986). These arguments are reminiscent of the discussions that centred around the institution of the NHS in 1948, and the escalating costs thereafter.

Case management models offer considerable benefits for older people and their carers, with potentially little cost increase. The government has declared that 'promoting choice and independence' underlies all their proposals (Department of Health, 1989a). The model of a multidisciplinary case management team working in collaboration with the primary health care team would seem to hold particular promise and to be flexible enough to meet the widely differing requirements of older people in the community. The philosophy of empowerment that underpins the case management approach is congruent with current concepts in nursing, such as advocacy, empowerment, promotion of independence, enhancing quality of life and client centred care.

Mental health and learning disability nurses have a strong tradition of acting in a keyworker role. Recent developments have resulted in a course leading to the dual qualification of social worker and registered nurse (learning disability). Existing community nursing courses devote a significant amount of time to social policy issues, so that little additional input would be required to equip district nurses or health visitors to successfully function in case manager roles. Comprehensive assessment is essential to create flexible suitable packages of care (Challis *et al.*, 1990). It has been suggested that this may require a considerable amount of staff training in order to provide case managers with the required skills (Carley *et al.*, 1987). However, community nurses have these skills and are experienced in working flexibly and managing care for frail older people. They have also worked in a case manager role on an *ad hoc* basis. Hospital at home schemes (Waters and Booth, 1991) are an example of how district nurses have worked in such a way without requiring further educational input. The recent changes in skill mix in nursing, particularly in relation to G grade district nurses, is forcing nurses to evaluate their roles. Developments in the organisation of community care offer scope for nurses to develop their roles in the case management arena.

Conclusion

There can be little doubt that it is preferable for people to live in a non-institutional environment, and that hospital care should be an inter-mission in their lives. The increasing numbers of older people requiring supportive care and assistance in caring for others will place considerable demands on the Health and Social Services. Nurses have a significant contribution to make in promoting the health of this age group, across the continuum from wellness to illness, not only in terms of directly provid-ing nursing care and health advice, but also in relation to the manage-ment and organisation of care.

Many nurse authors have written of the contribution that teaching makes to nursing care. Nursing is seen as a health promoting activity for patients and their significant others. Community nurses are ideally placed to utilise networking to improve the health of older people elderly within neighbourhoods or localities.

The literature suggests a conceptual separation between nursing care and health promotion/education. This is potentially very damaging for nursing. If we as nurses do not seize the opportunity to vocalise our contribution in promoting health, and nursing is seen as a series of tasks, the profession will be greatly diminished in terms of the benefits it has to offer and ultimately in the numbers of practitioners employed.

The transfer of patients between hospital and home remains a problem-atic area of care. The nurse's role as patient advocate and in documenting social histories is vital to ensure that appropriate arrangements are made. It is clear that developments to improve discharge planning can occur only when the process becomes patient/family centred, rather than service focused. Case management looks set to remain as a method of organising community care for the foreseeable future. Community nurses have the skills to act effectively as case managers and should seize the opportunity to embrace and develop the role.

References

Age Concern (1985) *Policies, Practices and Projects. Hospital Discharge and Aftercare Initiatives in London.* Age Concern, London.

Arnold D (1987) The broker model of long term care: a rose by any other name. *Home Health Care Services Quarterly* 8, 23–43.

Audit Commission (1992) *Lying In Wait: The Use of Medical Beds in Acute Hospitals.* HMSO, London.

Baker D (1978) Attitudes of Nurses to the Care of the Elderly. PhD thesis, University of Manchester.

Beardshaw V and Trowell D (1990) *Assessment and Case Management: Implications for the Implementation of Caring for People.* King's Fund Briefing Paper. King's Fund, London.

Benner P (1984) *From Novice to Expert: Excellence in Power and Clinical Nursing Practice.* Addison-Wesley, Menlo Park, California.

Bond J (1990) Living arrangements of elderly people. In Bond J and Coleman P (eds) *Ageing in Society, An Introduction to Social Gerontology,* pp. 161–80. Sage, London.

Bowling A and Betts G (1984) Communication on discharge. *Nursing Times* 80, 31–3.

Bowling A and Formby J (1991) Nurses' attitudes to elderly people: a study of nursing homes and elderly care wards in an inner-London health district. *Nursing Practice* 5, 16–24.

Carley M, Dant T, Gearing B and Johnson M (1987) *Care For Elderly People in the Community: A Review of the Issues and the Research.* Care for Elderly People at Home, Project Paper 1. Open University, Milton Keynes.

Challis D and Davis B (1986) *Case Management in Community Care: An Evaluated Experiment in the Care of the Elderly.* Personal Social Services Research Unit/ Gower, Aldershot.

Challis D, Chessum R, Chesterman J, Luckett R and Traske K (1990) *Case Management in Social and Health Care: The Gateshead Community Care Scheme.* Personal Social Services Research Unit, University of Kent, Canterbury.

Coutts LC and Hardy LK (1985) *Teaching for Health.* Churchill Livingstone, Edinburgh.

Dant T, Gearing B, Carley M and Johnson M (1989) *Care for Elderly People at Home. Project Paper Six. Keyworkers for Elderly People in the Community: Case Managers and Care Co-ordinators.* Open University/Policy Studies Institute, Milton Keynes.

Department of Health and Social Security (1986) *Neighbourhood Nursing – A Focus for Care.* HMSO, London.

Department of Health (1989a) *Caring for People: Community Care in the Next Decade and Beyond.* HMSO, London.

Department of Health (1989b) *Working for Patients.* London. HMSO.

Department of Health (1992a) *The Health of the Nation – A Summary of the Strategy for Health in England*. HMSO, London.

Department of Health (1992b) *The Patient's Charter*. HMSO, London.

Downie RS, Fyfe C and Tannahil A (1990) *Health Promotion: Models and Values*. Oxford University Press, Oxford.

Dunnell K and Dobbs J (1982) *Nurses Working in the Community*. HMSO, London.

Ebrahim S, Hedley R and Sheldon M (1984) Low levels of ill health among non-consulters in general practice. *British Medical Journal* 289, 1273–5.

Eng C (1987) Multi-disciplinary approach to medical care: the On-Lok model. *Clinical Report on Ageing* 1, 5–11.

English National Board (1985) *Consultation Paper. Professional Education/Training Courses*. English National Board, London.

Equal Opportunities Commission (1980) *The Experience of Caring for Elderly and Handicapped Dependents*. Survey Report. Equal Opportunities Commission, Manchester.

Evers H (1981) The creation of patient careers in geriatric wards: aspects of policy and practice. *Social Science and Medicine* 15A, 581–8.

Fielding P (1986) *Attitudes Revisited*. Royal College of Nursing, London.

Freer CB (1985) Geriatric screening: a re-appraisal of preventive strategies in the care of the elderly. *Journal of the Royal College of General Practitioners* 35, 288–90.

French J (1990) Boundaries and horizons, the role of health education within health promotion. *Health Education Journal* 49, 7–10.

Fry A (1992) A voice for an unsung army. *Care of the Elderly* 4, 444–5.

Fry J (1984) Checking on the elderly – should we bother? *Update* 29, 1029–31.

Gott M and O'Brien M (1990) Attitudes and beliefs in health promotion. *Nursing Standard* 3, 30–2.

Henderson V (1966) *The Nature of Nursing*. Collier Macmillan, London.

Hockey L (1968) *Care on the Balance*. Queen's Institute of Nursing, London.

Jackson MF (1994) Discharge planning: issues and challenges for gerontological nursing. A critique of the literature. *Journal of Advanced Nursing* 19, 492–502.

Jewell SE (1993) Discovery of the discharge process: a study of patient discharge from a care unit for elderly people. *Journal of Advanced Nursing* 18, 1288–96.

Johnson M, Gearing B, Dant T and Carley M (1987) *Care for Elderly People at Home, Project Papers*. Open University/Policy Studies Institute, Milton Keynes.

Jowett S and Armitage S (1988) Hospital and community liaison links in nursing: the role of the liaison nurse. *Journal of Advanced Nursing* 13, 579–87.

Kemper P, Applebaum R, and Harrigan M (1987) Community care demonstrations: what we have learned. *Health Care Financing Review* 8, 87–100.

Kennie DC (1993) *Preventive Care For Elderly People*. Cambridge University Press, Cambridge.

King C and Macmillan M (1994) Documentation and discharge planning for elderly patients. *Nursing Times* 90, 31–33.

King's Fund (1988) *Promoting Health Among Elderly People. A Statement from a Working Group*. Age Concern, Institute of Gerontology and the King's Fund Institute, London.

Luker KA (1981) Health visiting and the elderly. Occasional paper. *Nursing Times* 77, 33–5.

MacDonald B and Rich C (1983) Look me in the eye: old women, ageing and ageism. In Williams EI (ed.) *Caring for Elderly People in the Community,* 2nd edn. Chapman & Hall, London.

Macleod-Clark J and Webb C (1985) Health Education – a basis for professional nursing practice. *Nurse Education Today* 5, 210–14.

Malin N and Teasdale K (1991) Caring versus empowerment: considerations for nursing practice. *Journal of Advanced Nursing* 16, 657–62.

Mansfield K (1971) *Letters and Journals.* Pelican, London.

McBean S (1991) Health and health promotion – consensus and conflict. In Perry A and Jolley M (eds) *Nursing: A Knowledge Base for Practice,* pp. 52–92. Edward Arnold, London.

McGinnis P (1987) Teaching nurses to teach. In Davies B. (ed.) *Nursing Education: Research and Development,* pp. 106–21. Croom Helm, London.

Naylor MD (1990) Comprehensive discharge planning for the hospitalised elderly. *Nursing Research* 39, 151–61. Cited in Tierney A, Worth A, Closs SJ and Macmillan M (1994) Older patients' experiences of discharge from hospital. *Nursing Times* 90, 36–9.

Nightingale F (1859) *Notes on Nursing.* Churchill Livingstone, London.

O'Leary (1991) The realities of liaison. In Armitage SK (ed.) *Continuity of Nursing Care,* pp. 65–75. Scutari, London.

Orem DE (1980) *Nursing. Concepts of Practice,* 3rd edn. McGraw-Hill, New York.

Pearson A (ed.) (1988) *Preliminary Nursing.* Croom Helm, London.

Pilling D (1988) *The Case Manager Project: Report of the Evaluation.* Rehabitation Resource Centre, London.

Redman BK (1984) *The Process of Patient Education,* 5th edn. CV Mosby, St Louis.

Rissell C (1994) Empowerment: the Holy Grail of health promotion. *Health Promotion International* 9, 39–47.

Roberts I (1975) Discharged from Hospital. Royal College of Nursing, London.

Roper N, Logan W and Tierney A (1985) *Using a Model for Nursing.* Churchill Livingstone, Edinburgh.

Rorden JW and Taft E (1990) *Discharge Planning Guide for Nurses.* WB Saunders, Philadelphia.

Ross F (1990) Key issues in district nursing. Paper Two. In *New Horizons in community Care. Policy Perspectives for District Nursing.* District Nursing Association, London.

Roy C (1984) *Introduction to Nursing: An Adaption Model,* 2nd edn. Prentice-Hall, Englewood Cliffs, New Jersey.

Salvage A (1984) *Developments in Domiciliary Care for the Elderly.* King's Fund, London.

Salvage J (1990) The theory and practice of the 'new' nursing. *Nursing Times* 86, 42–5.

Schweer SF and Dayani EC (1973) The extended role of professional nursing – patient education. *International Nursing Review* 20, 174–5.

Seedhouse D (1986) *Health: The Foundations for Achievement.* Wiley, Chichester.

Skeet M (1970) *Home From Hospital.* Royal College of Nursing, London.

Slater J (1987) Data on Health Education. *Journal of District Nursing* 6, 5–10.

Smith T (1990) Poverty and health in the 1990s. *British Medical Journal* 301, 349–50.

Snape J (1986) Nurses' attitudes to care of the elderly. *Journal of Advanced Nursing* 11, 569–72.

Social Services Inspectorate (1992) *Social Services for Hospital Patients 1: Working at the Interface*. Department of Health, London.

Social Trends 24 (1994) HMSO, London

Steinberg RM and Carter GW (1983) *Case Management and the Elderly*. Lexington, Washington DC.

Tannahill A (1985) What is health promotion? *Health Education Journal* 44, 167–8.

Taylor RC, Ford G and Barber H (1983) *Research Perspectives on Ageing 6. The Elderly at Risk*. Age Concern Research Unit, London.

Tester S and Meredith B (1987) Ill informed? In *Information and Support for Elderly People in the Inner City*. Policy Studies Institute, London.

Tierney A, Worth A, Closs SJ, King C and Macmillan M (1994) Older patients' experiences of discharge from hospital. *Nursing Times* 9, 36–9.

Tones K, Tilford S and Robinson Y (1990) *Health Education: Effectiveness and Efficiency*. Chapman & Hall, London.

Townsend P (1986) Ageism and social policy. In Phillipson C and Walker A (eds) *Ageing and Social Policy*, pp. 15–44. Gower, Aldershot.

Turton P (1983) Health education and the district nurse. *Nursing Times Community Outlook*, 79, 222–30.

Turton P (1984) Nurses working in the community. *Nursing Times* 80, 40–2.

UKCC (1984) *Code of Professional Conduct for the Nurse, Midwife and Health Visitor*, 2nd ed. UKCC, London.

UKCC (1986) *Project 2000. A New Preparation for Practice*. UKCC, London.

UKCC (1989) *Exercising Accountability*. UKCC, London.

Vaughan B (1989) Autonomy and accountability. *Nursing Times* 85, 54–5.

Vetter NJ, Jones DA and Victor CR (1984) Effect of health visitors working with elderly patients in general practice: a randomised controlled trial. *British Medical Journal* 228, 369–72.

Victor CR and Vetter NJ (1984) DNs and the elderly after hospital discharge. *Nursing Times* 80, 61–2.

Victor CR, Young E, Hudson E and Wallace P (1993) Whose responsibility is it anyway? Hospital admission and discharge of older patients in an Inner-London district health authority. *Journal of Advanced Nursing* 18, 1297–304.

Waters KR (1987a) Discharge planning: an exploratory study of the process of discharge planning on geriatric wards. *Journal of Advanced Nursing* 12, 71–83.

Waters KR (1987b) Outcomes of discharge from hospital for elderly people. *Journal of Advanced Nursing* 12, 347–35.

Waters K and Booth J (1991) Home and dry. *Nursing Times* 87, 32–5.

Wells T (1980) *Problems in Geriatric Nursing Care*. Churchill Livingstone, Edinburgh.

Wheeler R (1986) Housing policy for elderly people. In Phillipson C and Walker A (eds) *Ageing and Social Policy: a critical assessment*. Gower, Aldershot.

Williams EI (1984) Characteristics of patients aged over 75 not seen during one year in general practice. *British Medical Journal* 288, 119–21.

Williams EI (1989) *Caring for Elderly People in the Community*, 2nd edn. Chapman & Hall, London.

Williams EI and Fritton F (1988) Factors affecting early unplanned readmission of elderly hospital patients. *British Medical Journal* 297, 784–7.

World Health Organization (1946) *Constitution*. WHO, New York.

World Health Organization (1978) *Alma Ata (1978) Primary Health Care*. WHO, Geneva.

World Health Organization (1979) *Formulating Strategies for Health for All by the Year 2000*. WHO, Geneva.

World Health Organization (1986a) *A Discussion Document on the Concept and Principles of Health Promotion*. Health Promotion. 1 January 1973.

World Health Organization (1986b) *Charter for Health Promotion*. WHO Health and Welfare, Ottawa.

Wright KG (ed.) (1979) Economics and planning the care of the elderly. In Wright KG (ed.) (1979) *Economics and Health Planning*. Croom Helm, London.

Wright S (1990) The practice of primary nursing. In Wright S (ed.) *My Patient – My Nurse*. Scutari, London.

Yeo M (1993) Toward an ethic of empowerment for health promotion. *Health Promotion International* 8, 225–35.

12

Care of the older person with a learning disability

David Sines

This chapter discusses the importance of working with people with learning disabilities and their families as partners in care. It emphasises the need for the development of inclusive services to meet the generic and specialist health and social care needs of this client group. It also describes a range of intervention strategies within the context of holistic and multi-agency care paradigms.

Older people with a learning disability have exactly the same needs as other members of society; their wants and ambitions are no different from those of their peers. In recognition of these similarities, and based on the principles of equity and justice, care for this client group is based on the 'ordinary life' model or on the principle of normalisation (Towell, 1988). However, there is no doubt that, when issues and consequences of ageing combine with those of learning disability, a more directed and specialist response may be demanded from the caring agencies.

An image commonly portrayed of older people is that of poor health, both physically and mentally, and of active disengagement from community life. Little acknowledgement is given to their life experiences and the contribution they can continue to make to society and to their peers.

The main problem faced by older people with learning disabilities is the persistence of a range of negative images that compare their status with that of younger persons. Consequently, it is the challenge of each carer to develop insight into and understanding of the needs of older persons and to do so with the aim of understanding the conditions (societal and physical) that affect them.

The rights of individuals in no way diminish with advancing years. The autonomy of the should be respected at all times and, for those with severe learning disabilities who are no longer autonomous, the views and opinions of their representatives (or advocates) should be sought regarding any aspect of their care. The 1992 *Patient's Charter* reinforces this principle (Department of Health, 1992). This chapter follows these concepts and emphasises the dynamic role that nurses may assume as they work in partnership with older people with learning disabilities and their families to promote valued lifestyles for service users in the community.

One other essential precept is that care for this client group is essentially grounded within the context of 'a mixed economy of care'. The contribution made by various agencies involved in the provision of care and support for this client group will be critically analysed.

For each older person requiring care or assistance, a responsive and individually designed assessment of need should be considered a right. Where there is a complexity of needs, the assessment should be carried out on a multidisciplinary basis within the care management and shared action planning structure (Brechin and Swain, 1987).

Outcome measures, designed to evaluate the effectiveness of our interventions, must no longer be directed solely by indices designed to measure the prevention of disability or disease. Rather, outcomes should be measured in terms of quality of life and client and carer satisfaction.

The nature of ageing and learning disability

Learning disability is now associated with longevity, which in turn has been influenced by improved social conditions and medical care (Hogg, Moss and Cooke, 1988). People are now much more likely to survive serious illness in old age than they were thirty years ago. Advances in perinatal care have resulted in a much greater proportion of children with learning disabilities surviving the first year of life. Fryers (1984) for example, reported, a death rate of 10 per cent among children with Down's syndrome compared with 50 per cent in 1958.

As a result of the increase in longevity, policy makers and planners now have to consider that at least half of all people with learning disabilities will survive into retirement (2.5 per 1000 live births among those with severe learning disabilities alone). Issues relating to social and economic dependence may therefore be regarded as being synonymous with those of other older members of society.

Elderly people with learning disabilities are, however, liable to be more disadvantaged than able minded peers. Dickerson *et al.* (1979) reported that by the age of 45–55 persons experience the death of their parents and may experience some degree of sensory deficit (and therefore require spectacles or hearing aids). The loss of a primary carer may have major consequences for life changes for the middle aged or older person with a learning disability who may find that they are forced to move. Changes of residence invariably (but not always) necessitate a move into some form of supported living home or residential accommodation.

Learning disability may present in a number of ways, but is always associated with difficulties in learning new skills and competences in society. Some users of services have experienced an upbringing from their families and carers that foster unnecessary dependence and which make assumptions about the limitations that may be made as new learning opportunities are presented. Some members of this client group have also been exposed to a sense of failure in their lives, which may be the result of inappropriate learning situations and high expectations by society.

No single definition of learning disability covers all of the people who may require access to specialist services at some time or another in their lives. There is, however, likely to be some degree of accord among lay and professional people about what constitutes either more severe or milder forms of learning disability. Many needs may be of a social nature and relate to competence in that area. People with mild learning disabilities, of whom the majority will be semiliterate, may have held down some form of employment in the ordinary labour market. Most will proceed normally to older life and may require few specialist services.

However, for people with severe learning disabilities, there may be associated physical problems such as epilepsy, sensory impairments, mental illness, diabetes and respiratory or circulatory dysfunction. The person with severe learning disability will also require more intensive (and often lifelong) support, which should be offered by a variety of professional (and lay) supporters at different times in their lives. The majority will not acquire total independence or competence in a range of basic self-help skills, and will require supervision in most areas of daily life. A typical high dependency clients may have multiple handicap associated with profound learning disabilities.

In the UK, information collected by Hogg, Moss and Cooke (1988) from hospital records suggests that there is general agreement about the incidence of various forms of physical illness among the older population

Table 12.1 Percentage of people with a learning
disability who have various medical conditions

	Age	
Condition	*Under 50*	*Over 50*
Epilepsy	34.8	15.2
Hearing impairment	5.6	9.3
Vision impairment	7.1	8.2
Mobility problems	19.6	24.6
Diabetes	0.8	2.8
Respiratory problems	0.0	1.2
Heart conditions	0.4	4.8

Source: Hogg, Moss and Cooke (1988: 85).

with learning disability. From Table 12.1, it can be seen that there is a
sharp drop in the number of people with epilepsy, while hearing impairment takes a sharp rise with increasing age. Mobility and vision problems
show only the most modest increase. Diabetes, respiratory and circulatory
diseases show an expected pattern of increase in accordance with that
found in older members of the general population. The increase in 'heart'
problems is marked.

Day (1987) surveyed the physical and mental health of people with a
learning disability over the age of 65 in one large mental hospital in the
north of England. He found that 23 per cent had no medical or surgical
problems, whereas 33 per cent had one or more conditions with an
average of 1.92 conditions. Day found, in the same study, that 87 per cent
of people aged 75 years or over had one or more conditions. Mobility
problems were found in 34 per cent of the group; 24 per cent had
cardiorespiratory conditions; 21 per cent had hearing problems; 21 per
cent were incontinent of urine.

Psychiatric disorders are also prevalent among older people with
learning disabilities. Eaton and Menolascino (1982) and Reiss (1982) have
reported surveys of people with a learning disability and the results of
their work suggest that these people are subject to a wide range of
emotional disturbances, and that the symptoms of mental illness are
essentially the same for people with and without learning disability.

Day (1985) confirmed that the incidence of mental illness among the
population with learning disability was higher than that in the general
population. Excluding alcohol and drug abuse, he found that the incidence was fifteen times higher than that in the ordinary population for
older people with learning disabilities.

Dementia is also prevalent among older people with learning disabilities. As the life expectancy for people with Down's syndrome has
increased, so has the risk that they will contract Alzheimer's disease.

There is considerable histopathological evidence that people with Down's syndrome aged 35 or over demonstrate changes in their brain structure which are commensurate with Alzheimer's disease (Thase *et al.*, 1982). Thase *et al.* (1982) compared 40 people with Down's syndrome living in long stay hospitals with a control group. They found that people with Down's syndrome performed worse on a battery of dementia scales, thus confirming their hypothesis that Down's syndrome is correlated with Alzheimer's disease.

The majority of older people with learning disabilities have the same range of physical and mental health needs as the rest of the population, but these often present with greater severity and prevalence. Health responses must therefore be planned specifically to meet the individual and collective needs of these older clients.

Health and social care

Following the implementation of the National Health Service and Community Care Act (1990), social service departments have assumed responsibility for the assessment and co-ordination of services for people with learning disabilities. For the majority, care will be provided in the community and clients will receive their services from both primary health care staff and specialist community learning disability nurses in health centres and social service departments. For many, their needs will be similar to those of any other member of the population, and the approaches required to provide individualised nursing care to meet their specific needs will require sensitive adaptation.

Specific health needs may also be present in addition to those mentioned above. Such needs may be physical, behavioural, emotional or psychological in both cause and nature, and in most cases specialist nursing care will be required as part of a multidisciplinary support service. The need for care usually has a physical or organic origin that demands an intensive and often specialist response from professional staff.

In some cases the requirement for specialist services may be transitory and there may not be a long term requirement for support (e.g. people with challenging behaviours may require intensive support to determine more appropriate coping or learning behaviours, but may not have a severe behavioural problem that persists over time). Most people who fall into this category have accumulated a history or biography that has been influenced by physical or psychological behaviours or needs, and these in turn have been influenced by life experiences received in the context of their family, care agency or the society within which they live. The need for health care may be determined by a variety of factors relating to their social world and by the responses that are demanded by society, which are in turn affected by government policies that determine the way in which services are provided.

People with behavioural problems often require considerable attention and support. The intensity of their behavioural presentation will determine the extent to which services are provided and will differ from person to person. The problems presented by these people often challenge the coping abilities of carers. Typical excessive behaviours include self injurious behaviours or aggressive outbursts and violent displays to others.

To match individual needs to specific service responses the 'care management' approach had been advocated within the spirit of the National Health Service and Community Act (1990).

Care management

Care management places an emphasis on providing individualised services for people, and requires that we design systems that are sensitive enough to take account of each person's needs (National Development Team, 1991).

Care management requires that each person with significant social or health care needs should have access to a named person who will be designated as a care manager. Care managers will usually be social workers, nurses or other community workers and they will be responsible for getting to know these individuals and their families. They will 'map' their day-to-day needs and requirements and formulate a clear action or care plan to take account of their needs, wants and ambitions.

The care management system requires that service users and their families are actively engaged in the identification of their needs; it does not necessarily restrict individual choice to the current range of services on offer at the time the assessment is made. Care management is essentially a way of ensuring that individuals are connected to all the services that they require irrespective of the source. It is a model based on the principle of providing the widest range of choice possible to clients without reliance on any one service agency.

Once the care manager has agreed a package of care to meet the needs of each individual, contracts will be assigned to one or more service providers who may be selected from statutory, voluntary or independent sector agencies. Contracts will identify the exact nature and cost of services to be offered and delivered and will contain clear statements of responsibility and accountability.

Each care package will also be costed and paid for from a complex system of allowances, which will be co-ordinated by the local authority social service department. Care packages are evaluated against a set of common standards and their effectiveness is judged in accordance with the extent to which they meet the actual needs of users (Brandon and Towe, 1989).

In order for care management to operate successfully, it will be necessary for health and social care agencies to work closely together both at a planning level (where major service decisions and strategic plans are made) and at the point of service delivery. In support of this approach it will also be necessary to demonstrate that multi-agency systems are in place to assess client needs and to measure their effectiveness. Shared training opportunities for nurses and social workers and joint participation in the design of both care packages and service systems will become an important feature of provision for people with learning disability in the future.

The principles of care management rely on the promotion of individually designed packages for people, and thus replace traditional models which fitted people into existing services (such as hostels, day services and long stay hospitals). It requires that a range of opportunities are provided to service users based on the principle of integration within normal communities, and requires that people have the right to adopt and to maintain an ordinary life and to have personal relationships and friendships.

These principles point to the need for a radical revision of the way in which nurses, doctors, social workers and psychologists assess people and plan to meet their needs. The care management process has been one attempt to improve the way in which we match services to people's needs. This approach requires that sensitive information is collected about individual choices and wishes and demands that an individual care package is designed in response. This is a very different approach to one which recommends that clients are made to 'fit' prescribed criteria for access to health or social service facilities.

Philosophy of care provision

According to government sources, over 30 000 people were resident in long stay mental handicap hospitals in the UK (Department of Health, 1988). Fortunately, nearly all of these people are now adults, and children appear to be able to live either in their family home or in small supported houses in the community.

As a result of government policy, there is an increasing pattern of change in the way in which residential care is provided for people with learning disabilities. Many of the large outdated hospitals are closing, and over 40 per cent are actively engaged in contracting their numbers as people are transferred to live in community residential facilities (Sines, 1995). These facilities may be provided by a variety of social and health care agencies and together they form what is now regarded as the 'mixed economy of care' (National Health Service and Community Care Act, 1990). The mixed economy of care refers to the broader context of care by the voluntary and private sectors, who are now responsible for the provision of 20 per cent of care for people with learning disabilities (Walker in McCarthy, 1989).

The philosophy of nursing care is based on the principle of normalisation (Wolfensberger, 1972). The characteristics of ordinary living underpin this approach, which aims to offer a range of choice and opportunities to people with learning disabilities from which they may be enabled to participate in real life experiences.

Community care is based on this principle and refers to the extent to which shops, public houses, leisure facilities and opportunities provided to the clients in the context of local neighbourhoods. The proximity of access to main public transport routes and the presence of community centres and local community groups also influence local perception of the community and its inhabitants.

Most local services now confirm that their published definition of community care will be based on the key principles presented above.

Good practice requires that services should publish a set of general principles that underpin the philosophy and values of their community provision. Such a statement of philosophy should ensure that staff and residents share space, activities, toilets, meals, recreation, holidays and interests, and should aim to encourage nursing staff to demonstrate appropriate behaviours and attitudes that will promote social acceptance and community integration.

All services should be as fully integrated into local neighbourhoods as possible. Staff care practices should emphasise the importance of involving service users in the planning of their lives and should aim to promote the concept of advocacy to encourage their participation in all decision making processes.

Essentially, most people's lives revolve around their homes, friends, work and families and the ways in which they choose to spend their time according to their personal choices and the demands made on their free time by others. Recognition of the need to maintain social activities and friendships is also of paramount importance for older people. Participation in integrated social and leisure activities should therefore be encouraged, and important social ties and connections should be maintained.

Older people also have the right to expect that their freedom of choice, integrity and status will be protected. In recognition of this, services should ensure that the following rights are explicitly upheld:

- The right to choose
- The right to dignity and respect
- The right to a home of one's own
- The right to a meaningful occupation for as long as one chooses

- The right to personal and sexual relationships (without limit of age)
- The right to advocacy and representation
- The right to independence
- The right to take calculated risks
- The right to make mistakes
- The right to say no
- The right to choose
- The right to maintain skills and continue to acquire new competences.

Older people with learning disabilities now receive increased opportunities to have their care in response to the principle of normalisation, and efforts have been taken to provide access to enable service users to enjoy ordinary lives. This aim requires some degree of commitment from staff to enter into contracts with service users to provide specific services in respect of their individual needs.

Care for this client group is essentially a multi-agency and interdisciplinary responsibility, and successful care planning will depend on the extent to which service responses are able to meet the actual needs of service users in partnership with a range of professionals and agencies.

The ordinary life philosophy referred to in this chapter provides valuable criteria against which to assess effectiveness of care delivery. Towell and Beardshaw (1991) suggest that through the provision of advocacy for service users new opportunities and partnerships may be developed to improve the quality of life of people. There are seven key accomplishments, which will be necessary if nurses are to achieve high quality care for their clients. The extent to which nurses are successful in providing high quality services to their clients may be evaluated in respect of the extent to which they provide opportunities for people to receive and to experience:

- Integration
- Choice
- Relationships
- Image and status
- Participation
- Rights and responsibilities
- Skill enhancement.

Towell *et al.* comment on the need to translate these value principles into real action if improvements are to be experienced and introduced into people's lives. Using the care management framework and the process of shared action planning, nurses are ideally placed to respond to this challenge. They have been able to demonstrate their versatility in responding to needs in a variety of settings, and as they assist people to move from large hospitals to the community their skills and competences adapt to meet new demands and responses from their client group.

Planning to meet individual needs

The problem solving approach associated with the profession of nursing is incorporated within a framework known as individual programme planning. The individual programme planning (IPP) system has become as much a part of care for nurses working with people with a learning disability as the nursing process has for their colleagues working in other specialties. There are many parallels between the two systems. Both require:

- A systematic framework and approach
- A detailed method to assess and to identify needs
- The involvement of clients and their carers in the planning and implementation of care programmes
- A method of recording and evaluating outcomes.

The following principles underpin the IPP system:

- People with learning disabilities should be involved in planning their own futures
- Desirable futures should be planned for people with learning disabilities
- All relevant people should be involved in the planning process
- Services should be co-ordinated to meet people's real needs
- Service deficiencies should be identified and used in the planning of future services.

Brechin and Swain (1987) provide an opportunity to further enhance the IPP system and introduce the concept of 'shared action planning', which emphasises the importance of relationships 'being the heart of the matter'. They start their analysis of shared action planning with the following passage (p. 3):

> Let us start from where you are: you are already a skilled person. The skills discussed and explored in this book are not just for 'experts', though many professionals would see them as crucial to their work. These skills are part and parcel of day to day living. They are used in friendships, family living, relationships at work and in mutual helping and caring. Such skills grow and develop through and within personal relationships. Relationships are, in this sense, the heart of the matter.

They introduce a new dimension into the personal planning process, which is based on the principle of the importance of the interactions that take place between the client and the carer (and their friends). They talk of the part that compassionate and supportive caring relationships play in determining the context of successful care planning and life experiences. They describe the shared action planning approach as having a focus on communication and relationship building, which are central to the process of growth and human development. It involves the sharing of key relationships and involves joint decisions and the pooling of ideas with the service user in order to challenge their environment by constructing an agenda of positive action. This agenda involves the formulation of shared plans of action about identified needs and includes safeguards to ensure that action plans are actually carried out: 'shared action planning happens when there is co-ordination, organisation and people know who is responsible for doing what' (p. 131).

Consequently, individualised approaches to care should provide a framework for people to express their wishes and desires through a shared process with named workers, which in turn should lead to valued outcomes for the individual. Individual programme planning uses the same four stages as the nursing process (assessment, planning, action and evaluation), but it is not a purely nursing method. It builds in inputs from every relevant discipline and carer on the basis of equality. It pays particular attention to clarifying the client's unique needs as the client sees them.

Shared action planning, like all other intervention techniques, will be successful only if the principles underpinning the approach are understood and practised to a standard of proficiency by the workforce.

Intervention strategies

The intervention strategy adopted will depend on the assessment of the person in their social context. Nurses must ask two questions:

- What intervention will enhance the health potential of the individual?
- What knowledge would support this intervention?

This requires an examination of the factors that impinge on a person's needs and lifestyle from natural science, social, interpersonal and political domains. This involves a retrospective examination of the person's biography and speculation about future health needs, which should aim to provide for maximum independence.

Care responses demand that practitioners acquire an understanding of personal and group psychology and the application of learning theory. This application implies the use of behaviour modification techniques (which rely on the use of operant conditioning) to enable people to develop appropriate behavioural responses and to facilitate new learning. Examples include one-to-one teaching in the acquisition of self help skills or social skills training in the community (teaching somebody to use public transport) and the reduction of inappropriate or challenging behaviour.

Responses must also respect individual social needs. Practitioners must be aware of the norms, values and social pressures that relate to such concepts as personal history, social class, and cultural and subcultural determinants and their influence on health and wellbeing. These factors remind practitioners that the delivery of care operates within a framework of politically inspired policies that need to be understood if not challenged. These social policies construct the systems within which care is provided and determine how clients will gain access.

The provision of nursing care demands that appropriate (and sensitive) communication is developed with service users in response to their perceived level of intelligence. (The level of intelligence may follow a normal distribution, although all have degrees of learning disability.) Nurses should also have regard to each person's potential for independence in an area where the individual can perform activities of daily living (such as dressing, feeding, washing and shaving) unaided.

Recently, much interest has been shown in the use of a range of alternative therapies such as reflexology, aromatherapy, deep massage and therapeutic touch. For older people who do not appear to respond well to external stimuli through normal channels of communication such as verbal reinforcement, touch, smell and physical contact may be alternative routes for stimulation. Practitioners are now engaged in the use of a variety of therapies for people with multiple handicaps (such as cerebral palsy) and also with people who require additional assistance to relax (for example, people with hyperactive behaviours).

Other responses include reminiscence therapy, psychotherapy and counselling (Scrutton, 1989).

Older people therefore have unique needs and problems. Many have one or more chronic conditions, which if left untreated may develop into acute illness and further disability. Practitioners therefore have a responsibility to provide effective, dynamic and high quality practice. Their actions should be permeated by the following principles:

- As key professionals working within the context of a multidisciplinary team, individuals should collaborate with clients and their carers to achieve mutually negotiated goals.
- All health and social care needs should be assessed as part of a comprehensive care package, using the principle of shared action planning, and at all times responding to the declared needs and rights of individuals.
  - Clients should be empowered to maximise their health and wellbeing.
  - Practitioners should develop and implement audit tools to measure the effectiveness of their actions.
  - Ethical and moral considerations should be appropriately deliberated and risk taking measures implemented to ensure that individual rights, status and dignity are upheld at all times.

- Practitioners should be committed to the principle of seeking to improve their practice through the process of reflection and supervision.

Interventions will also ensure that the following are provided:

- Respite for carers
- Perceptive assessment processes that are proactive and responsive to real needs
- Rehabilitation facilities that encourage and maximise active independence and participation in community life
- Arrangements for continuing care within an environment that encourages independent living.

Responding to these challenges demands that mental handicap nurses, social workers and other practitioners are able to work in a variety of domiciliary and residential care environments and teams. Thus a 'facility independent' model is required which ensures that practitioners are enabled to provide specialist care to older people with special needs (people who have multiple handicaps, people whose behaviour requires specific attention and intervention, people with superimposed mental health needs, people with medical and sensory impairments and others who require intensive nursing care). Practitioners will offer their skills on a contractual basis to their clients either through domiciliary support teams or by working with them in their new homes in the community.

Access to generic health care services

The government has recommended that, for the major part, people with learning disabilities should have access to generic health care services through primary health care teams and in general hospitals. People with learning disabilities are not immune from the trials and tribulations of day-to-day life, and as such are as likely as the next person to require access to general health services. In certain circumstances two areas might require specific attention whenever people with learning disabilities are admitted to hospital: the person as a patient may have anxieties, and the family at home may be concerned that the nurses will not be able to provide appropriate care.

Older people with a learning disability often like consistency and order, and may become anxious when confronted with changes in their routine (even ones of a minor nature). At times of crisis an increase in attention is sought by all of us, and avoidance of people in distress is seldom helpful. Like any person in a situation of acute stress, the individual may exhibit behaviour usually associated with an earlier age, and this needs to be recognised with warmth and understanding. The situation needs to be responded to tactfully, firmly and with compassion. The client's behaviour may be unintelligible to the uninitiated but it is likely to follow a particular pattern. Violence very rarely occurs, but aggressive outbursts are occasionally witnessed.

Avoidance of many of these problems can be achieved if time is taken to obtain a full history from family members or carers. Normal patterns of behaviour can be predicted, and if nurses are prepared in advanced precautions can be taken to ensure that the patient is settled in a manner that minimises anxiety and uncertainty. In particular, nurses should understand any form of communication system that the person uses. Communication will often be the most important aspect of care, and people with a learning disability may have developed elaborate systems of communication in the absence of verbal reasoning or speech. In such situations, reassurance and positive body language can be most helpful and may reduce anxiety. Conversely, vacillation and ambiguity on the part of the nurse are unhelpful: the situation needs to be managed with confidence, decisiveness and sensitivity.

Promoting positive health gain

The Strategic Intent of the NHS in Wales (Welsh Office/NHS Directorate, 1992) identifies three specific commitments for people with learning disabilities. Services should be:

- Health gain focused, adding years to life and life to years
- People centred, valuing people as individuals
- Resource effective, achieving a cost effective balance in its use of available resources.

The Welsh Office designed a protocol specifically for people with learning disabilities and, in keeping with government objectives, advised that appropriate specialist help from local communities and from health and local authorities should be made readily available when required.

The report summarises current trends affecting the specialism:

- The presence of learning disability in older age groups is likely to increase for at least the next thirty years owing to increased survival. There is little difference in mortality rate between this group and the general population.
- Improved life expectancy will bring attendant medical problems. Older people with learning disabilities are more vulnerable to age related physical and mental illness and high levels of physical and sensory impairment.

- There has been a marked reduction in institutionalised care throughout the UK (over an 80 per cent reduction in Wales alone during the past ten years). This has resulted in a major increase in people with learning disabilities expecting to have their health care needs met by community health services.

Four main areas of investment in health gain can be distinguished: the mainstream health services, including the primary health care team and the local acute hospitals; the large specialist hospitals; health services specifically designed to address learning disability, but with an emphasis on supporting people in the community; and other forms of support, which contribute to health in the wider sense, including housing associations and voluntary bodies.

Overall goals for health promotion may be summarised as:

- To reduce avoidable premature deaths
- To reduce preventable morbidity
- To achieve measurable improvements in health status
- To the development of support that maintains the health of carers.

Designing and implementing interventions to meet these goals should enhance the health status of clients with the aim of reducing the impact of any presenting handicap. For example, the high prevalence of sensory impairments requires investment in surveillance, accurate diagnosis and the supply of aids and equipment. For others with a propensity to acquire secondary handicaps, such as epilepsy and heart or respiratory defects, psychological support and introduction to healthy eating and exercise programmes will be necessary components of a health care regimen.

For others there will be a longer term investment need for intensive education to acquire enhanced self help and social skills. These should be accompanied by individually tailored communication programmes that provide opportunities for expressive language. Additionally, for people with multiple presentations that involve a physical disability, preventative treatment and passive exercises may reduce the impact of contractures and skeletal deformities.

Incontinence is another associated problem that can be reduced in the majority of cases, thus providing enhanced status and dignity as well as self respect. In such cases the combination of behavioural techniques and counselling often produce the desired effect for older people with learning disabilities.

Inclusive services

This chapter has considered the key issues confronting older people with learning disabilities. Selzer and Janicki (1991: 102) state that:

We believe that the integration of older persons with developmental disabilities is a goal in which we should be directing our efforts, but we do not know what service mix is the most effective in reaching this goal. We have not devoted enough critical thinking to answering the question of what we are trying to accomplish through these services. We consider as a fundamental premise the goal of maintaining the functional independence of older persons with developmental disabilities for as long as possible. However, when we enter service environments we find goals that are not as clearly defined.

The starting point for any consideration of the needs of older people with learning disabilities must therefore be the aim of including them in the mainstream of society. The quest for quality of life determinants (as well as indices to measure the effectiveness of care) must be regarded as the prime goal of our business as carers. However, we are reminded in the above quotation that service response are not always provided in such as a way as to realise these aims.

Quality of life also requires an investment in 'permanency planning'. This is a relatively new responsibility, which challenges previous orientations which are often reliant on residential alternatives to the family home. In their places are emerging new alternatives, which encourage people to move into supported living arrangements before they are forced into residential care following the death or loss of a primary carer. Supported living has been advocated by Kinsella (1993) and by McCallion (1994) and provides an exciting alternative to more institutionalised forms of care.

Four key statements also serve to remind us of key issues related to quality of life:

- Quality of life is not absolute
- Quality of life for individuals changes over time
- Quality of life varies within a culture
- Quality of life varies across cultures.

For older people there is a real need to build new alliances across care agencies and between professional and informal carers. Coalition building, networking and affiliation are considered as prerequisites for the maintenance of high quality service responses. These networks will need to bridge attitudinal barriers, which serve to segregate people with learning disabilities from generic health and social services. However, there is also a need to ensure that generic services are complemented by a range of discreet specialist responses provided by learning disability nurses and other specialist practitioners.

Older people with learning disabilities are therefore entitled to receive individually designed services in response to their individually diagnosed and assessed needs. They are also entitled to receive an assurance that their autonomy will be respected and that the quality of their lives will accord with their chosen preferences and expectations.

References

Brandon D and Towe N (1989) *Free to Choose – An Introduction to Service Brokerage*. Good Impressions, London.

Brechin J and Swain A (1987) *Changing Relationships – Shared Action Planning for People with a Mental Handicap*. Harper and Row, London.

Day K (1985) Psychiatric disorder in the middle aged and elderly mentally handicapped. *British Journal of Psychiatry* 147, 660–7.

Day K (1987) The elderly mentally handicapped in hospital: a clinical study. *Journal of Mental Deficiency Research* 17, 20–7.

Department of Health (1992) *The Patient's Charter*. Department of Health, London.

Department Health and Social Security (1988) *Health Service Development – Resource Assumptions and Planning Guidelines*, HC(88)43. HMSO, London.

Dickerson J, Hamilton J, Huber R and Segal R (1979) The aged mentally retarded: the invisible client: a challenge to the community. In Sweeney DP and Wilson TY (eds) *Double Jeopardy: The Plight of Aging and Aged Developmentally Disabled People in Mid-America*. Exceptional Child Centre, Logan, Utah.

Eaton LF and Menolascino FJ (1982) Psychiatric disorders in the mentally retarded: types, problems and challenges. *American Journal of Psychiatry* 139, 1297–303.

Fryers T (1984) *The Epidemiology of Severe Intellectual Impairment: The Dynamics of Prevalence*. Academic Press, New York.

Hogg J, Moss S and Cooke D (1988) *Aging and Mental Handicap*. Croom-Helm, London.

Kinsella P (1993) *Supported Living for People with Learning Disabilities*. National Development Team, London.

McCallion P (1994) Families and practitioners: differences in their views on permanency Planning. Paper presented at the Dublin Roundtable Conference on Aging and Mental Handicap, Dublin.

McCarthy M (ed.) (1989) *The New Policies of Welfare – An Agenda for the 1990s?* Macmillan, London.

National Development Team (1991) *The Andover Case Management Project*. National Development Team, London.

National Health Service and Community Care Act (1990) HMSO, London.

National Health Service Management Executive (1992) *Health Service Guidelines – Health Services for People with Learning Disabilities (Mental Handicap)*, HSG (92)42. NHS Management Executive, London.

Reiss S (1982) Psychology and mental retardation: survey of a developmental disabilities mental health program. *Mental Retardation* 20, 128–32.

Scrutton S (1989) *Counselling and Older People – A Creative Response to Ageing*. Edward Arnold, London.

Selzer MM and Janicki M (1991) Commentary and recommendations. In Janicki M and Selzer MM (eds) *Proceedings of the Boston Roundtable on Research Issues and Applications in Aging and Developmental Disabilities*. Boston, USA.

Sines DT (1995) *Community Health Care Nursing.* Blackwell Science, Oxford.

Thase ME, Liss L, Smelzer D and Maloon J (1982) Clinical evaluation of dementia in Down's syndrome: a preliminary report. *Journal of Mental Deficiency Research* 26, 239–44.

Towell D (1988) *An Ordinary Life in Practice.* King's Fund, London.

Towell D and Beardshaw V (1991) *Enabling Community Integration – The Role of Public Authorities in Promoting an Ordinary Life for People with Learning Disabilities in the 1990s.* King's Fund, London.

Welsh Office/NHS Directorate (1992) *Protocol for investment in Health Gain – Mental Handicap (Learning Disability).* Welsh Office Planning Forum. HMSO, Cardiff.

Wolfensberger W (1972) *The Principles of Normalisation in Human Services.* National Institute on Mental Retardation, Toronto.

13

Adapting to change

Lesley Wade

The title of this chapter may appear paradoxical. Whose adaptation are we talking about? Is it the older person's adaptation or, equally significantly, nursing's need to adapt to an older population? This chapter hopes to show that the older population has a positive synergistic effect on nursing. Developing an awareness in nursing as to the potential within older people to change alters gerontological nursing practice. Different pasts, traditions and life experiences have resulted in the most successfully aged population ever witnessed. It is therefore incorrect to think that growing old naturally creates problems in adapting to change. Using a gerontological perspective that combines knowledge about how older people themselves experience age is essential if we want a positive approach to ageing. This chapter uses research based nursing practice to illustrate the adaptability of older people. It also offers practical advice to nurses working within a changing but unstable political and social environment. Because the nature of nursing older people is a symbiotic relationship, how older people are valued reflects on nursing. Gerontological nursing's constant adaptation is evolutionary, but as the chapter concludes, requires a high degree of emotional labour.

Growth and development

It is important that anyone nursing older people considers and recognises that growing old is a period of growth and development (Sugarman, 1986). This positive approach towards growth and development has to be identified and reciprocated by growth and development within nursing itself. However, in preserving a successfully positive old age, nurses need to look at themselves: change within elderly care affects both the nurse and the nursed. Nursing shares with older people the dubious tradition of a work orientated culture, which relates often to status, success and power. An easily recognised feature of ageing is the clearly defined retirement from the work force. This creates problems for both sexes, particularly in adaptation and coping (Lackzo and Phillipson, 1991). From an internal psychological perspective, the maintenance of success and power requires complex psychological process and the successful resolution of several developmental tasks. The psychoanalyst Freud (who did not pay any attention to his own or anyone else's ageing) saw that the key to successful life was 'to love and to work' (Thompson, 1994). The key to successful ageing is to generate, maintain and create new opportunities for continual successful behaviours. This is illustrated by specific coping strategies that can sometimes be detected in colleagues and friends who are nearing retirement age. The first strategy is the demeaning of the person's present employment or lifestyle, which are then compensated for by finding new roles within voluntary bodies. This would be a successful strategy for nurses for example, as they would bring skills and a good chance of success to their new role. A further strategy in preserving self esteem is the growing awareness of investing in physical fitness, which brings with it new friends and new relationships. A problem for older people who have been employed in physical occupations is the loss of physical prowess, but again this can be adapted in developing new physical skills such as gardening. After retirement, therefore, everybody needs to find meaningful goal orientated tasks to replace work. A problem may be that if this is not achieved despair and depression can be produced. A case history that illustrates this point is of a 62-year-old former bank manager who felt forced to take early retirement and compensated by working a 12 hour day for various voluntary organisations. Despite being told to reduce his stress, he was admitted four times to the coronary care unit with irregular heart rhythms. Previous to this, the man had never been in hospital or felt ill in his life.

Whose adaptation? Teaching Columbus to fly

It is important to recognise that older people are actively reconstructing their lives. They are reconstructing not only the present and the future but also their past. Consider why there was a furore over the publication and screening of the television adaptation of Mary Wesley's *The Camomile Lawn* (1980), with its explicit account of sexuality during the second world war. Was it because it was written by a woman in her seventies, or that it destroyed the public's view of how a certain generation ought to behave? As nurses caring for older people, do we really recognise the abilities older people have in adapting and coping? Throughout their lives this group have adapted to new ways of seeing and doing what previously had never been considered. The group we call 'old' have lived in a state of flux that in many ways makes older people an authority in adapting and coping positively. Adapting and coping in old age has therefore become part of most older people's natures. George Bernard Shaw once observed that progress depended on the unreasonable person, in contrast to the reasonable person who adapts to the world. This unreasonable person persists in adapting the world to meet specific personal goals. Grimley-Evans (1993) sees that the first imperative for those wishing to be a healthy hundred is to be informed, to stay in command, and to be thoroughly obstreperous in refusing to be fobbed off with second rate care. Therefore the wilful and the cantankerous live longer than the more compliant sweet old folk, who so often appear to be the good patient. This assertive population is going to have different needs according to its age group, gender, class and ethnicity, so nursing requires new skills and roles in assisting certain types of adaptation. In fostering successful adaptation and coping, gerontological nursing needs to draw on different intellectual and technical skills. Older people are a diverse and complex group, taking part in social and economic changes that confirm age as one of the greatest period of discovery. The language, technology and environment will be new but this new age discoverer will triumph.

A simple litmus test in assessing younger people's ability to assimilate and cope with change can be demonstrated by asking a younger population to:

- Entertain a family without the television or video
- Preserve meat and poultry without a refrigerator
- Calculate how many farthings in half a crown
- Complete a dissertation without the aid of a typewriter or word processor.

No doubt after some adaptation and sharing of information a younger generation would learn to adapt and cope in the world our forefathers and foremothers lived in. Compounded by the stressors of normal ageing, older people additionally have to cope with being immobile, incontinent, bereaved and socially isolated, often simultaneously. To a certain extent, adapting to a rapidly changing environment by virtue of age carries with it inherent stressors and jeopardies. One of the quests of gerontological nursing is to recognise these individual responses to stress and adaptation, responding with appropriate nursing interventions. Before we move on to address specific nursing practices that may assist adaptation and coping, the concept of adaptation and stress within the older population needs some explanation.

Models of stress and coping

Coping is the immediate response of a person to stress; adaptation is the final response of a person to change that occurs. For a nurse to help a patient to cope and adapt, Bailey and Clarke (1989) say that an understanding of the models of stress and coping is essential.

They identify three broad approaches to defining stress:

- Stimulus or cause-and-effect models.
- Response models such as the general adaptation syndrome
- Transactional models, where the individual is seen as the active participant in the stress and coping relationship.

If we consider coping as a set of defence mechanisms, there are four main approaches:

- Ego defence mechanisms
- Coping that is characteristic of a particular personality type
- Coping that is related to a particular situation
- Coping that is a transaction between the individual and the environment.

Scrutton (1989) states that stress and coping can be highly individual and that the nurse needs to be sensitive to the different reactions and needs of clients. Admission to hospital may be perceived as a stressor and a threat to the older person (Bailey, 1989). In combination with ageism the experience of being an older *geriatric* may be demeaning, generating a loss of power and independence as well as being stressful (Robinson, 1979). Although it may be necessary and life saving, medical and nursing care can plummet older people into unfamiliar surroundings and often frightening environments out of their control. If gerontological nursing needed a guideline in helping older people to minimise anxiety and stress, areas to consider would be:

- Offering wider support of the client and family in the community
- Providing information on maintaining wellness in old age beginning with preretirement programmes
- Maintaining a therapeutic relationship with older people, who will increasingly require invasive nursing interventions

- Recognising that the clinical setting in which nursing takes place increases stress levels and that these areas of care may be in day care surgery or at home
- Understanding the fact that the act of nursing is often highly intimate and as such embarrasses and creates anxiety
- Recognising that the boundaries of care between social worker, health worker and nurse are increasingly becoming fuzzy.
- Being aware that in an organisation undergoing change there will be territorial inequalities and resulting conflicts of interest.

Adaptation as a concept in nursing older people

The concept of adaptation assumes that people are both open and closed systems, which respond to stimuli from both inside and outside the person. The response to such stimuli are termed adaptation. In its truest sense, it is neither positive nor negative; it is simply a response to any internal or external stimuli. In its application today, adaptation may be seen as a positive response, whereas a negative response is termed maladaptation. Physiological adaptation consists of homeostasis that maintains the stability of the internal environment of the person. Psychological adaptation is the possession of self esteem and identity. Illness and disease fall within the framework of maladaptations; mental illness and some purposed deviant behaviours are examples of maladaptation in the psychosocial realms. Older people, by virtue of the ageing process, draw on a number of physiological and psychological processes to adapt; this process is often compromised by numerous multiple stressors. Older people tend to collect diseases and it is not uncommon for them to be diagnosed as having six or seven (Wade, 1988). Together with the social and psychological losses attributed to old age (status, security, self image and bereavement), age alone brings with it a plethora of stimuli that require skilled adaption. Although models of nursing based on Roy's adaptation model have been used to explain how older people adapt and cope, models of nursing such as these often omit gerontological nursing knowledge. Nolan (1995) has suggested that a way forward for nurses working with older people should be built on three central premises:

- Knowledge building should begin from the perspective of the older person.
- The search for the correct model of nursing is as fruitless as searching for the holy grail.
- Nursing older people requires an eclectic approach, valuing and using knowledge no matter what its source.

Introducing new practices that adapt to older people's needs

It may be ironic that in a climate of limited resources nursing is spoilt for choice in the armoury of skills in helping older people to cope and adapt. Promoting health and wellness, focusing on rehabilitation skills, and assessing how specific health care deliveries contribute to care provides a logical pathway to assist with adaptation and coping in old age.

Promoting health and wellness

Within the concept of adaptation and coping, old age should not be associated with ill-health, decline and dependency. The Health and Life Style survey carried out in the mid-1980s found that the majority of people over 65 years felt healthier than their parents. However, the proportion who thought themselves healthier decreased with age (Victor, 1991).

One of the strategies nursing has to employ is to begin to alter older people's often pessimistic view of decline in older age, combined with positive health promotion and specific health education. In this context gerontological nurses need to sell health, recognising that the older person is a consumer. This can be achieved by a variety of people: health visitors, community nurses, practice nurses, diabetic and continence specialists, physiotherapists, doctors and self help groups. It can be developed in a variety of ways, using the local community, assessing local media and facilitating informal and formal groups. We need to take opportunities to target older groups who do not adapt to the ageing process. For example, particular emphasis is needed in motivating older men to recognise and understand about prostate cancer. Taking into account embarrassment and gender issues, posters and information leaflets could be displayed in football stadiums or other recreational and work environments to create a positive atmosphere that fosters inquiry.

Nurses also need to adapt their skills, exchanging information and competency in a facilitator's role outside of nursing's normal territory. For example, coping around the time of the menopause for older women requires adaptation within client and professional groups. Many nurses are familiar with menopausal clinics and their skills in promoting health could be transferred to gynaecological wards and specialist areas for older people. Preserving wellbeing and coping, particularly in relation to mental health, is a key area within gerontological nursing. Reminiscence therapy that aims to promote self esteem is an essential tool of any gerontological nurse. This is a specific clinical skill that helps older people who have been bereaved and are grieving. Raising self esteem, helping the client to keep physically as well as mentally fit, and assisting the individual to face and experience their different stages of grief are practical ways of helping the person to adapt and cope.

Rehabilitation

In what ever guise, rehabilitative skills are central in helping older people to adapt and cope, whether there is an uncomplicated single problem or a complex multifactorial one. For the stoic individual a degree of stress incontinence or a painful hip may not impinge too much on their coping mechanism: making sure they are near a toilet or not walking too far will be a minor modification. However, what is acceptable to one person may be totally unacceptable to another. Rehabilitation programmes therefore have to be individually tailored and jointly perceived by the nurse, the patient and other members of the multidisciplinary team. Rehabilitation signifies the whole process of restoring a disabled person to a condition in which they can resume a near normal life. This process may differ according to the nature of the disability. An older person with motor neuron disease will differ from a client who as a result of infection is temporarily incontinent. Within the older population, rehabilitation is often associated with cerebrovascular accident, amputation or other problems which reduce mobility, and specifically independence. Whatever the situation, rehabilitation has three kinds of activity which the gerontological nurse will be familiar with:

- *Reactivation*. This is the encouragement of the older person to be active within their surroundings. The type of environment and resources (including time) is important in determining this activity. For the older person recovering from a stroke, time is needed to form a relationship where trust and mutual respect is achieved. Constant assessment and feedback to the client and relatives with easily understood information assists in coping and adapting. Patient participation with specific functional assessments and rehabilitation techniques requires a well informed individual.
- *Resocialisation*. This is the encouragement of physical and verbal contact, by patients, with peers, families and others. For example, an older stroke patient needs to regain communication or compensate for communication problems. The use of language, touch, tone of voice and humour must be paralleled with an understanding of the individual's disordered physiology, recovery and adaptation level.
- *Re-integration*. At this stage there is a need to consider how that person will be restored and function, participating as much as possible in society. Body image, self esteem and a focus on normalisation should guide all three of these processes.

Rehabilitation is a fundamental part of helping older people to adapt and cope. This process begins as soon as possible and presently occurs within hospitals. In the future, however, a large part of rehabilitation may occur within specialised units or the patient's own home. Nursing will have to demonstrate its adaptive skills, increasing patient and carer teaching.

Health care delivery systems

Impacts of health care delivery systems need to be critically analysed for outcomes on care. Research examining the impact of primary nursing on a group of older women within a hospital setting exemplifies many of the key features that Nolan identifies as developing gerontological nursing (Wade, 1995). Using an ethnographic approach, this research analysed adoption of primary nursing in three wards. Evidence emerged to suggest that the lives of older women were not fully recognised. In an effort to adopt a universal model of ward organisation there was a lack of age and gender appropriate practice, and sociology, anthropology and life history were not taken into account. Significant issues that did arise from the research demonstrated that some nurses were able to recognise the culture and individual coping strengths of older people, recognising that individuals had an enormous reserve of coping and adaptive skills. As a consequence of listening to older women's biographies and focusing on older women's needs rather than *getting the work done*, a different image of the women emerged. This new image included their tenacity, risk taking and sense of adventure, challenging not only stereotypes but the delivery and priority of care. One of the key points to emerge within the research was how uniquely each woman reflected on and reviewed their life. In examining how nursing has tried to adapt to the individual needs of older people within a hospital setting the research suggests that nursing:

- Clarifies what skills are involved in nursing older people
- Challenges nursing roles, crossing traditional boundaries
- Moves away from traditional problem solving approaches that often mean cutting situations to fit limited professional knowledge
- Realise that other groups like friends, voluntary agencies and self help groups contribute to older people's wellness (Wade, 1992).

Adapting to change: individual responses

In keeping within a gerontological nursing perspective we will look at older people's experience of ageing. In helping older people to adapt and cope successfully, a gerontological perspective therefore needs to recognise the community in which the older person lives. Amy Jones, Dot McPhie and Ronald Rolf have been admitted as an emergency to their local hospital. The community they live in has changed a great deal over the last fifty years. Many of their neighbours are students and the small shops have long since gone. Amy is 90, Dot 78 and Ronald 71. They all have different lives, experiences and future expectations. They are similar in one respect and that is their dislike of the mixed sex ward they are on. Using a gerontological framework, we will draw on age appropriate practice, life span development and the specific health needs of each person to demonstrate their adapting and coping skills. It is important to consider that for some older people, such as this patient in a rehabilitation ward, the time and effort required in adapting may not enhance their quality of life:

> If I had time in tokens I would spend less time trying to dress and wash and more time sunbathing in the garden . . . after all, we get little sun and the effort it takes to wash and dress exhausts me for the rest of the day.

This was not a case of learned helplessness but of realistic wants and desires, which need to be included in care planning.

CASE STUDY 1: Problems with my waterworks

Ronald is the youngest patient, but not necessarily the most adaptable. He has a history of prostate enlargement but has ignored medical advice until his emergency admission last night. This may be a coping device for Ronald as he fears cancer of the prostate.

This type of cancer has been described as the quintessential cancer of old age (Thompson, 1994). It is a disease that rarely affects men below 50 and the average age of diagnosis is 73 (Karr and Murry, 1984). Carcinoma of the prostate is the fifth most common cancer in the world in men (OPCS, 1989). It is chiefly found in developed countries, and in the UK prostate cancer is the third most common cause of death. The prostate gland is small and hidden, and the majority of men and women appear unaware that it exists despite its vital role in the reproductive process. Sadler (1992) states that carcinoma of the prostate affects a generation of men who are not well informed about their bodies. Research by Maanen (1988) indicates that perceptions of health are determined by many dimensions. Ill-health is often unreported within the older population, as changes may often be put down to just getting old. Symptoms are often seen by older men as a normal consequence of ageing and not reported until a later stage, when it alters their patterns of daily life. Ronald's life history is firmly rooted in a background where bodily functions, particularly reproduction, were not openly discussed. He has a feeling of embarrassment about his symptoms and is reluctant to discuss problems such as incontinence with both strangers and friends. He may have denied his problem and, living alone, does not share it with anybody. Social support is a key element in assisting people to develop coping skills. It is interesting to note that the key confidants of older men are not men. Jerome (1990) states that older men's confidants are usually their wives, whereas older women tend to have confidantes outside their marriage. Widowhood and an increasing divorce rate mean that there is a significant number of older men living alone. Ronald's degree of social isolation, coupled with the lack of privacy and embarrassment afforded on a mixed ward, is going to reduce his and the nursing staff's ability to adapt and cope. Ronald has internal and external stressors that will raise his anxiety levels. The layout of most wards means that there is only a curtain or a partition separating one patient from another in the next bed. This means that there is little privacy, and patients and relatives know they can be heard in the next bed. If the other person is female, Ronald may feel unable to disclose specific information. In particular, the immediate nursing assessment with specific questions related to elimination may be avoided by both nursing staff and patients. It would seem that, in practice, assessments regarding elimination are often limited to whether a person is continent or not (Cheater, 1991). Similarly, the nurse undertaking the assessment may be embarrassed by asking personal and specific questions about bodily habits. Lawler (1991) identifies that intimate and invasive nursing care that centres around sexuality, genitalia or excreta is often ignored by nurses. An uneducated nurse may feel equally stressed and may fail to obtain a detailed history if not gerontologically orientated regarding her own and Ronald's attitudes to bodily functions. This is further complicated by Ronald's urgent admission into a mixed sex ward. *The Patient's Charter* statement that people have a right to single sex wards is negated if the patient is admitted as an acute admission case. A number of issues have arisen regarding the problems of dealing with an intimate aspect of care that is complicated by age, resources and specific nursing knowledge. Where once the workhouse environment was the subject of criticism, depersonalisation and institutional care (Evers, 1983), this has been superseded by the effects of mixed wards.

CASE STUDY 2: It doesn't matter at my age

Dot is a 78-year-old ex-nurse, who has been admitted with a provisional diagnosis of hyperglycaemia. Diabetes mellitus of the non-insulin-dependent type classically presents in late middle age with a history of being overweight, thirst, polyuria, tiredness and pruritus vulvae. Patients affected over a long time may also have foot ulcers (Watkins, Drury and Taylor, 1990). Dot trained in Jamaica in the early 1950s and she continued to practise when she emigrated to England in the 1960s. She has made several comments to her nurse about the new style of informality, which she admires in nursing today. However, she believes it is the doctors' responsibility to get her back to health.

In Dot's career the older population did not suffer a disproportionate amount of ill health in relation to diabetes, as life expectancy was lower and the quality of care was different. Dot is unaware of the risks of visual impairment and vascular disease and how a change in diet and lifestyle can cause changes to glucose tolerance (Alberti, 1993). Diabetes mellitus is unusual in that its management affects many important aspects of the way people live. It may involve major changes in eating habits and in lifestyle patterns as well as taking medications. Significantly for Dot, the major benefits of adapting and changing one's life style as a consequence of being a diabetic are not immediate. The diabetic control and complication trials (1994) have shown that good metabolic control over a mean of six years reduces the risks of retinopathy and neuropathic changes. Dot has conscientiously maintained her diet, but the recent death of her husband and her move into her son's house has created anxieties, grief and tensions. Due to her losses her technical skills in balancing medication, diet, exercise and lifestyle has been temporarily lost. Dot has told the nurses not to waste time on her, that it doesn't matter at her age. Dot is expected to assimilate a number of instructions from a number of different members of the multidisciplinary team, a task that drains her coping and adaptive skills.

There are a number of points that mitigate against Dot managing her diabetes successfully despite her life history of nursing and adapting to new cultures. Although nurses are in a good position to teach Dot, education is effective only if the multidisciplinary team communicates and understands the changes taking place in Dot's life. Before any education can be performed there is a need to recognise Dot's losses. These may include her husband and confidant, her house, her independence and degree of autonomy, and her new relationship with her son. A holistic approach is to achieve a balance between treatment regimens and lifestyle. The nursing staff need to recognise Dot's former career so that a relationship can be built up based on respect and trust, encouraging Dot to be involved in decision making. Patel (1993) suggests that one-to-one teaching can be effective, followed up by frequent but brief sessions, so that knowledge is not forgotten.

CASE STUDY 3: Fend for yourself

Amy is a 90-year-old woman who was a pawnbroker in the centre of a once densely populated part of the city. Amy does not conform to any stereotypes and can reflect back to when her mother was a navvy in the first world war and when she was the 'unofficial social worker' allowing families to pawn so that they could survive the weekend. Amy has been experiencing chest pains and is breathless on exertion. She is a popular lady, having great wit and determination, with tales to tell about the hardness of life before the National Health Service. On assessment it's clear that Amy has not been taking her medication at home because the tablets make her dizzy. However, Amy complains that she is bored just sitting in bed and her hospitalisation is doing her no good at all. Amy was unable to adapt and cope to slowing up: over the last month washing, going up stairs and cooking have become increasingly difficult. Amy had mentioned the dizziness to her health visitor, who said she would tell the doctors and ask the district nurse to call. Amy was very conscious of taking up valuable time, because in her day you had to fend for yourself. The difference now, she tells her nurse, is that the friends she once had have died or moved away. Still, as she says, she is used to fending for herself: perhaps a positive epigram for the future of older people's health.

Adapting to a changing population: a nursing response

Knowledge of epidemiology, cardiology and patient education needs to be married to the specific needs of older people. An older man admitted in bacteraemic shock needs more, not less, skill in assessment of peripheral shutdown. The older women who cries out in the night for the baby she lost in the blitz needs just as much emotional care as the younger woman on the gynaecology ward. Anti-embolytic treatment after myocardial infarction requires extra skills in electrocardiograph interpretation. Nursing older people is at the cutting edge of health care, so that changes in stimuli from external political pressure such as closure of hospitals and the use of mixed sex wards increases the amount of emotional labour required. Jobs that require a high degree of emotional labour involve the following:

- Face-to-face contact with the public
- Work that produces an emotional state in others

- Training and supervision exercising a degree of control over the activities of others.

Within the context of nursing older people, Kitson (1986) has identified that emotional labour is at the core of nursing older people therapeutically. The qualities identified were the ability to reflect on patient's predicaments contextually and the need to give fresh attention to the mundane. Kitson also argues that working in such a changing complex environment requires professionals to work towards mutual understanding. Nurses are faced with a number of stressors that were formerly seen to be out of their remit. The issue of health care priorities has become highly politicised. Decisions that were once the preserve of doctors and health authorities are now affecting nursing practice. As a norm, nursing older people requires a bewildering armoury of skills and adaptations. Central to practice will always be the concept of dignity and respect; this in turn enhances care and provides the impetus to continue caring.

The first step in successfully coping and adapting to the increasing demands of a changing older population and health service is to understand the changing context of contemporary care. Alterations in funding and restrictions on budgets are a reality that creates anxiety not only within nursing but for older clients and their relatives. As older people are often seen as non-productive within a market economy, nurses will have to fight for resources.

Clinically within our practice there are some techniques and practical approaches that we can use to assist in our own coping and adaptation.

Brainstorming

As a group, whether working in a hospital or in the community, we can use a brainstorming technique to explore the stresses of the area that we work in. What may emerge are considerable personal and cultural differences in stress, ways of coping and values. Meeting with colleagues for lunch or an away day, treating yourself with special gifts, and being extra caring to colleagues who are under pressure can all help.

Reflective practice

Reflective experience can be used for reviewing incidents that produced a great deal of emotional labour. Emotional labour, especially in nursing, is a rewarding experience; however, exposure to very high degrees (especially in a health service undergoing change) may produce burn-out. Using a critical incident technique, you may ask yourself three questions to assist your coping:

- What happened in the incident?
- How can it be explained?

- Are there any conceptual frameworks that may increase understanding of the situation?

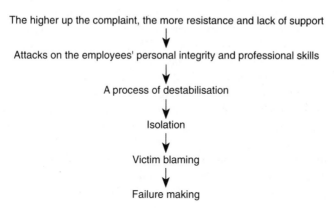

Figure 13.1 The ladder of emotional labour.

One of the ways in which nurses may have coped with an older population and an altering health service is by the increasing 'whistle blowing' – which has been accompanied by a corresponding management abuse. There is an easily recognised emotional labour ladder when coping and adaptive strategies fail (Figure 13.1). This is often accompanied by personal attacks, resulting in moral outrage and moral distress, which increases the degree of emotional labour even further. Such degrees of emotional labour also have repercussions for management: abuse of management positions now ranks highly in the UKCC league of misconduct. In preserving ethical caring within a health system undergoing change, a framework can be used which advocates:

- Building up a network of support
- Discussing issues with peers if changes are universally felt to be detrimental to practice
- Always using recognised channels and mechanisms to communicate above issues that are causing moral distress
- Documenting, signing, dating and posting in a sealed envelope communications about issues that need addressing.

Conclusion

This chapter challenges the idea that adaptation and coping with the older population lies solely with that population. The positive aspect of a gerontological approach is the receptiveness of nurses who know that in sharing with clients they too will adapt. Thus, both of the species will survive. The chapter has taken both a theoretical and clinical approach to adaptation. Emphasising growth and development and different models of stress, it demonstrates that older people face prejudice and disability but survive. In looking at appropriate nursing interventions a pathway has been outlined that considers health promotion, rehabilitation and appropriate care delivery systems; this pathway needs to be further explored. Older people's individual responses have been central in focusing how we help older people to age successfully. Equally, the cost of providing this quality of care is demonstrated by the emotional labour often encountered when nursing older people. The future will be as optimistic as nursing and older people allow it to be. Politically stronger year by advancing year, older people will choose who will co-ordinate and provide therapeutic care. No doubt they will choose the lateral thinking nurse who combines technical skills with compassion and can adapt quickly to new situations.

References

Alberti KG (1993) Problems related to definitions and epidemiology of type 2 (non-insulin dependent) diabetes mellitus: studies throughout the world. *Diabetologia* 9, 978–84.

Bailey, K and Clarke M (1989) *Stress and Coping in Nursing*. Chapman & Hall, London.

Bailey R (1989) *Coping with Stress in Caring*. Blackwell Scientific, Oxford.

Cheater F (1991) Attitudes towards urinary incontinence. *Nursing Standard* 26, 23–7.

Evers H (1983) Older women's self perception of dependency and some implications for service provision. *Journal of Epidemiology and Community Health* 38, 306–9.

Grimley-Evans J (1993) Can we live to be a healthy hundred? *Medical Research Council News* 64, 1–3.

Jerome D (1990) Intimate relationships, In Bond J and Coleman P (eds) *Ageing in Society*. Saga, London.

Karr J P and Murry SP (1984) Carcinoma of the prostate and its management. In Brocklehurst JC (ed.) *Urology in the Elderly*. Churchill Livingstone, London.

Kitson A (1986) Indicators of quality in nursing – an alternative approach. *Journal of Advanced Nursing* 11, 135–44.

Laczko F and Phillipson C (1991) *Changing Work and Retirement*. Open University, Milton Keynes.

Lawler J (1991) *Behind the Screens: Nursing Somology and the Problems of the Body*. Churchill Livingstone, Edinburgh.

Maanen HM (1988) Being old does not always mean being sick. *Journal of Advanced Nursing* 13, 701–9.

Nolan MR (1995) Geriatric nursing: an idea whose time has gone: a polemic. *Journal of Advanced Nursing* 99, 840–9.

OPCS (1989) *Cancer Statistics Registrations England and Wales.* Series MBI No. 22. HMSO, London.

Patel J (1993) Empowering of diabetes: a challenge for community nursing. *British Journal of Nursing* 2, 405–9.

Robinson, L (1979) *Sex, Class and Culture.* Methuen: New York.

Sadler C (1992) Men's hidden illness. *Nursing Times* 88, 18–19.

Scrutton, S (1989) *Counselling Older People (Age Concern Handbook).* Edward Arnold, London.

Sugarman L (1986) *Lifespan Development Concepts Theories and Interventions.* Routledge, London.

Thompson, E (1994) *Older Men's Lives.* Sage, New York.

Victor CR (1991) *Health and Health Care in Later Life.* Open University, Milton Keynes.

Wade L (1988) Promoting safety and comfort. In Wright SG (ed.) *Nursing the Older Patient.* Harper and Row, London.

Wade L (1992) The impact a health care delivery system (primary nurse) has on older women. Master of Arts Dissertation, University of Keele.

Wade L (1995) New perspectives on gerontological nursing. In Wade L and Waters K (eds) *A Textbook of Gerontological Nursing.* Baillière Tindall, London.

Watkins PJ, Drury PL and Taylor KW (1990) *Diabetes and Its Management,* 4th edn. Blackwell Scientific, Oxford.

14

Meeting psychosocial needs of elderly people

Kevin Hope

Each and every one of us enters into our relationship with patients and clients and is guided in how we care for them by a set of values, beliefs and attitudes. Such things influence our perception about what we do when we care which is good or bad, positive or negative, and helpful or unhelpful. As a consequence, each of us discharges our care in a unique way. However, at the same time, we are guided by other forces which strive to point us in the 'right' direction to improve our care. Many of these forces originate from external sources, particularly agencies charged with the responsibility of improving standards.

The term 'new nursing' has been used by Salvage (1990) to describe a change within nursing philosophy. Encapsulated within this term is the recognition that nursing, if it is to be effective, must use knowledge to provide a systematic delivery of care. In addition, a holistic approach to care, which encourages nurses to adopt a style that places greater emphasis on aspects of care that promote holism and include meeting psychosocial needs, is emphasised.

This chapter has been written to help direct nurses, specifically those who care for older people, to improve their practice by adopting the notion that for care to be truly effective it needs to be holistic. As a consequence, psychosocial needs must be addressed within any plan of care: anything less, according to Kershaw (1987), is not nursing – it isn't caring. According to De Raeve (1992), nurses should give more attention to their ability to be receptive, to 'tune in' to client messages.

How do nursing models address psychosocial needs?

The concept of need

What are psychosocial needs and how do nurses identify their own role in addressing them? A popular starting point is to look at dictionary definitions. In this case, need is described as:

* A condition of affairs placing one in difficulty or distress
* A condition of affairs marked by the lack or want of some necessary thing or requiring some extraneous aid or addition.

Psychology textbooks are also helpful and point out that the concept of need is closely aligned with that of motivation, having its base in humanistic philosophy wherein needs are viewed as an integral aspect of health maintenance. The most notable purveyor of such a view is Maslow (1954), who has described a hierarchy of needs. These fall into two groups: 'deficiency' needs and 'being' needs.

Nursing models

Immediately, nurses should begin to realise that the concept is related to what they do, as terms such as 'distress' and 'aid' register in their consciousness. However, in itself this is not enough to guide nursing intervention. We need to turn to nursing models to provide such a framework. A useful reference point is the human needs model of nursing (Minshull, Ross and Turner 1986) which, utilising Maslow's hierarchy, indicates that there are five categories of need which nurses should address:

* Physical
* Safety and security
* Affiliation
* Self esteem and dignity
* Self actualisation.

A model of nursing that aligns itself with Maslow's hierarchy in that it is founded on the notion of individuals being motivated to achieve self care is Orem's Model (Orem, 1980). Orem describes 'universal self care requisites' which include concepts such as activity and rest, isolation and company, the need to limit danger and the notion of normalcy.

Comparisons can be made with Neuman (1982), who focuses her model on the relationship between the individual and the environment. She aligns health with stability between the two, wherein tensions generated by stress (be they intrapersonal, interpersonal or extrapersonal) are harmonised by the individual's 'lines of resistance'. Similarly, Roy (1980) also conceptualises her model within a systems approach and describes four models of adaptation (physiological, self concept, role function and interdependence) which are activated in response to stimuli (focal, contextual and residual).

Health for these nursing theorists is clearly more than a physical attribute, and this is made clearer in the identification of the need for nursing intervention. Orem sees this as occurring at a point when illness generates demands that produce self care needs. When such demands outweigh self care abilities, nursing is required. For Neuman, nursing intervention is required when an individual's lines of resistance are failing to protect them from stressors, the important aspect being that the origin of such stressors lies in the three domains identified. Roy sees nursing as the reduction or removal of stimuli or the enhancement of an individual's adaptive response.

Systems models have been criticised for a mechanistic view of human needs, but the message is clearly repeated in other models. For example, Peplau (1952) sees nursing as a 'significant therapeutic interpersonal process', whereas Riehl (1980) utilises a symbolic interactionist framework to suggest that nurses need to strive to identify how clients make sense of their immediate experiences within three parameters (physiological, psychological and social).

What seems clear, then, is that there is a broad recognition that, if nursing intervention is to be holistic in nature, psychosocial needs of individuals must be addressed within the remit of nursing care. The utilisation of a model is recommended not only so that such needs remain in conscious thought but also because such an approach has been shown to influence the quality of care (McKenna, 1993).

Such frameworks are useful for conceptualising what, exactly, it is that nurses should be addressing when they give consideration to psychosocial needs. Minshull, Ross and Turner (1986) argue that other models commonly used in practice place too much emphasis on physical needs, citing Henderson (1961) and Roper, Logan and Tierney (1980) as exemplars.

Perhaps, at the end of the day, the most important message is that the model can only act as a guide for the nursing activity that follows. More important is the priority that each individual nurse attaches to the meeting of such needs and their own operational philosophy, a theme which will be returned to later.

What can nurses do to address psychosocial needs?

In addressing the issue of what it is that nurses can actually do, the human needs model of nursing has been chosen as a framework in which to organise the component parts. Physical needs and self actualisation will not be considered within this remit.

Safety and security needs

According to Minshull, Ross and Turner (1986) safety and security needs are those things that provide order and predictability in our lives. They include aspects such as the need for routine, for familiar and stable surroundings, and to be free from fear. We could include the need to be guided through health and ill-health. If needs are not met in this arena, the consequences can include anxiety, disorientation and abnormal behaviour. Orem (1980) suggests that the prevention of hazards to human life, human functioning and human wellbeing is a universal self care requisite. Importantly, an individual's age is cited as a factor that determines one's capacity for self care.

Control

Central to safety and security is the feeling of being in control. Nurses can facilitate such a feeling by structuring their intervention in such a way as to emphasise patient choice, participation and decision making. All of these things can only happen when the nurse actively pursues such outcomes. Although the following paragraphs attempt to identify specific examples, this is ultimately an artificial response because the nursing intervention that moves an individual towards independence is a function of that person at that point in time in the context in which he or she is nursed. The challenge is to reflect in and on your own practice and perhaps reconsider the activities you pursue that inhibit the amount of control a patient has.

There are, of course, many decisions that patients have little control over, yet this does not mean that special consideration cannot be given to older people. Within such a remit nurses could, for example, address issues such as when and why older people are exposed to different surroundings and the potential consequences of such action. The primary ageing effects on sight and hearing, which can lead to presbyacusis and presbyopia, respectively, mean that such changes in location can have significant effects on older people if their severity is not known. One example of such activity is the ritual movement of the beds so that patients with conditions considered more severe or liable to sudden change are nursed nearer the office or nurses' station. Of course, many manoeuvres of this type are necessary, and for good reasons (although much less so if one promotes primary nursing independent of ward geography), but in choosing who to move surely consideration can be given to preventing unnecessary disorientation to older people.

Rights versus risks

Maintaining a safe environment for older people in which the relative emphasis given to reducing risk and maintaining human rights can be problematic. There is a real danger that a professional agenda can become the overriding influence whereby the lowest common denominator determines nursing intervention. One such example is that of older people falling while in care. One incident can lead to unnecessary restrictions being applied carte blanche across a wide range of clients irrespective of individual capabilities. The endpoint is that restraint of patients becomes an active policy which is applied without true assessment or evaluation. At this level, concern is raised as to whether limiting risks takes on the form of abuse, and some groups have called for legislation to prevent this outcome (Tattam, 1992). Readers are urged to consult the Royal College of Nursing's guidelines for good practice (RCN, 1987) to aid policy development and serve as a basis to raise awareness as to what might constitute restraint.

Most nurses would balk at the suggestion that they might be involved in pursuing an active policy of restraint but this, perhaps, serves to minimise the pervasive effects that an underlying need to exercise control can give rise to. For example, there are a range of behaviours nurses are involved in which, when reflected on, can be viewed as a form of restraint. These include the obvious, like the use of cot sides and baffle locks, but also aspects such as the use of drugs, the positioning of furniture, the form of furniture (e.g. bean bags from which an older person cannot move themselves), and keeping people in night attire. Matteson and McConnell (1988) point out that such behaviours, as well as being dehumanising, can give rise to a false sense of security and indeed might raise the possibility of injuries to the person. The example of a patient falling an extra two feet over a cot side is a case in point.

It is of concern that many decisions to operationalise such forms of restraint are taken unilaterally by nurses, often without anyone else in authority or trust being aware of the action being taken to ensure the safety of patients. Indeed, family or important others may also be unaware. Good practice is consequently exemplified by a thorough assessment of the problem. The RCN (1987) suggests that justification for using any method of restraint should be provided, and that restraint should be a time limited intervention. The need to involve other members of the multidisciplinary team and the family at relevant stages is promoted as a way in which the delicate balance between rights and risks can be dealt with sensitively.

Sleep

Sleep falls within the remit of routine, and the promotion of a good night's sleep is worthy of specific nursing attention. Livingston, Blizard and Mann (1993) have highlighted the importance of sleep disturbance in older people and claim that it can be an important predictor of depression.

Cawthorn and Hope (1992) have identified nursing interventions to promote sleep. They include examining routines and questioning them, environmental concerns, promoting safety both physically and psychologically, and the use of complementary practices. Such interventions are not exclusively the remit of nurses working at night, and can be utilised to promote feelings of safety and security at other times. An important aspect to emphasise at this stage is the artificial notion of physical needs being considered as separate entities. Clearly, if some physical needs are not met, e.g. to be free from pain, there will be psychological sequelae.

Anxiety

Anxiety is an experience related to illness and the process of health care. For older people there are associated potential problems. For example, anxiety can become a self perpetuating phenomena due (according to Matteson and McConnell, 1988) to the tendency to enforce dependency on older people. The physiological sequelae can also exacerbate underlying pathology. As a consequence, it is important to be able to assess the degree, precedents and alleviating factors associated with anxiety so that planned nursing intervention can be delivered. Matteson and McConnell (1988) suggest that intervention can occur within four pathways. Environmental manipulation includes involving family and friends to assist in the development of a perceived securer environment. Behavioural aspects include the use of relaxation techniques such as aromatherapy. Psychotherapeutic interventions and medication are self explanatory. They go on to point out that less specific interventions, which emphasise the client's sense of mastery over a situation, are helpful, and they include the example of providing a consistent source of reference in the care giver. The notion of primary nursing then takes on further significance, as does the importance of clients retaining their dignity and self esteem, which will be discussed below.

Culture

Chapman (1987) points out that beliefs and attitudes determined or influenced by cultural factors are deeply intertwined with the notion of psychological safety. She gives examples of occupation, income, religion and ethnicity. It follows logically that nurses need to address such issues in planning and delivering individualised care. Of particular, and growing, concern is the health care experiences of older people from ethnic minorities who are ageing in a society where mechanisms and systems of care are not orientated towards their needs. Marr and Khadim (1993) have detailed examples of such shortfalls, such as how patients eating food with their fingers were occasionally viewed as having behavioural problems. They outline how a creative solution was found, i.e. the establishment of an ethnic liaison nurse, as a response to the identified needs of a changing population and the range of practical options available.

Affiliative needs

Minshull, Ross and Turner (1986) suggest that affiliative needs encompass the need for meaningful others and give examples of family, friends, pets and societal membership in this category. It encompasses the need to be accepted for what we are, to belong and to give and receive love. There are occasions in one's life when such needs come to the fore, and the experience of terminal or chronic illness or anxiety make this more likely.

Social interaction

The maintenance of a balance between solitude and social interaction is, for Orem (1980), a universal self care requisite. Of particular note when addressing the needs of older people is that being in someone else's company in a physical sense does not necessarily mean that social interaction is taking place. An example relates to a colleague who, undertaking the English National Board 941 Caring for Elderly People course, elected to find out what it would be like to spend a day as a patient in an elderly care area. After a relatively short period, unable to take the boredom any longer, he abandoned the experiment. Factors identified as generating this outcome included the layout of day rooms (with clients placed in such a way that eye contact is difficult), the utilisation of various items of furniture (tables, footstools, which acted as barriers), and the design of armchairs (with wide headpieces leading to isolation of the occupant). Of particular concern, though, was the fact that none of the older clients appeared to be actively engaged in any notable activity.

The experience motivated my colleague to do something about the situation, enroling on a course in creative therapy. The result has been the use of activity nursing in his own area.

Activity nursing

Affiliative needs can be met at several levels, as the case of activity clearly demonstrates. Activity is a concept which is noted in other models. Orem, in particular, suggests that individuals need to strike a balance between activity and rest. According to Turner (1993: 1727) activity nursing is 'a simple concept of therapeutic care which meets a patient's psychological and social needs through mental stimulation and individual care structured in the form of an activity programme'. This activity programme is dynamic in that it is individualised to fit the client's functional level and can incorporate a range of events such as physical, social and educational activity as well as more formalised therapeutic interaction such as reminiscence therapy, reality orientation and validation therapy. Turner's work in a continuing care environment indicates that the instigation of such a programme has positive influences on clients' cognitive functioning and their quality of life, as well as promoting better communication between staff and clients.

This is recognised as of benefit in other circles. A report from the charity Counsel and Care (1993) promotes activity, pointing out that 'active people are not invariably happy, but certainly bored people are often sad'.

Pet therapy

Specific forms of therapy can be utilised. Webb (1992) has demonstrated how, in the case of a lady recovering from a stroke, activity nursing was used within a care plan but, in particular, she highlights the use of pet therapy. Haggar (1992) has reviewed the literature and points out that, as well as a large amount of supportive anecdotal evidence, pet therapy has been found to have positive effects in relieving stress, promoting relaxation, improving recovery after myocardial infarction (Friedman, Katcher and Lynch, 1980), reducing systolic blood pressure (Baun, Bergstrom and Largston, 1984), improving the mood, alertness, reality orientation and interaction of patients with dementia (Furstenberg, 1988), and stimulating conversation. Hale (1989) reports how staff used animals as part of their overall aim of maintaining dignity, privacy, personal identity and choice. An important point to remember is that there are potential problems, which Haggar (1992) is keen to point out. Not least, the onus on individuality must be at the forefront of our minds: not everybody likes animals. However, these problems are not insurmountable and there are examples of creative thinking in avoiding some of the pitfalls. The example of proactive dog therapy is particularly appealing. This constitutes a register of dog owners who will volunteer their time and animal to visit inpatients or residents, and such a scheme can readily be seen to be a workable one.

Social networks

The notion of social networks also needs to be considered within the remit of affiliative needs. Family, friends and neighbours can take on particularly important roles for older people, and clarification of these roles is important. An intimate or confiding relationship can help in maintaining positive mental health (Murphy, 1982) and in coping with loss (Jerome, 1990a). Nurses must recognise that to meet affiliative needs others closer to the patient must be involved. Tate (1992) has demonstrated how inflexible ward procedures can get in the way of such an outcome. In her example, the focus was on a mother separated from her child by a rigid visiting policy. For older people, the potential for obstacles is no less, particularly if a relationship does not marry with the perceived norm. A case in point relates to older people who are not in a heterosexual relationship and the potential for their affiliative needs not being addressed because carers fail to recognise the individuality of that client's needs.

Utilising networks

Jerome (1990b) points out that there is a danger of overestimating the level of support available from family, friends and neighbours, arguing that policy documents have emphasised such agencies as substituting or compensating for other services. The reality is that there is a high degree of specialisation and division of labour within such groups. The nurse, then, is left with the task of filtering out the relevant information so that discharge planning makes full use of available resources but avoids making assumptions.

A related concern is the role of nurses in discharge planning, which promotes health or a movement towards better health when the patient leaves one's care. Consideration could be given to how older people who would benefit from integration into a social network can be assisted to do so. Follow-up services that promote psychosocial wellbeing may encounter some difficulty in the face of contemporary forces to promote efficiency and value for money, but this does not make them less valuable. The challenge is to demonstrate how, by giving attention to such areas, long term benefits accrue, for example in reducing readmission rates. Jackson (1994: 498) in reviewing the literature identifies that:

there is a lack of evidence that consultation occurs with patients and families about their concerns surrounding the discharge or about their own perceptions of needs. The inclusion of a family member on the discharge planning team does appear to increase caregiver understanding and satisfaction.

Dignity and self esteem needs

The category of dignity and self esteem includes being able to retain one's own identity as a unique human being, to have autonomy and to know and understand. The Social Services Inspectorate (1989) offers a definition which focuses on how the carer might perceive dignity. It is 'the recognition of the intrinsic value of people regardless of circumstances by respecting their uniqueness and their personal needs'. This slant is an important one because it highlights the role of carers as advocates. Gormally (1992) examines the philosophical basis of the value attached to human life and makes a case for the potential for older people, in particular those who lack cognitive and physical attributes held by the majority of a population, to be cast in the role of non-persons. He argues that older dependent people consequently have a greater reliance on others to attach value to their lives. Matteson and McConnell (1988) suggest that a possible outcome when such needs are not addressed is powerlessness which is defined (McLane, 1987) as 'the perception of the individual that one's own action will not significantly affect an outcome. Powerlessness is a perceived lack of control over a current situation or immediate happening'.

Advocacy

A formalised approach to advocacy has been used in a variety of settings. One such example is the work of the Beth Johnson Foundation who established the North Staffordshire Advocacy and Older People Project in 1991. The aims of the project were 'to help older people articulate their needs, wishes and preferences with regard to services provided by the statutory, voluntary and private sectors'.

Volunteer advocates, who have received training, visit wards and residential homes and, usually on a one-to-one level, offer their assistance in achieving the stated aims. Support is provided via an advocacy advisory panel. A key point is that initial evaluations revealed that this process was perceived as threatening by many professional carers, leading one to question what it is about the care currently on offer that generates such fears.

Attitudes

Self esteem can be promoted by external recognition (McCall, 1990) and nurses, potentially, occupy a central position in achieving such an aim. In particular, positive reinforcement, which emphasises individuals' abilities rather than their deficiencies, is a key strategy. This is worth emphasising in relation to older people and the perception that nurses may have of them. Johnson (1991) points out that a pathological model prevails wherein older people's problems are emphasised at the expense of their abilities. Hope (1994) found that there was a consistent trend in his subjects to score lower on an attitudinal rating scale (Kogans Old People Scale) with regards to positively worded statements about older people than they did on the same statements worded negatively. The suggestion is that nurses are readily able to react to negative statements but that the degree of internalisation of a positive attitudinal response is restricted because nurses are themselves exposed to the same forces that operate in society which discriminate against older people.

The role of nurses in fostering self esteem and dignity in older people is recognised in a joint publication from the British Geriatric Society, The Royal College of Psychiatrists and the Royal College of Nursing, entitled *Working with Older People* (RCN, 1993). The title is important (replacing its predecessor of 1987, *Improving Care of Elderly People in Hospital*), with its accent on partnership.

The document emphasises the patient's right to choose and the need for privacy, asking nurses to take opportunities to help those in their care to retain and regain skills of self care. Examples include self medication and the use of personalised clothing. The retention of personal possessions is helpful, and nurses can act as advocates by liaising with relatives and friends to help achieve such an outcome.

Another area receiving particular attention at present is that of mixed sex wards. Burgess (1994) has reviewed the literature and makes several pertinent points. In particular, the emphasis on efficiency and cost effectiveness appear to have generated pressures to introduce more mixed sex wards. Yet, evidence suggests that staff and patients have reservations.

Hope (1993) points out that, in his comparative study, there was a distinct difference in the profile of ward gender: only one medical nurse ($n = 38$) worked in a mixed sex ward, whereas twenty-three nurses in acute elderly care ($n = 38$) did so. The question is asked as to what factors may be operating when it would appear that when an individual is placed in a care of the elderly setting their individuality, in terms of sexuality, appears more likely to be compromised.

Reminiscence

Reminiscence therapy has been promoted as a viable method of helping older people to reaffirm their self identity and self esteem (Lewis, 1971). Fielden (1990) reports that a large body of empirical evidence is supportive of this notion, and reminiscence is being advanced for its positive effects on life satisfaction and psychosocial adjustment (Meriam and

Cross, 1981), integration of self concept (Lewis 1971), avoidance of depression (McMahon and Ruddick, 1964) and affect (Fallot, 1980). Unfortunately, much of the evidence is anecdotal or equivocal. Fielden (1990), a notable exception to this rule, investigated the effect of reminiscence therapy on two groups of older people in residential homes ($n = 31$) using an experimental design. The control group met weekly on nine occasions and participated in social interaction guided by a health promotion format. The experimental group met to reminisce using slides based on the years 1900–1980. Measures of morale, social interaction, general health and behaviour were collected before and after intervention.

The results indicated that reminiscence had a specific therapeutic effect, and that socialising alone was not sufficient to generate improvements. Fielden (1990) comments that, for the experimental group, 'the residents changed from a body of people seemingly unwilling to become involved with each other socially to a group of people requesting greater input from the warden and enjoying events organised'. She points out that reminiscence affords the opportunity for individuals to participate in a non-threatening manner because each person is an expert on their own past. However, not all reminiscing is painless. Coleman (1986) makes a call for sensitive use of the tool which is, perhaps, well demonstrated by Steve Goodwin's highly adventurous application wherein veterans of World War I revisited battlegrounds in Belgium. Goodwin (1989) recounts how often painful memories were harnessed, and refocused on the here and now. He argues that it is 'important that memories and thoughts lead back to the future, however short or uncertain that future may be'.

Most nurses will not have the opportunity to undertake a project as grand as Goodwin's, but the principles can be applied in all settings where older people are cared for. Norris (1986) is a strong advocate for reminiscence as a tool for promoting self esteem, particularly as it helps to focus on the abilities of older people rather than their disabilities, as well as helping to combat the stereotypes that we sometimes apply to 'the elderly'. Reminiscence therapy can be aligned with the philosophy of cosmic nursing (Goodwin, 1985), which challenges us to consider our clients as having a real past, present and future.

My personal belief is that the provision of photographs of older people who are in care, depicting themselves throughout their life cycle, would be particularly helpful in promoting individualised care because they would constantly act as a challenge to the stereotype. Adams, Prickett and Bornat (1993) offer some supportive evidence. They generated 'life story' books to analyse the effect of a specific intervention. They conclude that

> through the process of creating such books, nursing staff gained new insights into the previous life experiences, tastes, and significant relationships of patients for whom they had often been providing care for long periods of time.

Reminiscence, then, appears to afford huge potential in terms of meeting psycho-social needs. Boulton *et al.* (1988) have summarised as follows:

- Those who listen to life stories of older people whom they wish to help gain markedly different pictures of the person and their needs from those who administer traditional techniques.
- Self esteem can be greatly enhanced by skilful encouragement of reminiscence.

Psychosocial needs as a holistic concept

Addressing psychosocial needs has clearly been identified as falling within the remit of nursing practice. Models of nursing are characterised by their common message of promoting a holistic approach to care. It is evident, though, that the categorisation of nursing intervention into subgroups, as indicated above, is a simplistic view of the way in which such interventions may be used. Although helpful in delineating the areas to describe, the practical use of such interventions must be regarded as being supportive in many areas. For example, we cannot readily differentiate the beneficial effects that being involved in a reminiscence group can have on an individual's affiliative needs and their self esteem. A myriad of interconnections exist, and in dealing with one area we must automatically influence another.

The question is how do we begin to integrate such factors and, just as important, demonstrate that they are effective? A useful model is available in the form of the Social Services Inspectorate (1989) work into the quality of care in local authority and private residential homes. They identified six basic values that they felt underpin quality care: privacy, dignity, choice, independence, rights and fulfilment. Each of these has been considered with regard to a range of factors (e.g. physical environment, care practices, training and development) to produce a matrix composed of aspects of policy and practice that serve as a reference. Evaluation of the quality of care can then be made in relation to such criteria, and examples of documentation are provided.

Potential problems

Although the above highlights some aspects of how nurses may address psychosocial needs in older people, it has been argued that nurses must take on board further challenges if they are to be successful.

The value of older people

Deberry, Davis and Reinhard (1989) have described how older people are more susceptible to stressors due to a combination of a reduced ability to adapt and a raised level of vulnerability when exposed to the physio-logical sequelae of the stress response. This is an important factor for nurses to consider because it highlights the point that addressing psycho-social needs in older people may have more significant effect than in other groups in the population. Paradoxically, forces operating in wider society under the umbrella of ageism, and from which nurses themselves are not necessarily immune, tend to operate in such a way that less importance is attributed to older people's psychosocial needs.

Scrutton (1989) has examined the historical and philosophical roots of ageism and suggest that the work of founding fathers such as Freud (who didn't consider the over-50 age group as having therapeutic potential because of their (supposedly) fixed and unchanging cognitive processes) have polluted our thinking. Fortunately, contemporary theorists are suc-cessfully challenging such thinking, as exemplified by work in the field of reality orientation and reminiscence.

Green (1991) disguised herself as an older woman to compare how she would be treated in different circumstances. She vividly demonstrates how, when placed in the same situation, with the same people, older people were treated with less deference. The persistent and wearing pressures experienced in the mundane activities of life, such as shopping or travelling, strike at the very root of older people's self identity and esteem. The challenge for nurses is to combat the pressures that ageism in our society promote. Slevin (1991) argues that the profession has failed in this regard. What is needed is an emphasis on positive aspects of ageing wherein health orientated perspectives of care are promoted. Of particu-lar interest is Green's finding that the presence of an advocate has a particularly powerful effect in determining the nature of the interaction that older people experience. Certainly the notion of advocacy is one that professionals who aspire to holistic care can address.

The value attached to nursing older people

Closely related to the value attached to older people is the value that nurses attach to caring for older people and the notion of specialist knowledge and expertise. There is evidence that socialising influences may be reinforcing ageist attitudes. Bowling and Formby (1991) offer a range of examples in which professional groups are seen to perceive elderly care less positively than other activities. Snape (1986) suggests that geriatric (*sic*) nursing is seen as a stop gap, and anecdotal evidence supports the idea of nursing older people being used as a form of punishment for errant nurses.

Fortunately, things have changed: there is a growing swell of opinion that caring for older people affords the opportunity to develop and practise unique skills relating to a specialist field. Cheah and Moon (1993: 1614) have put such a case but point out that a 'more significant determinant of quality of care than specialism *per se* may be the carer's attitude towards elderly people'.

The document *Working with Older People* (RCN, 1993), cited above, is unequivocal about the central issues which will improve standards of care, and these are attitudes, education and training. Attitudes appear to be have been influenced in a positive direction. It has become increasingly evident that, within nursing, caring for elderly people has shed some of its worst attributes and is increasingly becoming the first choice for more nurses. For example, Kemp's follow-up study found that 22 per cent of the University of Hull's nursing graduates chose elderly care in comparison to 24 per cent choosing surgery (Kemp, 1988). Hope (1994) found that nurses' attitudes towards older people were generally positive, but that nurses working in acute elderly care areas held more positive attitudes than their counterparts in medical wards.

Booth (1991) has also put the case for nursing older people as a specialism and the resistance for its integration into acute services. This view has gained momentum, and a call for the establishment of a separate register of elderly care nurses has been a characteristic of the debates about the future of the profession.

The value attached to nursing

There is a challenge, then, for nurses to recognise the value of nursing elderly people, but there is an associated challenge of recognising the value of nursing itself. Kershaw (1992) has argued that, until nurses develop their own self awareness in relation to the themes inherent in any model, namely their values regarding humans, the environment, nursing and health, there will be an impedance to the delivery of high quality care. She points out that nurses need to value both themselves and the effect of nursing care. This is a theme gaining ground rapidly under the guise of therapeutic nursing, with an increasingly persuasive message. Proponents such as Pearson (1991) argue that the values integral to therapeutic nursing, i.e. holism and humanism, are increasingly gaining ground in society, and that the practice such approaches fuel (e.g. client autonomy, informed choice) actually make a difference to outcomes.

Nurses' individual responsibilities

What these threads inevitably lead us to consider is that it is a nurse's individual and unique operational philosophy which is perhaps the most decisive factor in determining the quality of care older people receive. Without an integral belief in the value of older people and the positive effect of nursing care, truly holistic care as promoted by the profession will not be within our grasp. Such a perspective raises issues beyond the scope of this chapter, although the implications for selection and recruitment of carers in an elderly care environment are central. One element to reinforce is the need for nurses to reflect on what they are doing and how they are doing it. Two forms of reflection are commonly identified. These are reflection *in* practice and reflection *on* practice. Atkins and Murphy (1993), following their review of the literature, suggest that an awareness of uncomfortable feelings or thoughts triggers the process of reflection which, through a process of constructive critical analysis, can lead to new perspectives on practice being developed.

Central to this process is the need for the individual nurses to have a level of self awareness that allows them to recognise those aspects of care which may be improved on, as well as an ability to be able to describe and articulate these concerns. Such activities are not necessarily integral to all nurses' personal qualities, and clinical supervision and mentorship is offered as a model by which professional development may be enhanced (Butterworth and Faugier, 1992).

Another important area to consider is what patients feel about the issue. Salvage (1990) is right to question whether the 'new nursing' philosophy is heading in the 'right' direction, and asks whether it aligns with patients' wishes, particularly important in our consumer led society.

Grau (1984) reports that older adults, when asked to write under the title 'what I expect from the nurse', rated the personal qualities of the nurse highest. Similarly, Webb and Hope (1995), utilising a structured interview schedule with a sample of 103 inpatients, found that, for these patients, listening to patients' worries was clearly the most important nursing activity. Indeed, for older people, this trend was more evident. In addition, the kind of nurse they preferred to engage in their care was distinguishable by the nurse's personal characteristics (e.g. kind and sympathetic).

It is interesting to observe the paradox in terms of what is promoted as a means of enhancing nurses' ability to address psychosocial needs and the systems, which are increasingly operationalised, that serve to make this more difficult. At the heart of this lies a tension between what the principle of holistic care asks us to do and the influence of the scientific management philosophy.

For example, De Raeve (1992) suggests that nurses can extend their capacity to deal with psychosocial needs by way of peer supervision, which focuses on reflection on practice. At the same time, many nurses are experiencing that the time spent in the company of peers (e.g. handover/overlap) is being eroded at the altar of cost efficiency. Bowman (1993) asks whether the money and commitment required to provide holistic care for older people are truly available.

Although immensely frustrating for many nurses, we must not automatically jump on any bandwagon that decries the theory–practice gap for, without such a gap, there is no tension in the system to serve as a force for improving practice. The challenge for nurses is for them as individuals to make a difference. This might mean revisualising one's goals, but a sweet and sour sauce analogy is useful. This views any therapeutic environment as consisting of ingredients which nurses have the ability to make sweeter or sourer by their individual contribution to the environment. The degree to which one can influence the overall taste is limited in terms of context, power and a wide range of other confounding variables. However, there will be times when you as an individual can make the difference. That may mean knowing when to stop 'doing' and to start 'being' with a client, or it may be when you decided actively to reminisce with a client. It may be when you know that your client feels unsafe and take the time to correct the situation, or when you let the client make the choice. It doesn't really matter: the important thing to realise is that you do have the potential to make a difference, and keeping hold of the theory is important if we are to make our caring environment sweeter, and therefore better, for those we care for.

Conclusion

Addressing psychosocial needs is an integral aspect of the delivery of holistic care. Such needs are identifiable within the framework of nursing models, and nurses are urged to encapsulate such needs within their own framework of nursing. Specific areas can be identified whereby such needs are addressed, but there is a danger that, in doing so, the significance of such actions may be seen to be reduced.

It is suggested that the issue of how psychosocial needs are addressed is dealt with in an integrated manner, central to which is the individual nurse's operational philosophy. This is decisive in determining the degree to which any nurse will take on such activities. The aim has been to reinforce the importance and degree of commitment that you, the reader, attach to these issues. You now have the opportunity to influence practice in such a direction.

References

Adams J, Prickett M and Bornat J (1993) Care planning and life histories. Paper presented at British Society of Gerontology Conference, Norwich.

Atkins S and Murphy K (1993) Reflection: a review of the literature. *Journal of Advanced Nursing* 18, 1188–92.

Baun M, Bergstrom N and Largston N (1984) Physiological effects of human/companion animal bonding. *Nursing Research* 33, 126–9.

Beth Johnson Foundation (1991) Advocacy in action. *Bulletin of the North Staffordshire Advocacy and Older People Project* Autumn, No. 1.

Booth B (1991) Nothing special? *Nursing Times* 87, 31.

Boulton J, Gully V, Mathews L and Gearing B (1988) *Developing the Biographical Approach in Practice with Older People*. Project Paper Seven. Open University/ Policy Studies Institute, Milton Keynes.

Bowling A and Formby J (1991) Nurses' attitudes to elderly people: a survey of nursing homes and elderly care wards in an Inner-London health district. *Nursing Practice* 5, 16–24.

Bowman C (1993) It's a dog's life in the sick world of the health supermarket. *Care of the Elderly* 5, 440.

Burgess L (1994) Mixed responses. *Nursing Times* 90, 30–4.

Butterworth CA and Faugier J (1992) *Clinical Supervision and Mentorship in Nursing*. Chapman & Hall, London.

Cawthorn A and Hope K (1992) Nursing interventions at night. In McMahon R (ed.) *Nursing at Night: A Professional Approach*. Scutari, London.

Chapman V (1987) Planning the nursing care of the patient. In Collins S and Parker E (eds) *Essentials of Nursing: An Introduction*, pp. 91–113. Macmillan, London.

Cheah Y and Moon G (1993) Specialism and nursing: the case for nursing care for elderly people. *Journal of Advanced Nursing* 18, 1610–16.

Coleman PG (1986) *Ageing and Reminiscence Processes: Social and Clinical Implications*. Wiley, Chichester.

Counsel and Care (1993) *Not only Bingo*. Counsel and Care, London.

Deberry S, Davis S and Reinhard K (1989) A comparison of meditation–relaxation and cognitive/behavioural techniques for reducing anxiety and depression in a geriatric population. *Journal of Geriatric Psychiatry* 22, 231–47.

De Raeve L (1992) Nurse patient relationships at night. In McMahon R (ed.) *Nursing at Night: A Professional Approach*. Scutari, London.

Fallot RD (1980) The impact of mood on verbal reminiscing in late adulthood. *International Journal of Aging and Human Development* 10, 385–400.

Fielden MA (1990) Reminiscence as a therapeutic intervention with sheltered housing residents: a comparative study. *British Journal of Social Work* 20, 21–44.

Friedman E, Katcher A and Lynch JJ (1980) Animal companions and first year surgical survival of patients after discharge from a coronary care unit. *Public Health Report* 95, 307–12.

Furstenberg FF (1988) Short term value of pets. *American Journal of Nursing* 88, 157.

Goodwin S (1985) Cosmic nursing. *Nursing Times* 81, 24–6.

Goodwin S (1989) Remembrance day. *Geriatric Nursing and Home Care* January, 18–19.

Gormally L (1992) The aged: non-persons, human dignity and justice. In Gormally L (ed.) *The Dependent Elderly: Autonomy, Justice and Quality of Care*, pp. 181–8. Cambridge University Press, Cambridge.

Grau L (1984) What older adults expect from the nurse. *Geriatric Nursing* January/ February, 14–18.

Green S (1991) A two faced society. *Nursing Times* 87, 26–9.

Haggar V (1992) Good companions. *Nursing Times* 88, 54–5.

Hale N (1989) Animal house. *Geriatric Nursing and Home Care* April, 12.

Henderson V (1961) *Basic Principles of Nursing Care*. International Council of Nurses, London.

Hope KW (1993) Attitudes towards older people: a comparison of nurses working in acute care of elderly areas with nurses working in acute medical areas. Unpublished MA dissertation. Keele University.

Hope KW (1994) Nurses' attitudes towards older people: a comparison of nurses working in acute medical and acute care of the elderly settings. *Journal of Advanced Nursing* 20, 605–12.

Jackson MF (1994) Discharge planning: issues and challenges for gerontological nursing: a critique of the literature. *Journal of Advanced Nursing* 19, 492–502.

Jerome D (1990a) Intimate relationships. In Bond J and Coleman P (eds) *Ageing in Society*, pp 181–208. Sage, London.

Jerome D (1990b) Frailty and friendship. *Journal of Cross-Cultural Gerontology* 5, 51–64.

Johnson M (1991) The meaning of old age. In Redfern S (ed.) *Nursing Elderly People*, 2nd edn., pp 3–18. Churchill Livingstone, Edinburgh.

Kemp J (1988) Qualified success. *Geriatric Nursing and Home Care* 10, 15.

Kershaw B (1987) Education for care. *Senior Nurse* 6, 28–9.

Kershaw B (1992) Nursing models. In Jolley M and Brykczynska G (eds) *Nursing Care: The Challenge to Change.* Edward Arnold, London.

Lewis CN (1971) Reminiscing and self concept in old age. *Journal of Gerontology* 21, 240–3.

Livingston G, Blizard B and Mann A (1993) Does sleep disturbance predict depression in elderly people? *British Journal of General Practice* 43, 445–8.

Marr J and Khadim N (1993) Meeting the needs of ethnic patients. *Nursing Standard* 8, 31–3.

Maslow AH (1954) *Motivation and Personality.* Harper and Row, New York.

Matteson MA and McConnell ES (1988) *Gerontological Nursing: Concepts and Practice.* WB Saunders, Philadelphia.

McCall J (1990) Fostering self esteem. *Surgical Nurse* 3, 4–10.

McKenna H (1993) The effects of nursing models on quality of care. *Nursing Times* 89, 43–6.

McLane AM (1987) *Classification of Nursing Diagnoses.* Proceedings of the seventh conference. CV Mosby, St Louis.

McMahon A and Ruddick P (1964) Reminiscing. *Archives of General Pyschiatry* 10, 292–8.

Meriam S and Cross L (1981) Aging, reminiscence and life satisfaction. *Activities, Adaptation and Ageing* 2, 39–50.

Minshull J, Ross K and Turner J (1986) The human needs model of nursing. *Journal of Advanced Nursing* 11, 643–9.

Murphy E (1982) Social origins of depression in old age. *British Journal of Psychiatry* 141, 135–41.

Neuman B (1982) *The Neuman Systems Model: Application to Nursing Education and Practice.* Appleton–Century–Crofts, Norwalk, Connecticut.

Norris A (1986) *Reminiscence and Elderly People.* Winslow Press, Bicester.

Orem DE (1980) *Nursing: Concepts of Practice.* New York. McGraw-Hill, New York.

Pearson A (1991) Taking up the challenge: the future for therapeutic nursing. In McMahon R and Pearson A (eds) *Nursing as Therapy.* Chapman & Hall, London.

Peplau H (1952) *Interpersonal Relations in Nursing.* Putnam, New York.

Riehl JR (1980) The Riehl interaction model. In Riehl JR and Riehl C (eds) *Conceptual Models for Nursing Practice*. Norwalk. Appleton–Century–Crofts, Norwalk, Connecticut.

Roper N, Logan WW and Tierney AJ (1980) *The Elements of Nursing*, 2nd edn. Churchill Livingstone, Edinburgh.

Roy C (1980) The Roy adaptation model. In Riehl JR and Riehl C (eds) *Conceptual Models for Nursing Practice*. Appleton–Century–Crofts, Norwalk, Connecticut.

Royal College of Nursing (1987) *Focus on Restraint: Guidelines on the Use of Restraint in the Care of Elderly People*. Royal College of Nursing, London.

Royal College of Nursing (1993) *Working with Older People*. Scutari, London.

Salvage J (1990) The theory and practice of the 'new nursing'. *Nursing Times* 86, 42–5.

Scrutton S (1989) *Counselling Older People – A Creative Response to Ageing*. Edward Arnold, London.

Slevin OD (1991) Ageist attitudes among young adults: implications for a caring profession. *Journal of Advanced Nursing* 16, 1197–205

Snape J (1986) Nurses' attitudes to care of the elderly. *Journal of Advanced Nursing* 11, 569–72.

Social Services Inspectorate (1989) *Homes are for Living in*. HMSO, London.

Tate S (1992) Visiting rules. *Nursing Times* 88, 26.

Tattam A (1992) Urgent call to curb abuse of restraint. *Nursing Times* 88, 8.

Turner P (1993) Activity nursing and the changes in the quality of life of elderly patients: a semi-quantitative study. *Journal of Advanced Nursing* 18, 1727–33.

Webb J (1992) A new lease of life. *Nursing Times* 88, 30–2.

Webb C and Hope K (1995) What kind of nurses do patients want? *Journal of Clinical Nursing* 4, 101–8.

15

Quality, audit and review

Mike Wafer

Today old people make greater use of health services than ever before. Approximately half of all hospital beds are occupied by people aged over 65 years, and nearly a third are occupied by people over the age of 75 years. This chapter is written with the belief that older people have a right to equity of care with the rest of the population, and that they have a right to a high quality of care. It will be argued that the issue of quality has always been important to nurses, but as a separate entity in itself it does not appear in the nursing literature in any substantial way until the early 1960s in the USA (Kitson and Harvey, 1991), with the first major text appearing in the UK in 1987 (Pearson, 1987).

Some difficulties arise when trying to understand the concept of quality. The term is used to cover a variety of activities including total quality management, quality assurance, standard setting, clinical audit, nursing audit, medical audit, *The Patient's Charter* and complaints monitoring. This is further complicated in that, although the terminology is used by all types of staff in their different settings, the emphasis and importance may be very different. For a chief executive in a trust, for example, the most important quality activity may be ensuring that the *Patient's Charter* standard (1995) 'that patients are seen within 30 minutes of their appointment time' is met because the consequence of not achieving this standard may mean that the trust does not receive income from the purchasers to provide services in the future. For a nurse working on a ward for older people, the most important quality issue might be that patients have a pair of knickers to put on that have not come from a common pool of clothing. The two issues may be directly related, as increased income for the unit as a whole may allow the opportunity to improve services such as laundry provision.

Defining quality

The word quality is derived from the Latin *qualis* which means 'of what sort'. In everyday language, for example, the words a 'quality product' would mean a product that is of a high standard. In writings about organisations, other definitions can be found, for example a quality product would be 'fit for its purpose or use', conforming to requirements, or meeting customers expectations (Parsley and Corrigan, 1994: 210). In the non-health literature, there is an explicit link between quality and price. Both a Lada car and a Rolls Royce can be regarded as a quality car because they conform to requirements and meet expectations for the price paid. In the health care and nursing literature there is little explicit discussion about the relationship between price and quality. However, historically it is evident that many older people have had to make do with the equivalent of the Lada, rather than the Rolls Royce.

Six features can be identified as constituting a quality service for older people (after Maxwell, 1984):

- *Accessibility*: that health services are accessible to all older people in the population being served
- *Relevance to need*: that services provided are relevant to the particular needs of older people in the community
- *Equity*: that all older people are treated equally regardless of race, religion or socioeconomic status
- *Social acceptability*: that services provided are acceptable to older people
- *Efficiency*: that services provided are cost effective
- *Effectiveness*: that services provided are effective and regular audits are implemented to ensure effectiveness.

Quality in health care is an especially difficult concept to define. Nursing care is difficult to describe because it is a human service, which must always hang on to an element of subjectivity and intuition (Pearson, 1987). It has been suggested that providing quality service is about achieving excellence, and that quality is dynamic – with the ultimate goal being perfection.

An extremely influential writer on health issues and quality is Donabedian (1980), who conceptualised quality as having three constituent parts:

- *Structure* covers 'concrete', and organisational factors such as physical environment, equipment, staffing levels and resources
- *Process* refers to what health professionals actually do, for example giving nursing care
- *Outcome* refers to what actually happens as a result of the health care system's interventions.

The idea of outcome measurement is especially important in relation to caring for older people, as this may be particularly difficult to define in a that may have multiple pathologies. In addition, older people may regard a higher quality of life as the most desirable outcome of any health care intervention, and this may be difficult to measure. The issue of outcomes will be discussed below.

Four perspectives of quality

It is useful to consider quality as having four dimensions:

- *The consumer perspective* is the most important perspective as all health services should focus on the recipient of care.
- *The professional perspective* is also of great importance, as professionals will have unique expertise and insights as to what constitutes quality care.
- *The organisation perspective* is quality viewed from a managerial point of view. To provide a high standard of care to the consumer, the organisation needs to run smoothly.
- *The health policy perspective* is quality as viewed by central government. This includes current initiatives such as *The Patient's Charter*.

These four dimensions should be viewed as interdependent and not mutually exclusive. Nurses working in clinical areas may not be able to see beyond the organisation's influence on quality. However, quality is considerably influenced at the health policy level as it is here that many decisions are made, such as those about allocations of funds for health. Ultimately, policy decisions are also influenced by politicians, who can be influenced by consumers, who decide how to use their votes in general elections.

Although consumers' views are extremely important, they are not always in a position to judge whether they are receiving expert care. In terms of nursing care, clients may judge quality on the basis of inter-personal skills, which are vital but may be superfluous if the wrong medication is being administered or an aseptic technique is being per-formed incorrectly. There may be conflicts of interest in relation to quality. The patient might regard as high quality care that he be allowed to stay in bed for several days following myocardial infarction, whereas the nurse will seek to mobilise the patient early to prevent the complications of immobility. General managers may put emphasis on efficiency (one of Maxwell's criteria of quality) and short stays in hospital, whereas health professionals may regard this as detrimental to the care of some patients.

Management of quality

Within health care organisations it is desirable that there is a named person who is responsible for facilitating quality improvement (Wilson, 1987, 1992). Historically, health service quality activities have developed in an *ad hoc* way, and initially focused on audit activities by separate professional groups. However, it is becoming increasingly recognised that, if one department breaks the quality chain, this will affect those receiving care (Sale, 1990: 51). Thus, for nurses to provide a high standard of nutritional care, they are dependent on the catering staff to provide high quality meals, porters to get the meals to the ward at the correct time, dietitians to give advice, and occupational therapists to assess and provide appropriate eating aids.

A managerial model which is being used successfully in health care is that advocated by Christopher Wilson (1987, 1992). He suggests that:

- The senior person in a unit or organisation should be committed to providing a quality service.
- There should be an identifiable central body that is responsible for quality, chaired by a senior member of the board or unit.
- Quality monitoring should be co-ordinated.
- There should be communication about quality activities across pro-fessional groups and departments.

It is suggested that quality activities should be

- *Focused on the needs of the client*
- *Built on trust*
- *Negotiable* between professional staff and managers
- *Driven by departments*
- *Action orientated*
- *Specific*
- *Efficient*

Three key concepts in Wilson's model are principal functions, important components and quality indicators.

Principal functions

A principal function is the end product that a department delivers. It is suggested that each department should be able to identify between four and six principal functions, which make up between 80 per cent and 90 per cent of a department's activities. Each function should take up at least 10 per cent of a department's work.

Thus, within the unit in which the author is employed (Medical Services for Older People), the principal functions are to provide:

- *Acute inpatient services* to older people with medical problems
- *Rehabilitation services* to older inpatients
- *Day care* medical and rehabilitation services to older people
- *Outpatient services* to older people with medical problems
- A regional and national resource as a *nursing development unit.*

Principal functions have potential value in the contracting process with purchasers of health care, as they allow units to articulate in a concise way the services that they provide. This allows purchasers to compare services of different provider units, and will assist them in decision making in placing contracts.

Important components

Important components are derived from principal functions and focus on activity. For example, important components of principal function that 'provide acute inpatient services to older people with medical problems' could be:

- A *full medical assessment* of all patients on admission to the unit
- A *full nursing assessment* on admission to the unit
- *Monitoring of clinical signs*, according to individual patients' needs and diagnosis during their stay in hospital.

Important components provide a useful tool for identifying areas on which standards (see below) can be written.

Quality indicators

Wilson describes an indicator as a quantity that tells us something about quality – it is always a number. These act as flags or signals, but should not be regarded as infallible: their meaning will not become clear until they are investigated. Examples of indicators of quality might be:

- *Readmission rates of patients* within two weeks of their discharge date.

- *Incidence of pressure sores* among hospital inpatients
- Average *length of inpatient stay.*

If pressure sore incidence is used as an indicator, it must be remembered that an increase in pressure sores could be caused by several factors, e.g. increase in the number of dependent patients, insufficient availability of pressure relieving aids, or insufficient number of nursing staff. It is important to emphasise that the number of pressure sores cannot automatically be taken as an indicator of the quality of nursing care alone.

The Audit Commission (1991) has recommended the use of indicators and has suggested that the following may be useful:

- The incidence and severity of pressure sores
- Incidence of hospital acquired infection
- Patient falls and other injuries to patients or staff
- Medication errors.

Arguments may be made against indicators, which may present an ambiguous message. A total absence of patient falls, for example, may indicate an unduly restrictive regime rather than ideal care. It is also possible that, in some instances, asking for data to be collected may increase awareness of some issues, and that this will in itself increase the number of reported incidents. Roberts (1985) in a study of accidents to hospital patients suspected that, as her study proceeded, nurses because more aware that she was collecting data on accidents to patients and that this increased the number of accidents documented.

Planning quality activities

Quality activities need to be planned and organised in a systematic way. A useful tool to achieve this is the quality calendar described by Wilson (1992: 102). (An example is given in Figure 15.1.) Using this, all the activities planned for a year are documented. Subjects for inclusion will be determined by professionals working within the area, by managers and by health policy. Some audits will be a one-off activity; others will be performed on regular basis. Typical activities in my workplace include:

- Patient satisfaction surveys
- Visitor satisfaction surveys
- Staff questionnaires
- Ward audits
- Infection control surveys
- Surveys by the Audit Commission and King's Fund Organisational Audit
- Audit of pressure sores

- Audit of patient falls and accidents
- Audit by the purchasing team
- Audit by the Community Health Council
- Equipment audits (e.g. accuracy of sphygmomanometers).

It is important that audits do not occur too frequently, as too many may result in poor quality audits (Wilson, 1992). Luther and Robinson (1993: 21) suggest an audit every three to six months in each ward and department. They also suggest flexibility in order to accommodate time lags in the collection of information and in the collation and presentation

QUALITY CALENDER
October 1996–September 1997

Month	Quality activity	Audit activity	Purchaser requirement
October 1996	*Patient's Charter* survey		*Patient's Charter* return
November 1996			
December 1996		Pressure sore audit	
January 1997	Infection control survey		*Patient's Charter* return
February 1997	Readmission survey	Ward audit	
March 1997			
April 1997			*Patient's Charter* return
May 1997		Discharge audit	
June 1997			
July 1997		Ward audit	*Patient's Charter* return
August 1997	Consumer satisfaction survey		
September 1997			

Figure 15.1 An example of a quality calendar.

of the data produced, and then time for implementing any changes and reassessing aspects of care delivery if necessary.

Responsibility for quality

Maintaining quality is the responsibility of everybody in a unit delivering care. Nurses must feel that they are personally responsible for the quality of care that they deliver, within the constraints of the resources available. Although managers within a unit and external auditors have a valuable part to play in the improvement of quality, genuine sustained quality improvements are more likely to be implemented if frontline staff are given support to monitor their own service. Wainwright (1987: 15) advocates the practice of peer review, defining it as 'the evaluation by practising nurses of the quality of nursing care performed by other nurses according to stated norms of the profession'.

A particularly useful form of peer review is the use of an audit tool in which nurses examine their own practice. An example of a documentation audit currently in use at Tameside is given in Figure 15.2. This audit tool is based on the unit standard for documentation (Nursing Development Unit, 1990) and allows the senior ward nurse to evaluate the documentation on their own ward.

Although it is useful for nurses working in clinical areas to evaluate their own practice, they will need support in the analysis and presentation of their findings. It is not usually possible for clinicians working in busy areas to produce high standard reports without the support of managers, particularly quality nurses/advisors if they are in post.

The purpose of the audit tool is to allow nurses to monitor their own documentation. It is suggested that the senior sister select at random ten *nursing notes*. Each set of nursing notes is assessed separately. Each item is given a score out of 5, i.e.

5 = Excellent
4 = Very good
3 = Adequate
2 = Less than adequate
1 = Very poor

There are ten items. Each care plan is scored out of 50 (10 $\times$ 5). The scores are then totalled to give a score out of 500 (50 $\times$ 10 nursing notes = 500).

Less than 300 = Cause for concern: action plan needed
300–400   = Adequate, but needs some improvement
400–500   = Documentation of high standard

Nurses should use their own professional judgement in assessing care plans. It it is recommended that primary nurses evaluate each other's nursing notes.

	5	4	3	2	1	
Admission sheet completed fully						Admission sheet incomplete
Documentation legible						Documentation illegible
All entries signed and dated						Entries not signed
No abbreviations used						Abbreviations commonplace
Documentation by named nurse/deputy						Documentation by nurse other than named nurse or deputy
Discharge plan documented						No evidence of discharge planning
Evidence of patient education						No evidence of patient education
Record of emotional need/feelings						No documentation of emotional needs or feelings
Evidence of multidisciplinary working						No evidence of multidisciplinary working
Care plan patient centred						Care plan not patient centred
Comments						Score =

Figure 15.2 Tameside Audit of Nurse Documentation.

Presentation of information

It is vital that the results of audit and quality activities are communicated. The first question that needs to be addressed is who needs to know the information. This will help in terms of deciding how to communicate information. In most instances it will be necessary to present some written

Do you receive information when you come to the ward? (please tick ✓ box)

Yes ☐
Sometimes ☐
Only if I ask ☐
Very rarely ☐
Never ☐
Please comment ....
....
....

Figure 15.3 An example of a question to elicit quantitative and qualitative data.

information on audit and quality activities. Information should be presented in as short and simple a manner as possible. Katz and Green (1992: 184) state that everyday language should be used that the audience will understand, and that jargon should, where possible, be avoided. It may also be necessary to write different reports on the same activity for different audiences. For example, the results of a report on nutrition may

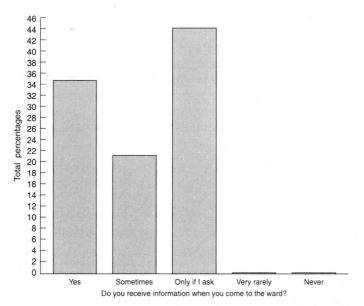

'When I asked for information everyone was frank and helpful'
'When a patient is seriously ill it is not easy for staff to decide how much information to give to relatives.'
'Mainly only if I ask, unless something exceptional happens.'
'Information freely given.'
'This is reasonable, staff are always very busy' (accompanying 'Only if I ask response').
'I appreciate the staff are pushed for time'.

Figure 15.4 Presentation of qualitative data together with quantitative data.

need to be communicated to the dietitian, consultant physician, ward sisters and unqualified staff.

Increasingly in the health service there is emphasis on presenting information quantitatively (i.e. in numbers, e.g. in graphs or pie charts). However, for many issues relating to clinical care, this may be very unsatisfactory. Presenting how patients felt about professionals' communication skills is unlikely to be expressed satisfactorily purely in quantitative terms.

A possible way around the quantitative/qualitative dilemma is to devise data collection instruments that produce both types of data. For example, questions within surveys can be framed in such a way that questions are asked and a choice of responses is given (see Figure 15.3), thus generating quantitative data; and within the same question the respondent can be asked to comment, thus generating qualitative data (e.g. Figure 15.3). Thus, examples of the qualitative data are written underneath graphs representing the quantitative data, as shown in Figure 15.4 (Wafer and Metcalfe, 1993).

Quality assurance

Quality assurance is an important part of any department's quality activities. It comes under the broad umbrella of quality, but is not synonymous with quality. It may include, for example, customer care courses, awareness training for special needs groups, and production of patient information in addition to quality assurance. Quality assurance is the promising, or making certain, of a certain standard of excellence. It has the following elements:

- The setting of standards
- Measurement
- Evaluation
- Acting on the evaluation.

Quality assurance programmes, it is suggested sceptically (Pollitt, 1992), are set up for the following reasons:

- As a *symbolic* action to protect a group, unit or organisation from external criticism
- To tighten *control over resources*
- To *strengthen managerial power* and influence
- To improve public *accountability*
- To generate more *systematic information* about quality and effectiveness, which may be useful in defending a service against economy drives
- To *enhance responsiveness* to service users/consumers
- As a type of *professional development and education.*

Quality assurance in nursing

There are two types of quality measurement currently being practised by nurses. Firstly there are the so called 'off the shelf' tools (Sale, 1990: 18) which include:

- *Phaneuf's Nursing Audit*. This is a retrospective documentation audit that identifies seven key functions of nursing. From these, Phaneuf (1972) identifies fifty components to help auditors to evaluate the quality of nursing (Pearson, 1987: 45). This tool, devised in the USA, was first published in 1972. Sparrow and Robinson (1992) suggest that the tool still has relevance for practice in the UK.
- *Qualpacs*. This is a tool devised by Wandelt and Ager in 1974. It is a concurrent review, which seeks to evaluate nursing care as it is being provided. It includes a review of the records, patient interviews, observation of patients and staff, and staff interview (Sale, 1990: 24). A good example of its use in practice is given by Pearson, Punton and Durant (1992) in their evaluation of the Nursing Development Unit in Oxford.
- *Monitor*. This is a UK adaptation of the Rush Medicus instrument devised in Chicago in 1972. Monitor has a patient orientated approach and is focused on individual patient care and patients' needs. It consists of 455 questions which are grouped into four sections: assessment and planning; physical care; non-physical care and evaluation (Sale, 1990: 30).

A second approach is that of practising nurses writing their own standards. This allows nurses to adopt a bottom-up approach to improving standards of care rather than being given standard tools by managers.

Setting standards in a nursing development unit for older people

A good example of nurses writing their own standards is provided by the nursing staff on the Nursing Development Unit for Older People at Tameside (Arnold and Wright, 1990). A working group of ward nurses and clinical specialists from within the unit was collected together to produce ideas and write a set of draft standards for the clinical areas. It was agreed with the unit managers that for the exercise to be beneficial the group should meet away from the hospital site because of the risk of interruptions.

As each draft standard was produced, this was circulated to the ward areas and, in response to their comments, the standard were revised by the working party. It was recognised when writing the standards that they were not 'written in stone' and would be revised on a regular basis. To facilitate this regular review, a standards validation group was convened, which met on a regular basis to review individual standards. This group consisted of ward based nurses who discussed whether standards were being met and, if they were not, drew this to the attention of managers within the unit. In all, a total of 27 standards were written. At Tameside a decision was made to document standards using a criterion approach (i.e. individual statements) as opposed to the structure–process–outcome approach adopted by Kitson (1990). This method was chosen after discussion with nursing staff and they felt that this was the best approach for them (Table 15.1).

Table 15.1 Standard relating to the giving of information to patients and significant others

It is accepted that all patients and significant others, as users of a public service, have the right to information regarding health problems and the services that are available to help resolve these. To this end:

1. The patient and significant others are given an information booklet which contains information regarding:

    - The hospital
    - The ward
    - The hospital and ward telephone numbers
    - The nursing philosophy
    - Personal items needed while in hospital
    - Times of meals and menu cards
    - Medication
    - Visiting
    - Portable telephones
    - The multidisciplinary team members
    - The patient's rights
    - The complaints procedure
    - The organisation of care
    - Smoking regulations
    - The ward/unit facilities available
    - Chaplaincy
    - Library services
    - The patient's shop
    - The hairdresser
    - Pensions/benefits
    - Valuables
    - Discharge arrangements

2. The named nurse explains to the patient and significant others what is involved in:

    - The admission procedure
    - Assessment
    - Goal setting

- Care planning
- Treatment facilities
- Evaluation of care
- Discharge preparation
3. Each ward/department has an 'information centre' displaying information to patients about the ward/department and community facilities.
4. Information on, and access to, complementary therapies is available for patients.
5. All information is available in languages other than English, and is written in a non-sexist non-racist manner and in terminology which the patient and significant others can comprehend.
6. A trained interpreter is available for patients and significant others.

To measure the twenty-seven standards of which the example given in Table 15.1 is one, an audit tool was devised. This consisted of:

- An *interview schedule for patients*. During the audit a minimum of ten patients are interviewed.
- An *interview schedule for the senior ward nurse*. As part of the audit the senior nurse is interviewed for approximately an hour.
- A *documentation audit*. Nursing documentation is examined using the unit tool (see Figure 15.2)
- A *postal questionnaire*. This is distributed to twenty visitors.
- An *observation schedule*. During the audit, the quality nurse undertook both participant and non-participant observation.

The responsibility for performing the audit is that of the clinical nurse specialist responsible for quality assurance.

It is important that clinical areas are given advanced warning of when audit activity is to take place and the tools that are to be used. This allows clinical areas to evaluate their practice critically and to seek improvements before the audit. It also means that, if areas are shown to need improvement, they genuinely need improvement and a poor audit is not just the result of an 'off day'. It is vital that the purpose of audit is not lost sight of. This is to measure current practice in order that improvements can be made to the benefit of the patient. It is not helpful if nurses see audit as a punitive activity; if they do, they may withhold information for fear of the consequences.

It is the practice at Tameside within the Nursing Development Unit for a report about the audit to be given to the ward sister for comment shortly before it is circulated to senior managers. Following this, it is recommended that copies of the audit are circulated to all ward nursing staff and interested parties, including other professionals working in the ward area. It may also be appropriate to send details to patients' representatives such as Age Concern, the Community Health Council, and purchasers of health care.

The report should include examples of good practice within the clinical area and, where appropriate, identify individuals who have been innovative, or who have made notable contributions. Typical examples of good practice might be as follows:

1. All of the patients interviewed were very positive about the nursing care that they received.
2. The ward is committed to primary nursing: the off duty was always written in such a way as to facilitate this. The majority of patients interviewed could name their primary nurse.

Recommendations/ comments	Action	Person(s) responsible
1. Some nursing admission assessments need to be more detailed	*Discuss at ward meeting* *Primary nurse to audit their own documentation using audit tool*	Support by CNS Ward Sister Primary/associate nurses
2. Nursing handover: lunchtime report seems unduly long: recommend a trial using taped reports for some information	*Raise a ward meeting* *Discuss at senior nurses' meeting* *Discuss with clinical director possibility of funding for taping equipment*	Clinical/Directorate manager CNS Ward Staff
3. Not all patients have been receiving primary nurse 'business card'	*Ensure all patients receive card on admission – ask ward clerk to include in admission pack*	Ward Clerk
4. On two shifts over the period monitored there was only one qualified nurse on duty	*Ensure off duty arranged so that there are always two qualified nurses on duty* *If insufficient staff to do this arrange bank nurses*	Ward Sister Directorate manager
5. Visitors say they are unable to get refreshments when visiting	*Discuss possibilitiy of vending machine* *Raise with catering manager* *Provide information about restaurant facilities within the hospital*	Directorate manager Catering manager Quality advisor
6 Ward has diminished supply of specialised eating aids (special cutlery, non-slip plates)	*Seek advice of occupational therapists as to most appropriate aides* *Contact supplies to order*	Ward Sister Occupational therapist Supplies manager
7. Ward needs further supplies of carrier and essential oils	*Order further oils with ward funds*	Ward Sister

Figure 15.5 An action plan.

3. Student nurses and the College of Nursing said that they felt the ward was an excellent learning environment. Students said they felt supported by ward staff and found staff very willing to share their expertise.
4. The ward staff have a strong interest in pain relief and have raised funds to purchase syringe drivers to administer analgesia. They are intending to begin a trial of self administration of p.r.n. oral analgesia.
5. The ward sister has helped to write the unit protocol on subcutaneous infusions, and is intending to be involved in the planned working party in educating nurses about initiating subcutaneous fluids as part of the extended role of the nurse.

An action plan at the end of the report should be included in which individuals at all levels in the unit are named to lead the appropriate action, and the date by which they need to act (see Figure 15.5). It is vital that it is recognised that acting on the audit is the responsibility not just of the ward sister but of all members of the ward team and the senior nursing staff and managers. An essential ingredient of successful audit activity is that of trust between those who are auditing and those being audited.

Issues in monitoring the quality of care of older people

Monitoring the quality of health care for older people may be problematic. For example:

- If we are to argue that part of quality care is meeting expectations, for some older people these may be low. The majority of older people today have memories of health care before the National Health Service was founded in 1948. Before 1948, much medical care was out of the question for low income families and hence, in many cases, any care, even if substandard, maybe gratefully received. Also, much of today's hospital care is provided in what was the old workhouse; and there may be a strong folklore in the local community that people entered only to die. (Happily, much of this accommodation is now being replaced.)
- Many older people are, or feel, very vulnerable in hospital. Hence, if they are asked about the standard of care they are receiving, they may be slightly less than honest because they fear that there may be reprisals against them if they are critical about care. In addition, it is my experience when interviewing inpatients that they are tremendously loyal to the staff, particularly the nurses, who are caring for them.

- Some older people have considerable communication problems and so may be unable adequately to articulate how they feel about the service being provided. These problems are particularly acute if the person comes from an ethnic minority whose first language is not English (see Marr and Khadim, 1993).
- Older people may not agree with the professionals' view of what is good practice. Hence, the professional view may be that good care involves early mobilisation, whereas the patient may regard this as less than ideal practice. They may have traditionalist views about the hospital ward hierarchy, for example, and may be perturbed by some of the attempts to break these down, such as nurses wearing their own clothes instead of a uniform (see Marr and Matthews, 1993) in order to facilitate a 'therapeutic relationship'. They may have difficulty with the idea of the primary nurse and may be nostalgic for the hospital Matron!

Outcome measures and the QALY

As a result of changes in health care and the restricted amount of resources available to health care, there has been an increased emphasis on monitoring the effectiveness of care through outcome measurements; that is, trying to determine the effect of health care interventions to see whether they have been successful, to judge cost effectiveness. Outcomes are extremely complex – they can be measured both directly and indirectly, over different periods of time and from different sources of information, and they vary according to perspective (Bond and Thomas, 1991). Many tools have been devised in an attempt to measure outcome; however, one tool has had particular dominance in recent years. This tool is the Quality Adjusted Life Year or QALY, which is unique in that it attempts to measure outcomes in terms of quality and quantity of life. This tool has been devised by health economists and puts a numerical value on life in which 0 = death and 1 = fit and healthy (Williams and Kind, 1992). Beneficial health care activities are regarded as those that generate large numbers of QALYs.

QALYs are said to have two main functions:

1. They allow more informed decisions to be made about the effectiveness of one form of treatment for a particular problem rather than another treatment for the same problem.
2. They can be used to judge priorities in health care (Mooney, 1992).

The use of QALYs in health care is very controversial, particularly as an outcome measure for older people. It is reasonable to use QALYs to choose between effective treatments, but they should not be used to decide which individuals are treated (Grimley-Evans, 1992). Mooney

(1992) has suggested that QALYs are a useful aid in giving information to patients about the potential outcome of different treatments. QALYs could be a cause of great concern for all individuals who care for older people, as if they are used to decide priorities in health care there is a risk that they will be used to discriminate against older people.

Outcome measures will become increasingly important in future years. It is important that outcomes should be judged on an individual basis, not for whole groups of people on the basis of stereotypical views. There is sometimes a view that with older people the emphasis is on ensuring quality of life, and that quantity is secondary, but for some survival and extension of life are equally important. The QALY debate reminds people caring for older people that all life should be given equal weight, and that an older life should be valued as highly as a younger one (Fletcher, 1992).

Conclusion

This chapter has given an overview of quality, and related it to nursing older people. Quality is difficult to define and can be viewed from different perspectives, some of which may appear to conflict with each other. What is important is that nurses caring for older people recognise all the influences that affect quality, and try to act on that information to improve care for older people. Management of quality has been discussed and a useful framework, Wilson's model, has been identified. It is vital that, if quality improvements are to be made, the most senior person in a care giving unit – whether it be the chief executive of a large provider unit or the owner of a 30 bedded nursing home – is committed to quality and identifies a named person to facilitate quality improvements. It is also important that all staff regard providing a high quality service as being of high priority and recognise that they are responsible for the quality of their own work. Support should be available for staff who identify deficiencies in care, so that staff are encouraged to report where improvements need to be made.

Examples have been given of quality monitoring in practice in the Nursing Development Unit for Older People at Tameside. It is important that nurses feel ownership of standards and that they feel that it has day-to-day relevance to their nursing practice, and is not something which is remote and the property of management. Trust between nurses and their managers is imperative if audit activities are to bring about genuine improvements in patient care. What is especially important in addition to discussing problem areas is that a positive approach is taken and areas of good practice are highlighted in audit reports.

Some issues have been discussed around special aspects of monitoring the quality of care of older people – a particular problem being that some may have relatively low expectations of the service. Finally, outcome measures have been discussed and concern expressed about the use of the QALY in evaluating health care interventions on older people. Ultimately, older people have a right to expect the same high quality health care as the rest of the population.

References

Arnold K and Wright SG (1990) Writing and using standards of nursing care. *Nursing Practice* 4, 10–14.

Audit Commission (1991) *The Virtue of Patients*. HMSO, London.

Bond S and Thomas L (1991) Issues in measuring outcomes in nursing. *Journal of Advanced Nursing* 16, 1492–502.

Department of Health (1995) *The Patient's Charter and You*. HMSO, London.

Donabedian A (1980) *The Definition of Quality and Approach to its Assessment*. Health Administration Press, Michigan.

Fletcher A (1992) Quality of life assessments in older people – discussion. In *Measures of Quality of Life*. Royal College of Physicians, London.

Grimley-Evans J (1992) Quality of life assessments in older people. In *Measures of Quality of Life*. Royal College of Physicians, London.

Katz J and Green E (1992) *Managing Quality: A Guide to Monitoring and Evaluating Nursing Services*. CV Mosby, St Louis.

Kitson A (1990) Setting standards. *Nursing Standard* 26, 55.

Kitson A and Harvey G (1991) *Quality Assurance and Standards of Care*. Scutari, London.

Luther J and Robinson L (1993) *The Royal Marsden Hospital Manual of Standards of Care*. Blackwell, Oxford.

Marr J and Khadim N (1993) Meeting the needs of ethnic patients. *Nursing Standard* 8, 31–3.

Marr J and Matthews T (1993) Change of a dress. *Nursing Standard* 7, 48–9.

Maxwell R (1984) Quality assessment in health. *British Medical Journal* 288, 1470–2.

Mooney G (1992) *Economics, Medicine and Health Care*, 2nd edn. Harvester Wheatsheaf, London.

Nursing Development Unit (1990) *Nursing Standards: older people*. Tameside Health Authority, Ashton-under-Lyne.

Parsley K and Corrigan P (1994) *Quality Improvement in Nursing and Health Care*. Chapman & Hall. London.

Pearson A (1987) *Nursing Quality Measurement*. Wiley, Chichester.

Phaneuf MC (1972) *The Nursing Audit*. Appleton-Century-Crofts, New York.

Pollitt C (1992) *Performance Evaluation in the Public Sector*. Paper given at Partnership in Audit Conference, York, 5 November 1992.

Roberts F (1985) Reported accidents to hospital patients. MSc thesis, Manchester University.

Sale D (1990) *Quality Assurance*. Macmillan, London.

Sparrow S and Robinson J (1992) The use and limitations of Phaneuf's nursing audit. *Journal of Advanced Nursing* 17, 1479–88.

Wafer M and Metcalfe S (1993) *Patient's Charter Survey. NDU for Older People.* Tameside. Health Authority, Ashton-under-Lyne.

Wainwright P (1987) Peer review. In Pearson A (ed.) *Nursing Quality Measurement.* Wiley, Chichester.

Wandelt MA and Ager JW (1974) *Quality Patient Care Scale.* Appleton-Century-Crofts. New York.

Williams A and Kind P (1992) The present state of play about QALYs. In Hopkins A (ed.) *Measures of the Quality of Life.* Royal College of Physicians, London.

Wilson C (1987) *Hospital Wide Quality Assurance.* WB Saunders, Toronto.

Wilson C (1992) *Strategies in Health Care Quality.* WB Saunders. Toronto.

Bibliography

Abrahams M (1978) *Beyond three-score and Ten: A First Report on a Survey of the Elderly.* Age Concern, London.

Abrahams M (1978) *Beyond Three-score and Ten: A Second Report on a Survey of the Elderly.* Age Concern, Surrey.

Adams J, Prickett M and Bornat J (1993) *Care Planning and Life Histories.* Paper presented at British Society of Gerontology Conference, Norwich.

Age Concern (1985) *Policies, Practices and Projects. Hospital Discharge and Aftercare Initiatives in London.* Age Concern, London.

Aggleton P and Chalmers H (1986) *Nursing Models and the Nursing Process.* Macmillan, Basingstoke.

Aitken LA (1995) *Ageing. An Introduction to Gerontology.* Sage, London.

Alberti KG (1993) Problems related to definitions of type 2 (non-insulin dependent) diabetes mellitus: studies throughout the world. *Diabetologia* 9, 978–84.

Allen I, Hogg D and Peace S (1992) *Elderly People: Choice, Participation and Satisfaction.* Policy Studies Institute, London.

Allen M (1989) The meaning of visual impairment to visually impaired adults. *Journal of Advanced Nursing* 14, 640–6.

Allen M (1991) Stigma and blindness. *Journal of Ophthalmology and Technology* 10, 147–52.

Altschul AT (1972) *Patient–nurse Interaction: A Study of Interaction Patterns in Acute Psychiatric Wards.* Churchill Livingstone, Edinburgh.

Arber S and Ginn J (1991) *Gender and Later Life.* Sage, London.

Argyle M (1972) Non verbal communication in human interaction. In Hine R (ed.) *Non Verbal Communication.* Cambridge University Press, Cambridge.

Argyle M (1978) *The Psychology of Human Interpersonal Behaviour.* Penguin, Harmondsworth.

Armstrong-Esther CA, Browne KD and McAfee JE (1994) Elderly patients still clean and sitting pretty. *Journal of Advanced Nursing* 19, 264–71.

Arnold D. (1987) The broker model of long term care: a rose by any other name. *Home Health Care Services Quarterly* 8, 23–43.

Arnold K and Wright SG (1990) Writing and using standards of nursing care. *Nursing Practice* 4, 10–14.

Atchley RC (1992) *Social Forces and Ageing.* Wadsworth, Belmont, California.

Atkins S and Murphy K (1993) Reflection: a review of the literature. *Journal of Advanced Nursing* 18, 1188–92.

Audit Commission (1986) *Making a Reality of Community Care.* HMSO, London.

Audit Commission (1991) *The Virtue of Patients.* Audit Commission. HMSO, London.

Audit Commission (1992) *Lying in Wait: The Use of Medical Beds in Acute Hospitals.* HMSO, London.

Bachelor I. (1980) *The Multi-disciplinary Clinical Team – A Working Paper.* King's Fund, London.

Bacon V and Lambkin C (1994) Mixed messages: day care design. *Health Service Journal* 30 June 1994, 20–1.

Bailey K and Clarke M (1989) *Stress and Coping in Nursing.* Chapman & Hall, London.

Bailey R (1985). *Coping with Stress in Caring.* Blackwell Scientific, Oxford.

Baker D (1978) Attitudes of Nurses to the Care of the Elderly. PhD thesis, University of Manchester.

Baker D (1993) Assessment in rehabilitation. *Reviews in Clinical Gerontology* 3, 169–86.

Barker P (1990) The philosophy of psychiatric nursing. *Nursing Standard* 5, 28–33.

Barnat J (1985) Exploring living memory: the uses of reminiscence. *Ageing and Society* 5, 333–7.

Barnett K (1972) A survey of the current utilisation of touch by health team personnel with hospitalised patients. *International Journal of Nursing Studies* 9, 195–209.

Barron C, Foxall MJ, Von Dolen K, Jones PA and Shull KA (1994) Marital status, social support and loneliness in visually impaired elderly people. *Journal of Advanced Nursing* 19, 272–80.

Barsa J, Jones J, Lantigua R and Curland B (1987) Ability of internists to recognise and manage depression in the elderly. *International Journal of Geriatric Psychiatry* 1, 57–62.

Baun M, Bergstrom N and Largston N (1984) Physiological effects of human/companion animal bonding. *Nursing Research* 33, 126–9.

Beardshaw V and Trowell D (1990) *Assessment and Case Management: Implications for the Implementation of Caring for People.* King's Fund briefing paper. King's Fund, London.

Beauchamp T and Childress J (1989) *Principles of Biomedical Ethics.* Oxford University Press, New York.

De Beavoir S (1973) *The Coming of Age.* Putnam, New York.

De Beauvoir S (1972) *Old Age.* Penguin, Harmondsworth.

Beck C and Heacock P (1988) Nursing interventions for patients with Alzheimer's Disease. *Nursing Clinics of North America* 23, 95–121.

Bell J (1992) In search of a discourse on ageing: the elderly on the TV. *Gerontologist* 32, 305–11.

Benner P (1984) *From Novice to Expert: Excellence in Power and Clinical Nursing Practice.* Addison-Wesley Menlo Park, California.

Benner P and Wrubel J (1989) *The Primacy of Caring: Stress and Coping in Health and Illness.* Addison Wesley, Menlo Park, California.

Bennet C (1994) Ending up. *The Guardian Weekend* October 8, 12–20.

Bennet G and Kingston P (1993) *Elder Abuse: Concepts, Theories and Interventions.* Chapman & Hall, London.

Bennett R and Eckman J (1973) Attitudes towards ageing: a critical examination of recent literature and implications for future research. In Eisdorfer C and Lawton MP (eds) *Psychology of Adult Development and Ageing*. American Psychological Association, Washington DC.

Berg S, Mellstrom D, Persson G and Svanorg A (1981) Loneliness in the Swedish aged. *Journal of Gerontology* 36, 342–9.

Berger R (1982) *Gay and Gray: the Older Homosexual Man*. University of Illinois Press, Urbana, Illinois.

Bernard M and Meade K (1993) *Women Come of Age*. Edward Arnold, London.

Berne E (1964) *Games People Play*. Penguin, Harmondsworth.

Beth Johnson Foundation (1991) *Advocacy in Action: The Bulletin of the North Staffordshire Advocacy and Older People Project* Autumn, No 1.

Biggs S (1990) Consumers, case management and inspection: obscuring social deprivation and need? Cited in: Williams D (1992) Social policy and provision. In Crompton A and Ashwin M (eds) *Community Care for Health Professionals*. Butterworth-Heinemann, Oxford.

Birdwhistell R (1970) *Kinesis and Context*. University of Pensylvania Press, Philadelphia.

Birren JE and Woods AM (1985) Psychology of ageing. In Pathy MSJ (ed.) *Principles and Practice of Geriatric Medicine*. Wiley, Chichester.

Bishop V (1994) Clinical supervision for an accountable profession. *Nursing Times* 90, 35–7.

Blake AJ, Morgan K, Bendall MJ, Dallosso H, Ebrahim SBJ, Arica THD, Fentem PH and Bassey EH (1988) Falls by elderly people at home: prevalence and associated factors. *Age and Ageing* 17, 365–72.

Blythe R (1987) *The View in Winter*. Penguin, Harmondsworth.

Bolam v Friern Hospital Management Committee (1957) 2. ALL ER 118.

Bond J (1990) Living arrangements of elderly people. In Bond J and Coleman P (eds) *Ageing in Society: An Introduction to Social Gerontology*. Sage, London.

Bond J, Coleman P, and Peace S (1993) *Ageing in Society: An Introduction to Social Gerontology*, 2nd edn. Sage, London.

Bond S and Thomas L (1991) Issues in measuring outcomes in nursing. *Journal of Advanced Nursing* 16, 1492–502.

Booth B (1991) Nothing special? *Nursing Times* 87, 31.

Bornat J, Pereira C, Pilgrim D and Williams F (eds) (1993) *Community Care: A Reader*. Macmillan Open University, London.

Bortz WM (1982) Disuse and ageing. *Journal of the American Medical Association* 248, 1203.

Bouchier C (1995) *Barrymore*. Granada TV, 12 March 95.

Boulton J, Gully V, Mathews L and Gearing B (1988) *Developing the Biographical Approach in Practice with Older People*. Project Paper Seven. Open University/Policy Studies Institute, Milton Keynes.

Bowling A and Betts G (1984) Communication on discharge. *Nursing Times* 80, 31–3.

Bowling A and Formby J (1991) Nurses' attitudes to elderly people: a survey of nursing homes and elderly care wards in an Inner-London health district. *Nursing Practice* 5, 16–24.

Bowman C (1993) It's a dog's life in the sick world of the health supermarket. *Care of the Elderly* 5, 440.

Brandon D and Towe N (1989) *Free to choose – An Introduction to Service Brokerage.* Good Impressions Publishing, London.

Brechin J and Swain A (1987) *Changing Relationships – Shared Action Planning for People with a Mental Handicap.* Harper and Row, London.

Broderick C (1978) Sexuality and ageing: an over-view. In Solnick R (ed.) *Sexuality and Ageing.* Ethel Perry Andrus Gerontology Center, University of Southern California Press.

Brown J, Kitson A. and McKnight T (1992) *Challenges in Caring.* Chapman & Hall, London.

Brunner LS and Suddarth DS (1989) *The Lippincott Manual of Medical–Surgical Nursing.* Harper and Row, London.

Burgess L (1994) Mixed responses. *Nursing Times* 90, 30–40.

Burnside IM (1973) Touching is talking. *American Journal of Nursing* 73, 2060–3.

Butler A and Tinker A (1983) Integration or segregation: housing in later life. In Butler A and Tinker A (eds) *Elderly People in the Community: Their Service Needs.* HMSO, London.

Butler R and Lewis M (1976) *Sex after Sixty.* Harper and Row, New York.

Butler RN (1969) Ageism: another form of bigotry. *Gerontologist* 9, 243–6.

Butler RN (1975) *Why survive? being old in America.* Harper and Row, New York.

Butler RN, Lewis M and Sunderland A (1991) *Ageing and Mental Health: Psychological and Biomedical Approaches.* Springer, New York.

Butterworth CA and Faugier J (1992) *Clinical Supervision and Mentorship in Nursing.* Chapman & Hall, London.

Byrne DS, Harrison SP, Keithley J and McCarthy P (1986) *Housing and Health: The Relationship between Housing Conditions and Health of Council Tenants.* Gower Press, London.

Callahan D (1987) *Setting Limits: Medical Goals in an Ageing Society.* Simon and Schuster, New York.

Carley M, Dant T, Gearing B and Johnson M (1987) *Care for Elderly People in the Community: A Review of the Issues and the Research.* Care for Elderly People at Home, Project Paper 1. Open University, Milton Keynes.

Carney S, Rich CL, Burke PA and Fowler RC (1994) Suicide over 60: the San Diego Study. *American Geriatrics* 42, 174–80.

Cass S (1978) The effects of the referral process on hospital in-patients. *Journal of Advanced Nursing* 3, 563–9.

Cawthorne A and Hope K (1992) Nursing interventions at night In McMahon R (ed.) *Nursing at Night: A Professional Approach.* Scutari, London.

Challis D and Davis B (1986) *Case Management in Community Care: An Evaluated Experiment in the Care of the Elderly.* Personal Social Services Research Unit/ Gower, Aldershot.

Challis D, Chessum R, Chesterman J, Luckett R and Traste K (1990) *Case Management in Social and Health Care: The Gateshead Community Care Scheme.* Personal Social Services Research Unit, University of Kent, Canterbury.

Chapman V (1987) Planning the nursing care of the patient. In Collins S and Parker E (eds) *Essentials of Nursing: An Introduction.* Macmillan, London.

Cheah Y and Moon G (1993) Specialism and nursing: the case for nursing care for elderly people. *Journal of Advanced Nursing* 18, 1610–16.

Cheater F (1991) Attitudes towards urinary incontinence. *Nursing Standard* 5, 23–7.

Chenitz W (1983) Entry into a nursing home as status passage: a theory to guide nursing practice. *Geriatric Nursing* 4, 92–7.

Chopra D (1993) *Ageless Body – Timeless Mind*. Harmony Press, New York.

Clancy J and McVicar A (1995) *Physiology and Anatomy: A Homeostatic Approach*. Edward Arnold, London.

Coffman T (1981) Relocation and survival of institutionalised aged: a re-examination of the evidence. *Gerontologist* 21, 483–500.

Cohen DR and Henderson JB (1988) *Health, Prevention and Economics*. Oxford, University Press, Oxford.

Coleman PG (1986) *Ageing and Reminiscence Processes: Social and Clinical Implications*. Wiley, Chichester.

Colton H (1983) *The Gift of Touch*. Sea View/Putnam, New York.

Comfort A (1976) *A Good Age*. Crown, New York.

Copstead LE (1980) Effect of touch on self appraisal and interaction appraisal for permanently institutionalised older adults. *Journal of Gerontological Nursing* 6, 747–52.

Cormack D (ed.) (1985) *Geriatric Nursing: A Conceptual Approach*. Oxford. Blackwell Scientific, Oxford.

Costello J (1994) The role of the nurse in the multidisciplinary team (1994) 4, 169–76.

Counsel and Care (1991) *Not Such Private Places*. Counsel and Care, London.

Counsel and Care (1992) *From Home to a Home*. Counsel and Care, London.

Counsel and Care (1993) *Not only Bingo*. Counsel and Care, London.

Counsel and Care (1993) *The Right to Take Risks*. Counsel and Care, London.

Coutts LC and Hardy LK (1985) *Teaching for Health*. Churchill Livingstone, Edinburgh.

Cumming E and Henry H (1961) *Growing Old: The Process of Disengagement*. Basic Books, New York.

Dale A, Evandrou M and Arber S (1987) The household structure of the elderly population in Britain. *Ageing and Society* 7, 37–56.

Dail PW (1988) Prime time TV portrayals of older adults in the context of family life. *Gerontologist* 28, 700–6.

Damrosh S (1984) Graduate nursing students' attitudes towards sexually active older person. *Gerontologist* 24, 299–302.

Dant T, Gearing B, Carley M and Johnson M (1989) *Care for Elderly People at Home*. Project Paper Six. *Keyworkers for Elderly People in the Community; Case Managers and Care Co-ordinators*. Open University/Policy Studies Institute, Milton Keynes.

Darby S *et al.* (1994) *Guidelines for Assessing Mental Health Needs in Old Age*. Royal College of Nursing, London.

Davies P (1994) Non verbal communication with patients. *British Journal of Nursing* 3, 220–3.

Davis RH and Davis A (1986) *Television's Image of the Elderly: A Practical Guide for Change*. Lexington Books, Lexington, Massachusetts.

Dawson PJ (1994). Philosophy, biology and mental disorder. *Journal of Advanced Nursing* 16, 587–96.

Day K (1985) Psychiatric disorder in the middle aged and elderly mentally handicapped. *British Journal of Psychiatry* 147, 660–7.

Day K (1987) The elderly mentally handicapped in hospital: a clinical study. *Journal of Mental Deficiency Research* 17, 20–7.

Day L (1988) How ageism impoverishes elderly care and how to combat it. *Geriatric Medicine* February 14–15.

Deberry S, Davis S and Reinhard K (1989) A comparison of meditation–relaxation and cognitive/behavioural techniques for reducing anxiety and depression in a geriatric population. *Journal of Geriatric Psychiatry* 22, 231–47.

Department of the Environment (1988) *English House Condition Survey 1986*. HMSO, London.

Department of Health (1989) *Working for Patients*. HMSO, London.

Department of Health (1989) *Caring for People: Community Care in the Next Decade and Beyond*. Cmmd. 849. HMSO, London.

Department of Health (1989) *Discharge of Patients from Hospitals*. HMSO, London.

Department of Health (1990) *Statistical Bulletin 2/90*. HMSO, London.

Department of Health (1992) *The Patient's Charter*. HMSO, London.

Department of Health (1992) *Residential Accommodation for Elderly and Younger Physically Handicapped People: Year Ending 31 May 1991*. Government Statistical Office, London.

Department of Health (1992) *The Health of the Nation – A Summary of the Strategy for Health in England*. HMSO, London.

Department of Health (1993) *A Vision for the Future*. HMSO, London.

Department of Health (1995) *The Patient's Charter and You*. HMSO, London.

Department of Health (1996) *Choice and Opportunity: Primary Care – The Future*. HMSO, London.

Department of Health and Social Security (1986) *Neighbourhood Nursing – A Focus for Care*. HMSO, London.

Department of Health and Social Security, (1988) *Health Service Development – Resource Assumptions and Planning Guidelines*. HC (88) 43. HMSO, London.

De Raeve L (1992) Nurse–patient relationships at night. In McMahon R (ed.) *Nursing at Night: A Professional Approach*. Scutari, London.

Dickerson J, Hamilton J, Huber R and Segak R (1989) The aged mentally retarded: the invisible client: a Challenge to the community. In Sweeney DP and Wilson TY (eds) *Double Jeopardy: The Plight of Ageing and Aged Developmentally Disabled People in Mid-America*. Exceptional Child Center, Logan, Utah.

Disabled Living Foundation (1990) *Clothing: A Quality Issue*. Disabled Living Foundation, Harrow.

Donabedian A (1980) *The Definition of Quality and Approach to its Assessment*. Health Administration Press, Michigan.

Downie RS, Fyfe C and Tannahil A (1990) *Health Promotion; Models and Values*. Oxford University Press, Oxford.

Dublin S (1992) The physiological changes of ageing. *Orthopaedic Nursing* 11, 45–50.

Dunn JE, Rudeberg MA, Furner SE and Cassel CK (1992) Mortality, disability, and falls in older persons: the role of underlying disease and disability. *American Journal of Public Health* 82, 395–400.

Dunnell K and Dobbs J (1982) *Nurses Working in the Community*. HMSO, London.

Eaton L (1993) Open to abuse. *Nursing Times* 89, 16.

Eaton LF and Menolascino FJ (1982) Psychiatric disorders in the mentally retarded: types, problems and challenges. *American Journal of Psychiatry* 139, 1297–303.

Ebersole P and Hess P (1990) *Towards Healthy Ageing: Human Needs and Nursing Response*. CV Mosby, St Louis.

Ebrahim S, Hedley R and Sheldon M (1984) Low levels of ill health among non-consulters in general practice. *British Medical Journal* 289, 1273–5.

Ekman P and Friessen WV (1975) *Unmasking the Face*. Prentice-Hall, Englewood Cliffs, New Jersey.

Elder G (1977) *The Alienated – Growing Old Today*. Writers and Readers Publishing Co-operative, London.

Elpoilos C (1993) *Gerontological Nursing*. JB Lippincott, Philadelphia.

Emery GF and Gatz M (1990) Psychological and cognitive effects on an exercise program for community residing older adults. *Gerontologist* 300, 184–8.

Eng C (1987) Multi-disciplinary approach to medical care: the On-Lok model, Clinical report on Ageing. In Dant T, Gearing B, Carley M and Johnson M (eds) (1989) *Care for Elderly People at Home*. Project Paper Six. *Keyworkers for Elderly People in the Community: Case Managers and Care Co-ordinators*. Open University/Policy Studies Institute, Milton Keynes.

English National Board (1985) *Consultation Paper. Professional Education/Training Courses*. English National Board, London.

Equal Opportunities Commission (1980) *The Experience of Caring for Elderly and Handicapped Dependents*. Survey Report. Equal Opportunities Commission, Manchester.

Estes CL, Swan JS and Gerard LE (1982) Dominant and competing paradigms in gerontology. *Ageing and Society* 2, 151–64.

Evers H (1981) The creation of patient careers in geriatric wards: aspects of policy and practice. *Social Science and Medicine* 15A, 581–8.

Evers H, Cameron E and Badger F (1988) *Community Care Project: Overview of Findings and Issues*. Working Paper Number 28. Department of Social Medicine, University of Birmingham, Birmingham.

Evers H (1983) Older women's self perception of dependency and some implications for service provision. *Journal of Epidemiology and Community Health* 38, 306–9.

Fallott RD (1980) The impact of mood on verbal reminiscing in late adulthood. *International Journal of Aging and Human Development* 10, 385–400.

Feezel D (1987) The language of ageing in different groups *Gerontologist* 22, 272–6.

Feil N (1992) *Validation: The Feil Method*. Edward Feil Productions, Cleveland.

Feil N (1993) *The Validation Breakthrough*. Health Professions Press, Baltimore.

Fenton S (1991) Ethnic minority populations in the United Kingdom. In Squires AJ (ed.) *Multicultural Health Care and Rehabilitation of Older People*. Edward Arnold/Age Concern, London.

Fielden MA (1990) Reminiscence as a therapeutic intervention with sheltered housing residents: a comparative study. *British Journal of Social Work* 20, 21–44.

Fielding P (1986) *Attitudes Revisited*. Royal College of Nursing, London.

Finch J (1989) *Attitudes Revisited*. Royal College of Nursing, London.

Fletcher A (1992) Quality of Life Assessments in Older People – Discussion. In *Measures of Quality of Life*. Royal College of Physicians, London.

Fletcher P (1991) *The Future of Sheltered Housing – Who Cares?* Policy report. London National Federation of Housing Associations, London.

Ford P and Walsh M (1994) *New Rituals for Old: Nursing Through the Looking Glass.* Butterworth-Heinemann, Oxford.

Fosbinder D (1994) Patient perceptions of nursing care: an emerging theory of interpersonal competence. *Journal of Advanced Nursing* 20, 1085–93.

Frantz RA and Ferrell Torry A (1993) Physical impairments in the elderly population. *Advances in Clinical Nursing Research* 28, 363–70.

Freer CB (1985) Geriatric screening: a re-appraisal of preventive strategies in the care of the elderly. *Journal of the Royal College of General Practitioners* 35, 288–290.

French J (1990) Boundaries and horizons, the role of health education within health promotion. *Health Education Journal* 49, 7–10.

Friedan B (1993) *The Fountain of Age.* Jonathan Cape, London.

Friedman E, Katcher A and Lynch JJ (1980) Animal companions and first year surgical survival of patients after discharge from a coronary care unit. *Public Health Report* 95, 307–12.

Friend R (1991) Older Lesbian and gay people : a theory of successful ageing. In Lee J (ed.) *Gay, Midlife and Maturity.* Haworth Press, New York.

Fry A (1992) A Voice for an Unsung Army. *Care of the Elderly* 4, 444–5.

Fry J (1984) Checking on the elderly – should we bother? *Update* 29, 1029–31.

Fryers T (1984) *The Epidemiology of Severe Intellectual Impairment: The Dynamics of Prevalence.* Academic Press, New York.

Furstenberg FF (1988) Short term value of pets. *American Journal of Nursing* 88, 157.

Gee E and Kimball M (1987) The double standard of ageing: images and sexuality. In Gee E and Kimball M (eds) *Women and Ageing.* Butterworths, Toronto.

General Household Survey (1985) In *Hansard* 15.03.88 Col. 552 and 21.04.88 Col. 547. HMSO, London.

Gibson H (1992) *The Emotional and Sexual Lives of Older People: A Manual for Professionals.* Chapman & Hall, London.

Gibson M (1984) Sexuality in Later Life. *Ageing International* 11, 8–13.

Gibson M (1990) Falls in later life. *Improving Health of Older People.* WHO, Geneva.

Giddens A (1993) *Sociology,* 2nd edn. Polity Press, Cambridge.

Gilhome-Herbst KR (1983) Psychological consequences of disorders of hearing in the elderly. In Hinchcliffe R (ed.) *Medicine in Old Age: Hearing and Balance.* Churchill Livingstone, London.

Gill G (1987) Health needs of the elderly. In *The Essentials of Nursing,* 2nd edn. Macmillan Education, London.

Gillon R (1992) *Philosophical Medical Ethics.* Wiley, Chichester.

Goffman E (1961) *Asylums: Essays on the Social Situation of Mental Patients and Other Inmates.* Doubleday, New York. (2nd edn, 1968).

Goodwin S (1985) Cosmic nursing. *Nursing Times* 81, 24–6.

Goodwin S (1989) Remembrance Day. *Geriatric Nursing and Home Care* January, 18–19.

Goodwin S and Mangan P (1985) Cosmic nursing: solitude and sanity. *Nursing Times* August, 7, pp. 45–6.

Goodinson S (1987) The biology of ageing: muscles, bones and joints. *Geriatric Nursing and Homecare* January, 13–19.

Gormally L (1992) The aged: non-persons, human dignity and justice. In Gormally L (ed.) *The Dependent Elderly: Autonomy, Justice and Quality of Care.* Cambridge University Press, Cambridge.

Gott M and O'Brien M (1990) Attitudes and beliefs in health promotion. *Nursing Standard* 3, 30–2.

Gould D (1987) The biology of ageing: the special senses. *Geriatric Nursing and Homecare* February, 15–19.

Grau L (1984) What older adults expect from the nurse. *Geriatric Nursing* January/ February, 14–18.

Green S (1991) A two faced society. *Nursing Times* 87, 26–9.

Greenberg BS, Korezenny F and Atken CK (1979) The portrayal of ageing trends on commercial TV. *Research on Ageing* 1, 319–34.

Grimley-Evans J (1992) Quality of life assessments in older people. In *Measures of Quantity of Life.* Royal College of Physics, London.

Grimley-Evans J (1994) Can we live to be a healthy hundred? *Medical Research Council News* 64, Autumn.

Grootenhuis C, Hawton K, Van Rooigen L and Fagg J (1994) Attempted suicide in Oxford and Utrecht. *British Journal of Psychiatry* 165, 73–8.

Guccione AA (ed.) (1993) *Geriatric Physical Therapy.* CV Mosby, St Louis.

Haggar V (1992) Good companions. *Nursing Times* 88, 54–5.

Hale N. (1989) Animal house. *Geriatric Nursing and Home Care* April, 12.

Hall GR and Buckwalter KC (1990) From almshouse to dedicated unit: care of institutionalised elderly with behavioural problems. *Archives of Psychiatric Nursing* 4, 3–11.

Hall JK (1966) *Nursing: Ethics and Law.* WB Saunders, London.

Hanks C (1986) The biology of ageing: digestion and nutrition in the elderly. *Geriatric Nursing* September/October 1986 12–15.

Hargreaves M, Fuller G, and Gazzard B (1988) Occult AIDS : *Pneumocystis carinii* pneumonia in elderly people. *British Medical Journal*, 297, 721–2.

Harper MS (ed.) 1991) *Management and Care of the Elderly: Psychological Perspectives.* Sage, London.

Hayflick and Moorhead PS (1961) The serial subcultivation of human cell strains. *Experimental Cell Research* 25, 585–621.

Hayslip B and Panek PE (eds) (1992) *Adult Development and Ageing,* 2nd edn. Harper Collins, New York.

Help the Aged (1995) *Living Alone – Sharing Responsibility.* Help the Aged, London.

Henderson V (1961) *Basic Principles of Nursing Care.* International Council of Nurses, London.

Henderson V (1966) *The Nature of Nursing.* Collier Macmillan, London.

Henwood M (1992) *Through a Glass Darkly: Community Care and Elderly People.* Research Report 14. King's Fund, London.

Herbert R (1986) The biology of ageing: maintenance of homeostasis. *Geriatric Nursing* May/June, 14–16 and July/August, 16–18.

Herbert R (1991) The normal ageing process reviewed. *Nursing Standard* 5, 36–9.

Hesse K and Campian E (1983) The geriatric patient for rehabilitation. *Journal of the American Geriatric Society* 31, 586–9.

Hilgard ER, Atkinson RL and Atkinson RC (1979) *Introduction to Psychology.* Harcourt Brace Jovanovich, New York.

HM Treasury (1991) *The Government's Expenditure Plans 1991–1992 to 1993–1994.* Department of Social Security Cm 1514. HMSO, London.

Hockey L (1968) *Care in the Balance.* Queen's Institute of Nursing, London.

Hodges JR (1994) *Cognitive Assessment for Clinicians.* Oxford University Press, Oxford.

Hogg J, Moss S and Cooke D (1988) *Ageing and Mental Handicap.* Croom-Helm, London.

Holden UP and Woods RT (1984) *Reality Orientation: Psychological Approaches to the 'Confused' Elderly.* Churchill Livingstone, Edinburgh.

Hollis M, Kitchen SS, Sandford B and Waddington PJ (1989) *Practical Exercise Therapy,* 3rd edn. Blackwell, London.

Holmen K, Ericsson K, Andersson L and Winblad B (1992) Loneliness among elderly people living in Stockholm: a population study. *Journal of Advanced Nursing* 17, 43–51.

Home Office (1968) *Report of the Committee on Local Authority and Allied Personal Social Serivces (Seebohm Report).* HMSO, London.

Hope KW (1993) Attitudes towards older people: a comparison of nurses working in acute care of elderly areas with nurses working in acute medical areas. Unpublished MA dissertation, Keele University.

Hope KW (1994) Nurses' attitudes towards older people: a comparison of nurses working in acute medical and acute care of the elderly settings. *Journal of Advanced Nursing* 20, 605–12.

Hunt A (1978) *The Elderly at Home: A study of people aged 65 and over living in the Community in England in 1976.* OPCS, London.

Hutchinson J (1991) Living with a visual handicap. In Hawker M and Davis M (eds) *Visual Handicap – A Distance Learning Pack for Physiotherapists, Occupational Therapists and other Health Care Professionals.* Disabled Living Foundation, London.

Institute of Actuaries (1993) *Financial Long-term Care in Great Britain.* Institute of Actuaries, Oxford.

Jackson C (1988) Now hear this. *Geriatric Nursing and Home Care* 8, 19.

Jackson J (1987) Don't shout nurse. *Geriatric Nursing* 6, 12–13.

Jackson MF (1994) Discharge planning: issues and challenges for gerontological nursing. A critique of the literature *Journal of Advanced Nursing* 19, 492–502.

Jacques A (1992) *Understanding Dementia.* Churchill Livingstone, Edinburgh.

Janus S and Janus C (1993) *The Janus Report on Sexual Behaviour.* Wiley, Chichester.

Jewell SE (1993) Discovery of the discharge process: a study of patient discharge from a care unit for elderly people. *Journal of Advanced Nursing* 18, 1288–96.

Jerome D (1990) Intimate relationships. In Bond J and Coleman P (eds) *Ageing in Society.* Sage, London.

Jerome D (1990) Frailty and friendship. *Journal of Cross-Cultural Gerontology* 5, 51–64.

Johnson M (1991) The meaning of old age. In Redfern S (ed.) *Nursing Elderly People at Home,* 2nd edn. Churchill Livingstone, Edinburgh.

Johnson M, Gearing B, Dant T, and Carley M (1987) *Care for Elderly People at Home Project Papers.* Open University/Policy Studies Institute, Milton Keynes.

Jones D and Lester C (1994) Hospital care and discharge: patients' and carers' opinions. *Age and Ageing* 23, 91–6.

Jones G and Miesen BML (1992) *Caregiving in Dementia: Research and Application.* Routledge, London.

Joseph J (1991) 'Warning'. In Martz S (ed.) (1991) *When I am an old woman I shall wear purple.* PMP, Watsonville.

Jowett S and Armitage S (1988) Hospital and community liaison links in nursing: the role of the liaison nurse. *Journal of Advanced Nursing* 13, 579–87.

Kaas M (1978) Sexual expression of the elderly in nursing homes. *Gerontologist* 16, 39–44.

Kagan AR and Levi L (1974) Health and environment. Psychosocial stimuli – a review. *Social Science and Medicine* 8, 225–241.

Karr JP and Murry SP (1984) Carcinoma of the prostate and its management. In Brocklehurst JC (ed.) *Urology in the Elderly.* Churchill Livingstone, London.

Kassell VC (1966) Polygamy after 60. *Geriatrics* 21, 214–18.

Katz J and Green E (1992) *Managing Quality: A Guide to Monitoring and Evaluating Nursing Services.* CV Mosby, St Louis.

Kaufmann T (1993) *A Crisis of Silence: HIV, AIDS and Older People.* Age Concern, London.

Kausler DH (1991) *Experimental Psychology and Human Ageing,* 2nd edn. Springer-Verlag, New York.

Kastenbaum R (1987) Gerontology's search for understanding. *Gerontologist* 18, 59–63.

Kemp J (1988) Qualified success. *Geriatric Nursing and Home Care* 10, 15.

Kemper P, Applebaum R and Harrigan M (1987) Community care demonstrations: what we have learned. *Health Care Financing Review* 8, 87–100.

Kenney RA (1989) *Physiology of Ageing: A Synopsis.* Year Book Medical Publishers, Chicago.

Kennie DC (1993) *Preventive Care for Elderly People.* Cambridge University Press, Cambridge.

Kershaw B (1987) Education for care. *Senior Nurse* 6, 28–9.

Kershaw B (1992) Nursing models. In Jolley M and Brykczynska G (eds) *Nursing Care: The Challenge to Change.* Edward Arnold, London.

Khan R.L. and Antonucci TC (1984) *Social Supports of the Elderly: Family/Friends/ Professionals.* Final Report to the National Institute on Ageing, Hyattsville, Maryland.

King C and Macmillan M (1994) Documentation and discharge planning for elderly patients. *Nursing Times* 90, 31–33.

King's Fund (1988) *Promoting Health Among Elderly People. A Statement from a Working Group.* London. Age Concern Institute of Gerontology/King's Fund, London.

Kinsella P (1993) *Supported Living for People with Learning Disabilities.* National Development Team, London.

Kimmell DC (1988) Ageism, psychology and public policy. *American Psychologist* 43 175–8.

Kitson A (1986) Indicators of quality in nursing – an alternative approach. *Journal of Advanced Nursing* 11, 135–44.

Kitson AL (1987) Raising standards of clinical practice: the fundamental issues of effective nursing care. *Journal of Advanced Nursing* 12, 321–9.

Kitson A (1990) Setting standards. *Nursing Standard* 26, 55.

Kitson A and Harvey G (1991) *Quality Assurance and Standards of Care.* Scutari, London.

Kitwood T (1993) Towards a theory of dementia care: the interpersonal process. *Ageing and Society* 13, 51–67.

Kitwood T and Bredin K (1992) *Person to Person: A Guide to the Care of those with Failing Mental Powers.* Gale Centre, Loughton.

Kitwood T and Bredin K (1992) Towards a theory of dementia care: personhood and well-being. *Ageing and Society* 12, 269–87.

Kitwood T and Bredin K (1993) *Evaluating Dementia Care: The DCM Method.* Bradford Dementia Research Group, Bradford.

Knowles R (1987) Who's a pretty girl then? *Nursing Times* 23, 58–9.

Kyriazis M (1994) Age and reason. *Nursing Times* 90, (18) 61–3.

Kuhn M (1976) Sexual myths surrounding the ageing. In Oaks W *et al.* (eds) *Sex and the Life Cycle.* Grune and Stratton, New York.

La Vecchia C, Lucchini F and Levi F (1994) Worldwide trends in suicide mortality 1955–1989. *Acta Psychiatrica Scandnavica* 90, 53–64.

Laczko J and Phillipson C (1991) *Changing Work and Retirement.* Open University Press, Milton Keynes.

Lader M (1977) *Psychiatry on Trial.* Penguin, Harmondsworth.

Laflin M. (1985) Sexuality and the elderly. In Lewis C (ed.) *Ageing: The Health Care Challenge.* FA Davies, Philadelphia.

Laing W and (1993) *The Care of Elderly People Market Survey 1992/3,* 6th edn. Laing and Buisson, London.

Laing W and Hall M (1991) *The Challenges of Ageing: A Review of the Economic. Social and Medical Implications of An Ageing Population.* Association of the British Pharmaceutical Industry, London.

Langelaan D (1986) The biology of ageing: an introduction. *Geriatric Nursing* March/April, 16–19.

LaRue A, Dessonville C and Jarvik LF (1985) Ageing and mental disorders. In Birren JE and Schaie KW (eds) *Handbook of Ageing and the Social Sciences,* 2nd edn. Van Nostrand, New York.

Langer E (1982) Old age: an artifact? In Kiesler S and McGaugh J (eds.) *Biology, Behaviour and Ageing.* National Research Council, New York.

Law CM and Warnes AM (1982) The destination decision in retirement migration. In Warnes AM (ed.) *Geographical Perspectives on the Elderly.* Wiley, Chichester.

Lawler J (1991) *Behind the Screens: Nursing Somology and the Problems of the Body.* Churchill Livingstone, London.

Leather P and Wheeler R (1988) *Making Use of Home Equity in Old Age.* Building Societies Association, London.

Lee J (ed.) (1991) *Gay, Midlife and Maturity.* Haworth Press, New York.

Levi P (1969) *If this is a Man.* Orion Press, London.

Levi P (1986) *Moments of Reprieve.* Michael Joseph, London.

Levin J and Levin W (1980) *Ageism: Prejudice and Discrimination about the Elderly.* Wadsworth, Belmont, California.

Lewis CB and Bottomley JM (1990) *Musculoskeletal Changes with Age: Clinical Implications,* 2nd edn. FA Davies, Philadelphia.

Lewis CN (1971) Reminiscing and self concept in old age. *Journal of Gerontology* 21, 240–3.

Little J (1986) *Mental Disorder: Its Care and Treatment*. Baillière Tindall, London.

Livingston G, Blizard B and Mann A (1993) Does sleep disturbance predict depression in elderly people? *British Journal of General Practice* 43, 445–48.

Long CA, Holden R, Mulkerrin E and Sykes D (1991) Opportunistic screening of visual acuity in elderly patients attending out patient clinic. *Age and Ageing* 20, 392–5.

Long RG, Reiser RR and Hill EW (1990) Mobility in individuals with moderate visual impairment. *Journal of Visual Impairment and Blindness* 84, 111–18.

Lookinland S and Anson K (1995) Perpetuation of ageist attitudes among present and future health care personnel: implications for elder care. *Journal of Advanced Nursing* 21, 47–56.

Lowell W, Gerson D and McCord G (1987) Risk of imbalance in elderly people with impaired hearing or vision. *Age and Ageing* 18, 31–4.

Lowenthal M (1965) Interaction and adaption, intimacy as a crucial variable. *American Sociological Review* 33, 20–30.

Ludlow JW, DeCaprio JA, Huang CM, Lee WH, Paucha E and Livingstone DM. (1989) SV 40 larte T antigen binds preferentially to an under phosphorylated member of the retinoblastoma susceptibility gene product family. *CELL* 56, 57–65.

Luker KA (1981) Health visiting and the elderly. Occasional paper. *Nursing Times* 77, 33–5.

Luther J and Robinson L (1993) *The Royal Marsden Hospital Manual of Standards of Care*. Blackwells, Oxford.

Lyon S (1993) Alone in a crowd. *Geriatric Medicine* 23, 5 (commentary).

Maanen HM (1988) Being old does not always mean being sick. *Journal of Advanced Nursing* 13, 701–9.

Macdonald AJD (1986) Do general practitioners 'miss' depression in elderly patients? *British Medical Journal* 292, 1365–7.

Macdonald B and Rich C (1983) Look me in the eye: old women, ageing and ageism. In Williams EI (1989) *Caring for Elderly People in the Community*, 2nd edn. Chapman & Hall, London.

MacFarlane A (1994) On behalf of an older disabled woman. *Disability and Society* 255–6.

Macleod-Clark J (1983) Nurse–patient communication: an analysis of conversations from surgical wards. In Wilson-Barnett J (ed.) *Nursing Research: Ten Studies in Patient Care*. Wiley, Chichester.

Macleod-Clark J and Webb C (1985) Health education – a basis for professional nursing practice. *Nurse Education Today* 5, 210–14.

Malin N and Teasdale K (1991) Caring *versus* empowerment: considerations for nursing practice. *Journal of Advanced Nursing* 16, 657–62.

Mallick M and McHale J (1995) Support for advocacy. *Nursing Times* 91, 28–30.

Mansfield K (1971) *Letters and Journals*. Pelican, London.

Manthey M, Ciske K, Robertson P *et al.* (1970) Primary nursing. *Nursing Forum* 9, 64–83.

Manthey M (1992) *The Practice of Primary Nursing*. King's Fund, London.

Marr J and Khadim N (1993) Meeting the needs of ethnic patients. *Nursing Standard* 8, 31–3.

Marr J and Matthews T (1993) Change of a dress. *Nursing Standard* 7, 48–9.

Marshall M (1993) Designing for confused old people. In Arie T (ed.) *Recent Advances in Psychogeriatrics*. Churchill Livingstone, London.

Maslow A (1954) *Motivation and Personality*. Harper and Row, New York.

Mason A (1988) Massage. In Rankin-Box D (ed.) *Complementary Health Therapies: A Guide for Nurses and the Caring Professions*. Croom Helm, London.

Masters W and Johnson V (1966) *Human Sexual Response*. Little, Brown, Boston.

Matteson MA and McConnell ES (1988) *Gerontological Nursing: Concepts and Practice*. WB Saunders, Philadelphia.

Maxwell R (1984) Quality assessment in health. *British Medical Journal* 288, 1470–2.

McBean S. (1991) Health and health promotion – consensus and conflict. In Perry A and Jolley M (1991) *Nursing: A Knowledge Base for Practice*. Edward Arnold, London.

McCaffery M (1983) *Nursing the Patient in Pain*. Harper and Row, London.

McCall J (1990) Fostering self esteem. *Surgical Nurse* 3, 4–10.

McCallion P (1994) *Families and Practitioners: Differences in their Views on Permanency Planning,*. Paper Presented at the Dublin Round Table Conference on Ageing and Mental Handicap, Dublin.

McCarthy M, (ed.) (1989) *The New Politics of Welfare – An Agenda for the 1990s?* Macmillan, London.

McCormack B (1992) A case study identifying nursing staff's perception of the delivery of method of care in practice on a particular ward. *Journal of Advanced Nursing* 17, 187–97.

McCormack B (1996) Life transition. In Ford P and Heath H (eds) *Older People and Nursing: Issues of Living in a Care Home*. Butterworth-Heinemann, Oxford.

McCracken A (1988) Sexual practice by elders: the forgotten aspect of functional health. *Gerontological Nursing* 14, 13–17.

McGinnis P (1987) Teaching nurses to teach. In Davis B (ed.) *Nursing Education: Research and Development*. Croom Helm, London.

McKenna H (1993) The effects of nursing models on quality of care. *Nursing Times* 89, 43–6.

McKenzie AJ, Chawla HB and Gordon D (1986) *The Special Senses*. Churchill Livingstone, London.

McLane (1987) *Classification of Nursing Diagnoses*. Proceedings of the Seventh Conference. CV Mosby, St Louis.

McMahon A and Ruddick P (1964) Reminiscing. *Archives of General Psychiatry* 10, 292–8.

Mead GH (1934) *Mind, Self and Society*. University of Chicago Press, Chicago.

Merriam S and Cross L (1981) Ageing, reminiscence and life satisfaction. *Activities, Adaptation and Ageing* 2, 39–50.

Midwinter E (1991) *British Gas Report on Attitudes to the Ageing*. Centre for Policy on Ageing, London.

Midwinter E (1991) *Out of Focus: Old Age, the Press and Broadcasting*. Centre for Policy on Ageing, London.

Mikhail M (1992) Psychological responses to relocating to a nursing home. *Journal of Gerontological Nursing*, March, 35–9.

Minshull J, Ross K and Turner J (1986) The human needs model of nursing. *Journal of Advanced Nursing* 11, 643–9.

Mithacht S and Weinberg RA (1991) G1/S phosphorylation of the retinoblastoma protein is associated with an altered affinity for the nuclear compartment. *CELL* 65, 381–93.

Moody RH (1988) Towards a critical gerontology: the contribution of the humanities to the thoughts of ageing. Cited in Birren JE and Schaie JW (eds) *Emergent Theories of Ageing*. Springer–Verlag, New York.

Mooney G (1992) *Economics and Health Care*, 2nd edn. Harvester Wheatsheaf, London.

Mulley GP (1988) Everyday aids and appliances – provision of aids. *British Medical Journal* 296, 475–6.

Mulley GP (1990) Everyday aids and appliances: walking frames. *British Medical Journal* 300, 925–7.

Mulley GP (1994) Principles of rehabilitation. *Reviews in Clinical Gerontology* 4, 61–9.

Murphy E (1982) Social origins of depression in old age. *British Journal of Psychiatry* 141, 135–41.

Murphy K (1987) Problems of impaired hearing. *Geriatric Nursing and Home Care*, 7, 9–11.

Naidoo J and Willis J (1994) *Health Promotion*. Baillière Tindall London.

National Association of Health Authorities (1989) *Will You Still Love Me?* Society of Family Practitioner Committees, London.

National Development Team (1991) *The Andover Case Management Project*. National Development Team, London.

National Health Service and Community Care Act (1990) HMSO, London.

National Health Service Management Executive (1992) *Health Service Guidelines – Health Services for People with Learning Disabilities (Mental Handicap)*. HSG (92) 42. NHS Management Executive, London.

National Health Service Management Executive (1993) *Dementia*. Department of Health, London.

Nay R (1995) Nursing home residents' perceptions of relocation. *Journal of Clinical Nursing*, 4, 319–25.

Naylor MD (1990) Comprehensive discharge planning for the hospitalised elderly. *Nursing Research* 39, 151–61. Cited in Tierney A, Worth A, Closs SJ and Macmillan M (1994) Older patients' experiences of discharge from hospital. *Nursing Times* 90, 36–9.

NCHS (1977) Vital statistics of the United States. *Suicide Rates in the USA by Age*.

Neal M. (1994) An ethnographic study into the experience of five nurses importing the communication technique known as validation into their work with clients experiencing dementia. Thesis, Leeds Metropolitan University.

Neugarten BL (1977) Personality and ageing. In Birren JE and Schaie KW (eds) *Handbook of the Psychology of Ageing*. Reinhold, New York.

Neugarten BL (1993) Social and psychological characteristics of older person. In Guccione AA (ed.) *Geriatiric Physical Therapy*. CV Mosby, St Louis.

Neuman B (1982) *The Neuman Systems Model: Application to Nursing Education and Practice*. Appleton–Century–Crofts, New York.

Nightingale F (1859) *Notes on Nursing*. Churchill Livingstone, London.

Nolan P (1991) Looking at the first 100 years. *Senior Nurse* 11, 22–5.

Nolan MR (1989) Geriatric nursing: an idea whose time has gone: a polemic. *Journal of Advanced Nursing* 99, 840–9.

Norman A (1982) *Mental Illness in Old Age: Meeting the Challenge.* Centre for Policy on Ageing, London.

Norman A (1985) *Triple Jeopardy: Growing Old in a Second Homeland.* Centre for Policy on Ageing, London.

Norman A (1987) *Aspects of Ageism: A Discussion Paper.* Centre for Policy on Ageing, London.

Norman AJ (1980) *Rights and Risk.* Centre for Policy on Ageing, London.

Norris A (1986) *Reminiscence and Elderly People.* Winslow Press, Bicester.

Nuessel F (1987) The language of ageism. *Gerontologist* 27, 527–31.

Nursing Development Unit (1990) *Nursing Standards: older people.* Tameside Health Authority, Ashton-under-Lyne.

O'Brien, J and Lyle C (1987) *Framework for Accomplishment.* Responsive Service Systems Associates, Georgia.

O'Leary (1991) The realities of liaison. In Armitage SK (ed.) (1991) *Continuity of Nursing Care.* Scutari, London.

O'Loughlin JL, Robitaille Y, Boivin JE and Suissa S (1993) Incidence of and risk factors for all and injuries falls among the community-dwelling elderly. *American Journal of Epidemiology* 137, 342–54.

Oakley A (1985) *The Sociology of Housework.* Blackwell, Oxford.

Office of Population Censuses and Surveys (1982) *General Household Survey 1980.* HMSO, London.

Office of Population Censuses and Surveys (1988) *General Household Survey 1985.* HMSO, London.

Office of Population Censuses and Surveys (1989) *Cancer Statistics Registrations England and Wales.* Series MBI No 22. HMSO, London.

Office of Population Censuses and Surveys (1991) *Population Trends.* HMSO, London.

Office of Population Censuses and Surveys (1992) *Population Trends Autumn 1992.* HMSO, London.

Office of Population Censuses and Surveys (1993) *The 1991 Census: Persons Aged 60 and Over, Great Britain.* HMSO, London.

Ogden V (1992) Advocates for the elderly. *Journal of Community Nursing* 6, 8–9.

Oliver S and Redfern SJ (ed.) (1991) Interpersonal communication between nurses and elderly patients: refinement and observation schedule. *Journal of Advanced Nursing* 16, 30–8.

Olshansky SJ, Carnes BA and Casel C (1990) In search of Methuselah: estimating the upper limits to human ingenuity. *Science* 250, 634–40.

Orem DE (1980) *Nursing: Concepts of Practice.* McGraw-Hill, New York.

Organisation for Economic Cooperation and Development (1988) *Ageing Populations. The Ageing Policy Implications.* OECD, Paris.

Overstall PW, Exton-Smith AN, Imms FJ and Johnson AL (1977) Falls in the elderly related to postural imbalance. *British Medical Journal* 1, 261–4.

Paffenbarger RS, Wing AL and Hyder T (1978) Physical activity as an index of heart attack risk in College of Alumni. *American Journal of Epidemiology* 108, 161–75.

Palmore E (1971) Attitudes towards ageing as shown by humour. *Gerontologist* 11, 81–187.

Parker G (1990) *With Due Care and Attention: A Review of Research on Informal Care.* Family Policy Studies Centre, London.

Parsley K and Corrigan P (1994) *Quality Improvement in Nursing and Health Care.* Chapman & Hall, London.

Patel J (1993) Empowering of diabetes: a challenge for community nursing. *British Journal of Nursing* 2, 405–9.

Payton OD and Poland JL (1983) Ageing process. *Physical Therapy* 63, 41–7.

Peace S (1988) Living environments for the elderly 2: promoting the 'right' institutional environment. In Wells N and Freer C (eds) *The Ageing Population: Burden or Challenge.* Macmillan, Basingstoke.

Peace S (1993) The living environments of older women. In Bernard M and Meade K (eds) *Women Come of Age: Understanding the Lives of Older Women.* Edward Arnold, London.

Pearson A (1987) *Nursing Quality and Measurement.* Wiley, Chichester.

Pearson A (1988) *Preliminary Nursing.* London, Croom Helm, London.

Pearson A (1991) Taking up the challenge: the future for therapeutic nursing. In McMahon R and Pearson A (eds) *Nursing as Therapy.* Chapman & Hall, London.

Pearson A, Punton S and Durrant I (1992) *Nursing Beds: An Evaluation of the Effects of Therapeutic Nursing.* Scutari, London.

Pearson A and Vaughan B (1986) *Nursing Models for Practice.* Heinemann Nursing, Oxford.

Peplau H (1952) *Interpersonal Relations in Nursing.* Putnam, New York.

Peplau H (1994) Challenge and change. *Journal of Psychiatric and Mental Health Nursing* 1, 3–7.

Perry PW (1974) The night of ageism. *Mental Health* 58, 13–20.

Persson G (1980) Sexuality in a 70 year old urban population. *Journal of Psychosomatic Research* 24, 335–42.

Pfeiffer E, Verwoedert A and Wang H (1968) Duke longitudinal studies: aged men and women. *Archives of General Psychiatry* 19, 753–8.

Phaneuf MC (1972) *The Nursing Audit.* Appleton–Century–Crofts, New York.

Phifer J and Murrell S (1986) Etiological factors in the late onset of depressive symptoms in older adults. *Journal of Abnormal Psychology* 95, 282–91.

Phillips J (1992) *Private Residential Care: The Admission Process and Reactions of the Public Sector.* Avebury Press, Aldershot.

Phillipson C (1982) *Capitalism and the Construction of Old Age.* Macmillan, London.

Phillipson C and Walker A (1986) *Ageing and Social Policy: A Critical Assessment* Gower, Aldershot.

Pilling D (1988) *The Case Manager Project: Report of the Evaluation.* London Rehabilitation Resource Centre, Department of Systems Science, City University. In Dant T and Gearing B (1993) Keyworkers for elderly people in the community. In Bornat J, Pereira C, Pilgrim D and Williams F (eds) (1993) *Community Care: A Reader.* Macmillan/Open University, London.

Pitt B (1988) Characteristics of depression in the elderly. In Gearing B *et al.* (eds) *Mental Health Problems in Old Age.* Open University/Wiley, Milton Keynes.

Pollitt C (1992) Performance evaluation in the public sector. Paper given at the Partnership in Audit Conference, York, 5 November 1992.

Porrit L (1984) *Communication: Choices for Nurses* Churchill Livingstone, Melbourne.

Power Smith O (1992) Encounters with older lesbians in psychiatric practice. *Sex and Marital Therapy* 7, 79–86.

Pratt MW, Diessner R, Hunsberg B *et al.* (1991) Four pathways in the analysis of adult development and ageing: comparing analyses of reasoning about personal-life dilemmas. *Psychology and Ageing* 6, 666–75.

Prosiner SB (1991) The molecular biology of prion diseases. Science 252, 1515–22.

Public Health Laboratory Service (1993) *AIDS/HIV Quarterly Surveillance Tables No. 20.* Communicable Disease Surveillance Centre, June 1993.

Ram Dass (1995) *Conscious Ageing,* a collection of tapes available from the Hanuman Foundation, New Mexico. A book is currently in press.

Raphael S and Robertson M (1980) Lesbians and gay men in later life. *Generations* 6, 16.

Redfern SJ (ed.) (1991) *Nursing Elderly People,* 2nd edn. Churchill Livingstone, Edinburgh.

Redman BK (1984) *The Process of Patient Education,* 5th edn. CV Mosby, St Louis.

Reiss S (1982) Psycholology and mental retardation: survey of a developmental disabilities mental health program. *Mental Retardation* 20, 128–32.

Rickford F (1993) Longstay beds for elderly cut by 40 per cent. *The Guardian,* 5 August.

Riehl JR (1980) The Riehl interaction model. In Riehl JR and Roy C (eds) *Conceptual Models for Nursing Practice.* Appleton–Century–Crofts, Norwalk, Connecticut.

Rissell C (1994) Empowerment: the holy grail of health promotion. *Health Promotion International* 9, 39–47.

Robb B (1968) *Sans Everything: A Case to Answer.* Nelson, London.

Roberts F (1985) Reported accidents to hospital patients. MSc thesis, Manchester University.

Roberts I (1975) *Discharged from Hospital.* Royal College of Nursing, London.

Robinson P (1983) The sociological perspective. In Weg R (ed.) *Sexuality in the Later Years: Roles and Behaviour.* Academic Press, New York.

Rockwood K (1994) Setting goals in geriatric rehabilitation and measuring their attainment. *Reviews in Clinical Gerontology* 4, 141–9.

Rogers C (1951) *Client-centred Therapy: Its Current Practice, Implications and Theory.* Constable, London.

Rogers JC (1980) Advocacy – The key to assessing older client. *Journal of Geriatric Nursing* 6, 33–6.

Rogstad K and Bignell C (1991) Age is no bar to sexually acquired infection. *Age and Ageing* 20, 377–8.

Roper N, Logan W and Tiernay AJ (1980) *The Elements of Nursing,* 2nd edn. Churchill Livingstone, Edinburgh.

Roper N, Logan W and Tierney A (1985) *Using a Model for Nursing.* Churchill Livingstone, Edinburgh.

Rorden JW and Taft E (1990) *Discharge Planning Guide for Nurses.* WB Saunders, Philadelphia.

Rosenhan DL (1973) On being sane in insane places. *Science* 179, 250–8. Also in Gross RD (ed.) (1994) *Key Studies in Psychology.* Hodder and Stoughton, London.

Ross F (1987) District nursing. In Littlewood J (1987) *Recent Advances in Nursing. Community Nursing* 15, 132–6.

Ross F (1990) Key issues in district nursing. Paper two. *New Horizons in Community Care, Policy Perspectives for District Nursing.* District Nursing Association, London.

Roy C (1980) The Roy adaptation model. In Riehl JR and Roy C (eds) *Conceptual Models for Nursing Practice.* Appleton–Century–Crofts, Norwalk, Connecticut.

Roy C (1984) *Introduction to Nursing: An Adaptation Model,* 2nd edn. Prentice-Hall, Englewood Cliffs, New Jersey.

Royal College of Nursing (1987) *Focus on Restraint: Guidelines on the Use of Restraint in the Care of Elderly People.* RCN, London.

Royal College of Nursing (1993) *Working with Older People.* Scutari, London.

Royal College of Nursing (1993) *The Value and Skills of Nurses Working with Older People.* RCN, London.

Royal National Institute for the Blind (1992) *Ten Things You Should Know About Visual Handicap.* RNIB, London.

Ruuskanen JM and Ruoppila I (1995) Physical activity and psychological well-being among people aged 65–84 years. *Age and Ageing* 24, 292–6.

Sadler C (1992) Men's hidden illness. *Nursing Times* 88, 18–19.

Sale D (1990) *Quality Assurance.* Macmillan, London.

Salthouse TA (1991) *Theoretical Perspectives on Cognitive Ageing.* Erlbaum, Hillsdale, New Jersey.

Salvage A (1984) *Developments in Domiciliary Care for the Elderly.* King's Fund, London.

Salvage J (1990) The theory and practice of the 'new nursing'. *Nursing Times* 86, 42–5.

Salvage J and Wright S (1995) *Nursing Development Units – A Force for Change.* Scutari, London.

Sarton M (1967) *As We Are Now.* Women's Press, New York.

Saxby J (1993) Jane Saxby. In Jones B (ed.) *Three Lives.* NFCO, London.

Schachter S and Singer JE (1962) Cognitive, social and psychological determinants of emotional state. *Psychological Review* 69, 379–99. Also in Cross RD (ed.) (1994) *Key Studies in Psychology.* Hodder and Stoughton, London.

Schultz R and Brenner G (1977) Relocation of the aged – a review and theoretical analysis. *Journal of Gerontology* 32, 323.

Schultz NR and Moore D (1984) Loneliness: correlates, attributions and coping among older adults. *Personality and Social Psychology Bulletin* 10, 67–77.

Schweer SF and Dayani EC (1973) The extended role of professional nursing – patient education. *International Nursing Review* 20, 174–5.

Scrutton S (1989) *Counselling and Older People – A Creative Response to Ageing.* Edward Arnold, London.

Seedhouse D (1986) *Health: The Foundations for Achievement.* Wiley, Chichester.

Seedhouse D and Lovett L (1992) *Practical Medical Ethics.* Wiley, Chichester.

Selzer MM and Janicki, M (1991) Commentary and recommendations. In Janicki M and Selzer MM, *Proceedings of the Boston Roundtable on Research Issues and Applications in Ageing and Developmental Disabilities,* Boston, USA.

Silver M (1986) The dental problems of elderly people. *Geriatric Nursing and Home Care* 6, 31–2.

Simmons S (1994) Social networks: their relevance to mental health nursing. *Journal of Advanced Nursing* 18, 281–9.

Sines DT (1995) *Commmunity Health Care Nursing*. Blackwell Science, Oxford.

Sixsmith AJ (1986) Independence and home in later life. In Phillipson C, Bernard M and Strang P (eds) *Dependency and interdependency in old age – theoretical perspectives and policy alternatives*. Croom Helm, London.

Sixsmith AJ (1990) The meaning and experience of 'home' in later life. In Blytheway B and Johnson J (eds) *Welfare and the Ageing Experience*. Avebury Press, Aldershot.

Skeet M (1970) *Home From Hospital*. London.

Skelly M (1975) Aphasic patients talk back. *American Journal of Nursing* 75, 1104–6.

Slater J (1987) Data on health education. *Journal of District Nursing* 6, 5–10.

Slevin OD (1991) Ageist attitudes amongst young adults: implications for a caring profession. *Journal of Advanced Nursing* 16, 1197–205.

Smith P and Leigh N (1986) The biology of ageing: body temperature regulation. *Geriatric Nursing* July/August, 16–18.

Smith P and Leigh N (1986) The biology of ageing: the ageing brain. *Geriatric Nursing and Homecare* November/December, 20–5.

Smith T (1990) Poverty and health in the 1990s. *British Medical Journal* 301, 349–50.

Smythe M and Browne F (1992) *General Household Survey 1990*. HMSO, London.

Snape J (1986) Nurses' attitudes to care of the elderly. *Journal of Advanced Nursing* 11, 569–72.

Social Services Inspectorate (1989) *Homes are for Living In*. HMSO, London.

Social Services Inspectorate (1993) *Standards for the Residential Care of Elderly People with Mental Disorders*. Department of Health, London.

Social Services Inspectorate (1992) *Social Services for Hospital Patients. 1: Working at the Interface*. Department of Health, London.

Social Trends 24 (1994) HMSO, London.

Sogyal Rinpoche (1992) *The Tibetan Book of Living and Dying*. Ryder London.

Sontag R (1978) The double standard of ageing. In Carver V and Liddiard P (eds) *An Ageing Population*. Hodder and Stoughton, London.

Sparrow S and Robinson J (1992) The use and limitations of Phaneuf's nursing audit. *Journal of Advanced Nursing* 17, 1479–88.

Spencer R (1988) Transitions. Reflections on being blind in a sighted world. *Journal of Ophthalmic Nursing and Technology* 7, 220–2.

Starr B and Weiner M (1981) *The Weiner Report on Sex and Sexuality in the Mature Years*. McGrath, New York.

Steinberg RM and Carter GW (1983) *Case Management and the Elderly*. Lexington, Washington DC.

Stevenson O (1989) *Age and Vulnerability: A Guide to Better Care*. Arnold, London.

Stokes G (1992) *On Being Old: The Psychology of Later Life*. Falmer Press, London.

Stokes G and Goudie F (1988) Dealing with confusion. *Nursing Times* 85, 35–7.

Sugarman L (1986) *Lifespan Development Concepts Theories and Interventions*. Routledge, London.

Tannahill A (1985) What is health promotion? *Health Education Journal* 44, 167–8.

Tate S (1992) Visiting rules. *Nursing Times* 88, 26.

Tattam A (1992) Urgent call to curb abuse of restraint. *Nursing Times* 88, 8.

Taylor RC, Ford G and Barber H (1983) *Research Perspectives on Ageing 6. The Elderly at Risk.* Age Concern Research Unit, London. In Williams EI (1989) *Caring for Elderly People in the Community,* 2nd edn. Chapman & Hall, London.

Tester S and Meredith B (1987) Ill informed? *Information and Support for Elderly People in the Inner City.* Policy Studies Institute, London.

Thase ME, Liss L, Smelzer D and Maloon J (1982) Clinical evaluation of dementia in Down's syndrome: a preliminary report, *Journal of Mental Deficiency Research,* 26, 239–44.

Thompson H (1989) An old problem. *Geriatric Nursing and Home Care* 9, 20.

Thompson I, Melia K and Boyd K (1994) *Nursing Ethics.* Churchill Livingstone, Edinburgh.

Thompson J, Gibson J and Jagger C (1989) An association between visual impairment and mortality in elderly people. *Age and Ageing* 18, 83–8.

Tierney AJ and Worth A (1995) A review: readmission of elderly patients to hospital. *Age and Ageing* 24, 163–6.

Tierney A, Worth A, Closs SJ, King C and Macmillan M (1994) Older patients' experiences of discharge from hospital. *Nursing Times* 90, 36–9.

Tinker A (1984) *Staying at Home: Helping Elderly People.* London HMSO, London.

Tinker A (1991) *Elderly People in Modern Society.* Longman, Harlow.

Tinker A, McCreadie C, Wright F and Salvage AV (1994) *The Care of Frail Elderly People in the United Kingdom.* HMSO, London.

Tones K, Tilford S and Robinson Y (1990) *Health Education. Effectiveness and Efficiency.* Chapman & Hall, London.

Towell, D (1988) *An Ordinary Life in Practice.* King's Fund Institute, London.

Towell D and Beardshaw V (1991) *Enabling Community Integration – The Role of Public Authorities in Promoting an Ordinary Life for People with Learning Disabilities in the 1990s.* King's Fund, London.

Townsend P (1986) Ageism and social policy. In Phillipson C and Walker A (eds) *Ageing and Social Policy.* Gower, Aldershot.

Treharne G (1990) Attitudes towards the care of elderly people: are they getting better? *Journal of Advanced Nursing* 15, 777–81.

Turner P (1993) Activity nursing and the changes in the quality of life of elderly patients: a semi-quantitative study. *Journal of Advanced Nursing* 18, 1727–33.

Turton P (1983) Health Education and the District Nurse. *Nursing Times. Community Outlook* 79, 222–30.

Turton P (1984) Nurses working in the community. *Nursing Times* 80, 40–2.

United Kingdom Central Council for Nurses Midwives and Health Visitors (1992) *Code of Professional Conduct for the Nurse, Midwife and Health Visitor.* UKCC, London.

United Kingdom Central Council for Nurses, Midwives and Health Visitors (1986) *Project 2000. A New Preparation for Practice.* UKCC, London.

United Kingdom Central Council for Nurses, Midwives and Health Visitors (1989) *Exercising Accountability.* UKCC, London.

United Kingdom Central Council for Nurses, Midwives and Health Visitors (1992) *The Scope of Professional Practice.* UKCC, London.

Ungerson C *Why do Women Care?* In Finch J and Groves D (eds) *A Labour of Love.* Routledge and Kegan Paul, London.

Vaughan B (1989) Autonomy and accountability. *Nursing Times* 85, 54–5.

Verwoerdt A (1976) *Clinical Gerontology.* Williams and Wilkins, Baltimore.

Vetter NJ, Jones DA and Victor CR (1984) Effect of health visitors working with elderly patients in general practice: a randomised controlled trial. *British Medical Journal* 228, 369–72.

Victor C (1987) *Old Age in Modern Society*. Chapman & Hall, London.

Victor CR (1991) *Health and Health Care in Later Life*. Open University Press, Milton Keynes.

Victor CR and Vetter NJ (1984) DNs and the elderly after hospital discharge. *Nursing Times* 80, 61–2.

Victor CR and Vetter NJ (1988) Preparing the elderly for discharge from hospital: a neglected aspect of patients' care? *Age and Ageing* 17, 155–63.

Victor CR, Young E, Hudson E and Wallace P (1993) Whose responsibility is it anyway? Hospital admission and discharge of older patients in an Inner-London district health authority. *Journal of Advanced Nursing* 18, 1297–304.

Vincent S (1994) Exits. *Guardian Weekend* Special Report, pp. 6–10.

Wade L (1988) Promoting safety and comfort. In Wright SG (ed.) *Nursing the Older Patient*. Harper and Row, London.

Wade L (1992) The impact a health care delivery system (primary nurse) has on older women. Unpublished Master of Arts Dissertation. University of Keele.

Wade L (1995) New perspectives of gerontological nursing. In Wade L and Waters K (eds) *A Textbook of Gerontological Nursing*. Baillière Tindall, London.

Wafer M. and Metcalfe S. (1993) *Patient's Charter Survey. NDU for Older People*. Tameside Health Authority, Ashton-under-Lyne

Wagner Report (1988) *Residential Care – A Positive Choice*. HMSO, London.

Wagstaff P and Coakley D (1988) *Physiotherapy and the Elderly Patient: Therapy in Practice*. Croom Helm, London.

Wainwright P. (1987) Peer review. In Pearson A (ed.) *Nursing Quality Measurement*. Wiley, Chichester.

Walsh M and Ford P (1989) *Nursing Rituals*. Butterworth-Heinemann, Oxford.

Wandelt MA and Ager JW (1974) *Quality Patient Care Scale*. Appleton–Century–Crofts, New York.

Warner N (1994) *Community Care: Just a Fairytale?* Carers' National Association, London.

Waters KR (1987) Discharge planning: an exploratory study of the process of discharge planning on geriatric wards. *Journal of Advanced Nursing* 12, 71–83.

Waters KR (1987) Outcomes of discharge from hospital for elderly people. *Journal of Advanced Nursing* 12, 347–35.

Waters K and Booth J (1991) Home and dry. *Nursing Times* 87, 32–5.

Watkins PJ, Drury PL and Taylor KW (1990) *Diabetes and Its Management*, 4th edn. Blackwell Scientific, Blackwell.

Watson J (1992) *Medical–Surgical Nursing and Related Physiology*. WB Saunders, London.

Watson JD and Crick F (1953) *Psalm 90 v. 10* SPCK, London.

Watson R. (1993). *Caring for Elderly People*. WB Saunders, London.

Watson WH (1975) The meaning of touch: geriatric nursing. *Journal of Communication* 25, 104–12.

Webb C (1992) Expressing sexuality. In Redfern S (ed.) *Nursing Elderly People*. Churchill Livingstone, Edinburgh.

Webb C and Hope K (1994) What kind of nurses do patients want? *Journal of Clinical Nursing* 4, 101–8.

Webb J (1992) A new lease of life. *Nursing Times* 88, 30–2.

Webber-Jones J (1992) Doomed to deafness. *American Journal of Nursing* November.

Weg R (ed.) (1983) *Sexuality in the Later Years, Roles and Behaviour*. Academic Press, New York.

Weinberg RA (1992) The retinoblastoma gene and gene product. *Cancer Surveys* Vol 12, *Tumour Suppressor Genes, the Cell Cycle and Cancer*, pp. 45–7.

Weisz JR (1983). Can I control it? The pursuit of veridical answers across the life-span. In Baltes PE and Brim O (eds) *Life-span Development and Behaviour*. Academic Press, New York.

Wells T (1980) *Problems in Geriatric Nursing Care*. Churchill Livingstone, Edinburgh.

Welsh Office/NHS Directorate (1992) *Protocol for Investment in Health Gain – Mental Handicap (Learning Disability)*. Welsh Office Planning Forum. HMSO, Cardiff.

Wenger GC (1995) A comparison of urban with rural support networks: Liverpool and North Wales. *Ageing and Society* 15, 1 March.

Wenger GC (1996) *Support Networks for Older People and the Demand for Community Care Services*. Centre for Social Policy Research and Development, University of Wales, Bangor.

West B (1993) The essence of aromatherapy. *Elderly Care* 5, 24–5.

Wheeler R (1986) Housing policy for elderly people. In Phillipson C and Walker A (eds) *Ageing and Social Policy: A Critical Assessment*. Gower, Aldershot.

Whitehouse MJ (1992) The physiology of ageing. *Journal of Intravenous Nursing* 15 (suppl) S7–S13.

Whitaker P (1991) The dangers of ageism in clinical decision-making. *Geriatric Medicine* October 51–5.

Windmill V (1992) *Caring for the Elderly*. Pitman, London.

Willcocks D, Peace S and Kellaher L (1987) *Private Lives in Public Places: A Research-based Critique of Residential Life in Local Authority Old People's Homes*. Tavistock, London.

Williams A and Kind P (1992) The present state of play about QALYs. In Hopkins A (ed.) *Measures of the Quality of Life*. Royal College of Physicians, London.

Williams EI (1984) Characteristics of patients aged over 75 not seen during one year in general practice. *British Medical Journal* 288, 119–21.

Williams EI (1989) *Caring for Elderly People in the Community*, 2nd edn. Chapman & Hall, London.

Williams EI and Fritton F (1988) Factors affecting early unplanned readmission of elderly hospital patients. *British Medical Journal* 297, 784–7.

Williams TF (ed.) (1984) *Rehabilitation in the Ageing*. Raven Press, New York.

Wilson C (1987) *Hospital Wide Quality Assurance*. WB Saunders, Toronto.

Wilson C (1992) *Strategies in Health Care Quality* WB Saunders, Toronto.

Windmill V (1992) *Caring for the Elderly*. Pitman, London.

Wolfensberger W (1972) *The Principles of Normalisation in Human Services*. National Institute on Mental Retardation, Toronto.

Wolfensberger W and Thomas S (1983) *Program Analysis of Service Systems Implementation of Normalisation*. Canadian National Institute on Mental Retardation, Toronto.

Woods B, Portnoy S and Jones G (1992) Reminiscence and life review with persons with dementia: which way forward? In Jones G and Miesen BML (eds) *Caregiving in Dementia*. Routledge, London.

Woods N (1978) Human sexuality and the healthy elderly. In Brown M (ed.) *Readings in Gerontology*. CV Mosby, St Louis.

Woods RT and Britton PG (1985) *Clinical Psychology with the Elderly*. Croom Helm, London.

World Health Organization (1946) *Constitution* WHO, New York.

World Health Organization (1978) *Alma Ata (1978) Primary Health Care*. WHO, Geneva.

World Health Organization (1979) *Formulating Strategies for Health for all by the Year 2000*. WHO, Geneva.

World Health Organization (1986) *A Discussion Document on the Concept and Principles of Health Promotion*. WHO, Geneva.

World Health Organization (1986) *Charter for Health Promotion*. WHO, Health and Welfare, Ottawa.

Wright KG (1979) Economics and planning the care of the elderly. In Wright KG (ed.) (1979) *Economics and Health Planning*. Croom Helm, London.

Wright S (1988) *Nursing the Older Patient*. Harper and Row, London.

Wright S (1989) *Changing Nursing Practice*. Edward Arnold, London.

Wright S (1990) The practice of primary nursing. In Wright S (ed.) *My Patient – My Nurse*. Scutari Press, London.

Wyke A (1994) The Future of Medicine – Peering into 2010. *The Economist* 330, suppl. 10/3.

Yeo M (1993). Toward an ethic of empowerment for health promotion. *Health Promotion International* 8, 225–35.

Yura H and Walsh MB (1973) *The Nursing Process*. Appleton–Century–Crofts, New York.

Yurick AG, Spier BE, Robb SS and Ebert NJ (1989) *The Aged Person and the Nursing Process*. Appleton and Lange, California.

Index